Bodies under Siege

Bodies under Siege

Self-mutilation, Nonsuicidal Self-injury,
and Body Modification in Culture and Psychiatry

THIRD EDITION

ARMANDO FAVAZZA, M.D.
Emeritus Professor, Department of Psychiatry
University of Missouri–Columbia School of Medicine

The Johns Hopkins University Press
Baltimore

© 1987, 1996, 2011 The Johns Hopkins University Press
All rights reserved. Published 2011
Printed in the United States of America on acid-free paper
2 4 6 8 9 7 5 3 1

The Johns Hopkins University Press
2715 North Charles Street
Baltimore, Maryland 21218-4363
www.press.jhu.edu

Library of Congress Cataloging-in-Publication Data
Favazza, Armando R.
Bodies under siege : self-mutilation, nonsuicidal self-injury, and body
modification in culture and psychiatry / Armando Favazza. — 3rd ed.
p. ; cm.
Includes bibliographical references and index.
ISBN-13: 978-0-8018-9965-2 (hardcover : alk. paper)
ISBN-10: 0-8018-9965-6 (hardcover : alk. paper)
ISBN-13: 978-0-8018-9966-9 (pbk. : alk. paper)
ISBN-10: 0-8018-9966-4 (pbk. : alk. paper)
1. Self-mutilation. 2. Cultural psychiatry. 3. Psychiatry, Transcultural. I. Title.
[DNLM: 1. Self Mutilation—ethnology. 2. Self Mutilation—therapy. 3. Body
Modification, Non-Therapeutic. 4. Cross-Cultural Comparison.
5. Ethnopsychology. WM 165 F272b 2011]
RC552.S4F38 2011
616.85M'82—dc22   2010025284

A catalog record for this book is available from the British Library.

*Special discounts are available for bulk purchases of this book. For more information,
please contact Special Sales at 410-516-6936 or specialsales@press.jhu.edu.*

The Johns Hopkins University Press uses environmentally friendly book
materials, including recycled text paper that is composed of at least 30 percent
post-consumer waste, whenever possible. All of our book papers are acid-free,
and our jackets and covers are printed on paper with recycled content.

To the patient who wrote the following to me:
Thank you for the opportunity to express my feelings
and for the attention you are paying to my problem.
I believe there is a larger truth at work in the riddle of self-harm
which is important for society as a whole to penetrate.
May you find the answers which you seek.

CONTENTS

The awakened and knowing say: body am I entirely, and nothing
else; and soul is only a word for something about the body.
—Nietzsche, *Thus Spoke Zarathustra*

My introduction to the first edition (1987) of *Bodies under Siege* was only four
pages long. Its opening paragraphs are worth repeating:

In the vast repertoire of human behaviors, self-mutilation ranks among the least
understood and the most puzzling. Is it possible to strip away the mysterious aura
that surrounds it? What could possibly motivate people to alter and destroy their
body tissue or to consent to the mutilation of their bodies by others?

In an attempt to answer these questions, this book explores the many variations
of self-mutilative acts across cultures and through time, utilizing the perspective of
cultural psychiatry. Just as culture strives to organize a society into a logically integrated, functional, sense-making whole, so too cultural psychiatry strives to integrate the components of complex, problematic behaviors such as self-mutilation
and to make sense out of what may appear to be senseless. Thus, we shall examine
the wide variety of forces—ranging from congenital insensitivity to pain to hyper-
secretion of adrenal hormones, from castration anxiety to intolerable guilt, from the
experience of child abuse to confused perceptions of maleness and femaleness—
that may impel or compel people to mutilate themselves. Further, we shall examine the vast array of cultural practices, attitudes, and beliefs—ranging from religion
and mythology to folk healing, from infibulation to initiation rites, from artistic
and literary depictions to blood customs—that form the theater within which self-
mutilation is performed.

My preface to the second edition (1996) was much longer. I related how I became interested in bodily harm, including an encounter with a Sudanese graduate student's wife who as a child had had her clitoris ritually removed and then became depressed when her American girlfriends described the joy of orgasmic sexuality that she would never experience. I later discovered self-mutilation as a therapeutic tool among Moroccan mystics, who slashed open their own heads and offered bits of bread drenched in their own healing blood to the sick. And then there was my opportune reading about the first reported case of repetitive nonsuicidal self-injury in the fifth chapter of the Gospel of Mark, which describes a demon-possessed man chained in a cemetery, who, night and day, cried and cut himself with small stones. Jesus exorcised the demons, who then entered a herd of swine, which committed suicide by drowning in a river (was it possible that the man had suicidal urges that were kept in check by his repeated skin cutting?).

I described the exciting discoveries about self-mutilation that I uncovered as I wrote the book as well as my loneliness because so few others seemed interested. I praised the Johns Hopkins University Press for allowing Fakir Musafar to write an epilogue. Fakir, the guru philosopher of the "modern primitives" movement, is a man of great artistic talents and exceptional knowledge about body modification. He is my good friend and has personally experienced many types of body modification. His new epilogue recounts his discoveries about the possibilities, the rewards, and the dangers of these practices. When I was asked by the president of the American College of Psychiatrists, in 1999, to provide a "San Francisco experience" for society members, I, in turn, invited Fakir to make a presentation. The august audience was stunned. Some thought he was bonkers but most were mystified and intrigued. At that time, body modification was a cottage industry and the spirituality movement was beginning to gear up. Along came Fakir, who talked about things that were foreign to most psychiatrists and that brought them out of their comfort zone. Nowadays, the "San Francisco experience" has become a global one with Fakir at its epicenter. And, although psychiatry is focused on the primacy of cellular, genetic, and neuronal approaches, there is growing recognition that culture cannot be ignored. For a scholarly discussion of Fakir's work, see Graver (1995).

Fakir follows a universally noble tradition in which spirituality is gained by taming the bonds of the flesh. By conquering pain and transforming his body, he walks on the path to enlightenment. He places his practices outside of Christian culture, but had he lived in earlier centuries, he might well have found soul mates among the company of the Desert Fathers, the athletes of God who sought salvation through mortification. Properly speaking, Fakir does not truly mortify his body but rather attempts to transcend pain. Even with the proper spiritual training, those who would emulate him do so at grave personal peril. I for one cannot even think about putting holes in my body without shuddering, yet there are many persons who carve and cut themselves. As an uncontrollable behavior, the morbidity may be high. As a controlled behavior, however, it may have its rewards. In this edition, Fakir discusses the astonishing growth of the body modification community, which contains both shallow poseurs and, sad to say, frightening extremists.

I also recounted the lifting of my spirits because of the favorable reviews of the book in professional journals. One reviewer described his reaction to my presentation of the new Deliberate Self-Harm syndrome as "a sense of sharing in a clarifying discovery, as I imagine an early reader of Gull's description of anorexia nervosa might have felt." Another reviewer wrote in the *British Journal of Psychiatry*: "A comprehensive, lucid, and interestingly written book which is likely to become a classic on the subject."

Given that the book has remained in print since 1987, that it is still referenced in both professional and lay publications, that it has resulted in my appearing on many major television and radio shows and lecturing at a large number of prestigious universities both at home and abroad (Columbia, Harvard, the Karolinska Institution, Mayo Clinic, Yale, etc.), and that it is now available in a third edition, I suppose that it might be considered a "classic."

In preparing for this third edition, I no longer felt lonely. The literature has grown enormously, and I have selectively included several hundred new references. I have offered advice to many students who have written master's and doctoral theses on the topic. The term self-mutilation is still used in some psychiatric journals but has been replaced by the more precise nonsuicidal self-injury (NSSI) in recent years. Although NSSI is an inclusive term, I have decided to retain "self-mutilation" when referring to major acts of self-injury, such as eye enucleation and amputation of body parts. I do use "NSSI" when referring to moderate/superficial acts, such as skin-cutting and burning, which are the most common form of self-injury as well as the major focus of current research and treatment.

Special praise should be given to Karen Conterio for her enduring efforts in educating the public about self-injury and developing "S.A.F.E." therapeutic programs. Praise is also due to three psychologists: Matthew Nock of Harvard University and Janis Whitlock of Cornell University, for their work and leadership in the scientific study of self-injury, and Barent Walsh, for producing practical guides for treatment. Although the new literature (Nock 2009a) significantly expands and clarifies our knowledge about self-injury, provides models for understanding it, and offers more hopeful treatments, the fundamental findings in the first two editions of *Bodies under Siege* remarkably remain valid.

It is instructive to compare two articles that were published twenty years apart: my article "Why patients mutilate themselves" (1989), and Nock's "Why do people hurt themselves?" (2009b). The titles are telling. I, as a physician, focus on patients, while Nock, a psychologist, focuses on "people." I use the term *mutilate*, while he uses the term *hurt*.

In my article, I considered self-mutilation as a product of mental illness and as a morbid act of self-help behavior that is inherent in the repertoire of human activity. I discussed biological, psychological, social, cultural, and patients' explanations for its occurrence. Patients' explanations for their acts of major self-mutilation were divided into two main themes: religious (a psychotic reading of the biblical injunction to tear out an offending eye or to become a eunuch for the kingdom of heaven's sake, atonement for sins, etc.) and sexual (a man's desire to become a woman, repudiation of one's sexual organs, etc.). Patients' explanations for moderate self-mutilation, such as skin cutting, included a host of themes, such as the release of tension, the cessation of feelings of emotional deadness and estrangement from the environment, and influencing the behavior of other persons. I discussed a number of psychological explanations, which included psychodynamic theories (the blood produced by cutting may serve as a solacing, transitional object; relief of sexual guilt in persons who were abused during childhood, etc.); an attempt to emotionally blackmail others or to force them to provide a caring, mothering response; a means for terminating episodes of depersonalization (the shock of seeing blood directs attention to the difference between the self and the environment); a response to command hallucinations or a preemptive gesture to forestall imaginary paranoid attacks; one form of impulsive behavior; and behavioral theories (e.g., self-mutilation is maintained by terminating or avoiding aversive stimuli and by positive reinforcement, or may represent "a morbid type of problem-solving in persons who have a low tolerance for distress, inadequate coping resources, and self-harm expectancies"). Under social explanations, I discussed endemic and epidemic self-mutilation in repressive settings such as prisons. As for cultural explanations, I provided details about my statement in the first edition of *Bodies under Siege* that "self-mutilation is not alien to the human condition; but rather it is culturally and psychologically embedded in the profound, elemental experiences of healing, religion, and social amity." I noted that the weakest link in our chain of knowledge is the biological one and that no simple explanation can be applied to all patients.

Two decades later, Matthew Nock, the most prolific and astute current researcher on self-injury, published his article on the same topic. He used the new terminology, nonsuicidal self-injury (NSSI), and conceptualized it not as a symptom of mental illness but rather as a "harmful behavior" that can serve several functions both internally within a person and externally in a person's relationships with others. This approach holds that NSSI is maintained by four functions through positive and negative reinforcement: NSSI may decrease internal aversive (unpleasant) thoughts or feelings, may generate desired feelings and stimulation, may facilitate help-seeking, and may provide an escape from undesired social interactions.

Nock then provided an integrated theoretical model of the development and maintenance of NSSI in a person. He starts with background distal factors such as experiencing childhood abuse, maltreatment, and familial hostility and criticism and having a genetic predisposition for high emotional and cognitive reactivity. These distal factors can affect persons who are vulnerable for NSSI because they have high levels of aversive emotions and thoughts as well as poor communication skills, problem-solving abilities, and tolerance in dealing with distress. In persons who possess these distal and vulnerability factors, experiencing a stressful event may trigger responses of underarousal or overarousal or may present unmanageable social demands. The final factor that results in engaging in NSSI is the interaction of a person's stress response with that person's NSSI-specific vulnerability factors, such as observing or learning about NSSI being used by others; a need for self-punishment resulting from repeated abuse or criticism by others; a need to signal personal distress dramatically because the usual methods of talking or yelling fail; a choice to use NSSI to achieve a desired goal or function because it is a fast and readily accessible method; an ability to experience NSSI with little or no pain; and a propensity to identify with NSSI and to value it as an effective means of achieving one of the desired functions, such as the regulation of a distressing social situation or of disturbing affects.

At first glance, there seems to be a wide gap between my consideration of NSSI as a product of mental illness and Nock's contention that it is a harmful behavior, but both perspectives are useful in different ways. My knowledge about NSSI comes from patients who, by the time they arrive at my office, are usually in dire straits and clearly have a mental illness (ranging from schizophrenia to generalized anxiety disorder to borderline personality disorder) or mental retardation. I am trained, as a physician and psychiatrist, to recognize, diagnose, and treat patients who are mentally ill. Psychiatry has a formal *Diagnostic and Statistical Manual of Mental Disorders*, updated periodically, that lists obligatory criteria and associated symptomatic features for arriving at a diagnosis of a mental illness. Unfortunately, this manual does not deal with NSSI meaningfully; that is, it is a criterion only for borderline personality disorder (although this diagnosis can be made without the presence of NSSI) and for trichotillomania (pulling out body hairs), which, by definition, is a form of NSSI. One of my contributions has been to point out that NSSI may be an associated feature of many mental disorders. The manual is descriptive and does not deal with causality (e.g., it lists "dementia due to head trauma" but does not explain the processes by which head trauma may result in dementia). The reason for this is obvious: we simply do not understand the processes fully. Unlike many medical illnesses for which the processes are known, mental illnesses are just too complicated.

Good psychiatry operates on a model that considers all the biological, psychological, social, and cultural factors that cause people to become mentally ill. Nock (2009b) is correct when he writes that "suggesting that people engage in NSSI because it is a symptom of a disorder provides little explanatory power," but a good psychiatrist observes a symptom of a mental disorder, such as NSSI, and then attempts to understand the biopsychosociocultural factors that have resulted in the symptom. It is unfortunate that nowadays many psychiatrists, urged by insurance companies to provide only "medication checks" services, do not make full use of the biopsychosociocultural model in evaluating and treating patients.

Both *Bodies under Siege* and my 1989 article derived from my clinical experience. I attempted to bring together a lot of disparate information, adding my unique cultural perspective, and through my classification to present the universe of culturally sanctioned and deviant deliberate self-harm behaviors as an integrated whole. I believe that my approach has succeeded in several ways. It has provided clinicians with a framework for conceptualizing self-injury, albeit within the context of mental illness. I have never suggested that labeling deviant self-injury as a symptom is an endpoint, but rather have urged clinicians to make use in their formulations of the various explanations that I provided in their formulations. I specifically mentioned explanations such as positive and negative reinforcement, low tolerance for distress, inadequate coping resources, and self-harm expectancies even though these factors were not widely discussed in the self-harm literature of the 1980s. My approach also succeeded in calling attention to the phenomenon of self-injury and to the plight of chronic injurers, as well as in legitimizing the study of self-injury as a topic worthy of academic research.

Over the years, psychologists have become the main students of self-injury. Nock, for example, has taken the importance of positive and negative reinforcements in NSSI far beyond my relatively brief mention of them. His theoretical model of the development and maintenance of NSSI is integrative and far more advanced than mine. I took the first major step and he has taken the second. He and others have clarified, expanded, and made explicit what was implicit in my work, and for this I am grateful. This is not to say that we now fully understand self-injury. As Nock (2009b) noted, his model is not entirely satisfactory in dealing with the comorbidity of NSSI behaviors and mental illness. Additionally, many of the vulnerability factors in his model are relevant to NSSI but also increase the risk of differing psychiatric disorders. "If NSSI and some psychiatric disorders share an etiologic pathway and represent different forms of behavior that can serve the same function, one is left wondering why some people select NSSI rather than another pathological behavior to regulate their affective and social experience."

The short answer to the question "Why do patients deliberately harm themselves?" is that it counterintuitively provides temporary relief from distressing situations and from a host of painful symptoms, such as anxiety, depersonalization, and desperation. The long answer is that it also touches on the profound human experiences of salvation, healing, and orderliness. Self-injury is a morbid form of self-help. In the hands of special individuals who are able to control the behavior, it provides some benefit. However, the training, discipline, and courage needed to attain such positive results is not my cup of tea, nor would it appeal to most people. Self-mutilation and NSSI are nothing to trifle with. For individuals who cannot control the behavior, it provides short-term relief but at a great cost, such as the loss of an eye or unsightly scars. It is encouraging that new understandings of NSSI have entered into clinical treatment via cognitive, interpersonal, and dialectic behavioral therapies, but a breakthrough in biological treatments remains elusive.

The numerous examples of self-injury in this book are painful to comprehend. The culturally sanctioned modification rituals may seem strange at first glance, but they are no stranger than going to church and worshiping a crucified god. *Bodies under Siege* is more than a catalog of horrors. It goes beyond mere description to search for meaning. Ultimately, it celebrates not death but rather the will to live. It chronicles the struggle of humankind to maintain equilibrium in the face of adversity. Therefore, dear reader, empathize if you can with the poor souls who are the victims of self-injury, but save your grieving for the dead.

PART ONE

MUTILATIVE BELIEFS, RELIGION, EATING, AND ETHOLOGY

To understand better the complex behavior of abnormal self-mutilation, we need to examine beliefs, attitudes, practices, and images relating to mutilation in general. Many blood customs, for example, pertain to healing practices and to the sealing of pacts. Sexual mutilation provides opposing images of psychotic monsters and of pleasurable self-indulgence. Literary accounts range from uncontrolled mob violence to the exquisitely painful machinations of Kafka's famous penal colony.

Cosmogonic myths demonstrate the origins of social order from the body parts of dismembered primal beings. In shamanism, imagined self-mutilation of the healer leads to wisdom and to the capacity to heal oneself and others. Mutilative images are central to disparate religions, as demonstrated by Tibetan Tantric meditation, North American Plains Indian mysticism, and the iconography of Christ's Passion. Indeed, the best-known and most widely revered religious symbols are the cross on which Christ was tortured and the stone lingam representing the phallus of Siva, who castrated himself out of anger. The claims of some mentally ill self-mutilators that they are gods or godly agents become more understandable in the light of the interconnectedness of religious sentiments, violence, suffering, sacrifice, and the sacred.

The relationship between eating disorders and nonsuicidal self-injury is special. It may be described clinically in terms of impulsivity and issues of control over one's body. From a different standpoint, however, the experience of learning to eat may underlie a basic propensity for self-injury. Cannibalism, a fundamental form of institutionalized aggression, provides a unique, gut-level perspective on the inherent nature of self-harm.

Automutilation among animals is also examined in this section. Medical science often uses animal models, and this approach is being tried in the study of self-mutilation. By environmental manipulation, surgical procedures, and administration of drugs, researchers can induce laboratory animals to injure themselves. The difficulties associated with comparing animal and human nature impose limits on the relevance of ethology for understanding self-injury, but some leads from such studies hold promise.

CHAPTER ONE

Mutilative Beliefs, Attitudes, Practices, and Images

Beliefs, attitudes, practices, and images diffuse across latitudes and longitudes and centuries. Our perceptions of self-mutilation as grotesque or beautiful, heroic or cowardly, awesome or pitiful, meaningful or senseless, derive in great part from the perceptions of those who have lived before us. They are passed on in great paintings and statues and folk art, in novels and fairy tales, in history books and travelers' accounts, in religious rituals and secular customs, in the waging of war and the punishment of criminals, in popular songs and theatrical performances, in the ways we heal the sick and bury the dead, in the rearing of children and the handling of animals.

Self-mutilation cannot be totally divorced from the more general concept of mutilation directed against others; the perceptions and practices of the one are intimately linked to the other. However, the mutilation of unwilling victims is less intellectually troublesome because it usually can be explained or rationalized in fairly simple terms, such as revenge or a method of instilling fear. Even when persons mutilate others for idiosyncratic reasons, a reasonable response traditionally has been either to lock them in a jail or mental hospital or to kill them. Self-mutilation, however, is a profound phenomenon that defies ready comprehension and rational response.

A major goal of this book is to strip away the aura of mystery that surrounds self-mutilation. This is not an easy task because our perceptions are often unconsciously linked not only with the fear, revenge, mob violence, and governmental power associated with mutilation in general but also with concepts such as sacredness, self-knowledge, and the power of blood to heal and to bind individuals together. Let us, then, begin this task by examining some beliefs, attitudes, practices, and evocative images of mutilation.

Decapitation and Scalping

Decapitation as a punishment has been popular throughout history and reached its apotheosis with the use of the guillotine in France. The ghoulish image of Salome dancing around the severed head of John the Baptist has long fascinated

Westerners, the scene even being set to music in Strauss's popular opera. A most curious Chinese legal ritual held that a man was at liberty, upon surprising his wife in the act of adultery, to slay the couple. To substantiate the truthfulness of the situation, however, he had to cut off their heads and bring them to a magistrate. The heads were placed in a tub of water, which was then violently stirred so that the heads would revolve and meet in the middle. If the heads met back to back, the victims were pronounced innocent and the husband killed. If they met face-to-face, the husband's story was accepted. He was then gently beaten to teach him to watch over a future wife more closely.

Decapitation has long been used as a technique of terrorism in warfare. Victors would cut off the heads of the vanquished and display them on poles to demoralize remaining enemy forces. Such tactics were commonly employed during the Christian-Muslim wars. The biblical account of the Maccabean revolt ends with the mutilation of Nicanor. His vanquishers put his head on public display as evidence that the Lord had helped them.

Carroll (1982) gathered data on the "rolling head" myth among many Native American tribes. In the most common story, a man's wife has illicit sexual relations with a snake lover. The husband then kills both the wife and the lover, severing the wife's head. The head pursues her children—predominantly her sons—who eventually destroy it. Carroll interpreted these stories to be ultimately concerned with castration anxiety, the severed head symbolizing a severed penis.

Head taking was a preoccupation among the Slavs, Turks, and Albanians. Sworn brethren would cut off the head of a dead or dying comrade to prevent it from being taken by the enemy. In the pan-Balkan custom of head shaving, persons left a large hairy lock intact so that, upon decapitation, their heads could be carried by using the lock of hair as a handle. Both Muslims and Christians shuddered at the thought of having infidel fingers in their mouths.

In border fights between Montenegrins and Turks in 1912 a new fad emerged of taking noses instead of heads. This was possibly related to the fact that the Montenegrin soldiers were no longer issued the *handzhar*, a large knife well suited for head taking. Durham (1928) recounted a conversation with a professor who, at the news of the fighting, gleefully stated, "Now you will see plenty of noses! Even baskets full!" When told that such behavior would disgust all of Europe, the enraged professor declared that nose cutting was a national custom and that Turks were not human beings. Just as heads were carried by the hair-lock, so too noses were carried by the mustache.

North American Indians practiced scalping, as did the Visigoths, Anglo-Saxons, and Franks. Herodotus mentions it, as does the second book of Maccabees. Native American warriors willingly engaged in activities that they knew would lead to the loss of their own or the gain of another's scalp. The scalp was removed to provide evidence of having killed an enemy even though the operation was not always fatal and many lived through the procedure (Nadeau 1941). Eastern tribes removed the entire scalp. Nadeau wrote: "They remove it as nicely as we would the skin of a rabbit. First they cut the skin to the bone all around the head with a knife and peel off the scalp as easily as one would a glove from the hand" (p. 180).

The Chinooks practiced a more radical form, sometimes pulling off the ears, eyes, or all of the facial skin with the scalp. Plains Indians favored partial scalping. The nineteenth-century traveler George Catlin noted: "The scalp is procured by cutting out a piece of the skin of the head, the size of the palm of the hand or less, containing the very center or crown of the head, the place where the hair radiates from a point, and exactly over what the phrenologists call self-esteem" (Nadeau 1941, p. 183).

Scalping was also done by European settlers. Catlin noted that settlers paid for the scalp of their enemies, both Indian and Caucasian. In fact, a type of knife made in Sheffield, England, was popular for scalping and was traded to the Indians for horses.

The Zuni Indians of the American Southwest had a scalp "house" in each town. In Zuni theology, dead persons are often considered rainmakers, thus the scalp ceremonial was performed not only to propitiate the dead enemy but also to ensure rainfall and abundant crops.

Blood Customs, Healing, and Corpse Abuse

Blood customs are among the oldest known to mankind. Blood has awesome symbolic and physiologic powers, as evidenced by its role in religious sacrifice, healing, the formation of brotherhoods, and blood feuds. When harvested properly, it can alter the course of personal and communal history. It is my contention that some mentally ill persons mutilate themselves as a primitive method of drawing on their blood's ability to foster bonds of loyalty and union among members of their social network, to demonstrate their hatred of and conquest over real and imaginary enemies, to heal their afflictions, and, as is discussed in chapter 2, to set right their relationship with God.

Although blood customs have a worldwide distribution, they were especially important in the everyday life of people living in the Balkans (Boehm 1984). Union could be achieved, for example, by feasting on an enemy's blood. Balkan pirates displayed the mutilated corpse of the Holy Roman emperor's envoy in a church. Wives then demonstrated solidarity with their husbands by licking the bloody body.

Human blood and fragments of flesh and bone have been prized as healing agents. In book 28 of his monumental *Natural History*, Pliny writes: "Thus epileptics even drink the blood of gladiators out of living goblets. . . . They consider it the most effective method of cure to swallow down the blood when it is still warm and bubbling out of the man himself, and thus simultaneously to swallow the very breath of life from the mouth of the wound." A sympathetic magic belief in the efficacy of the blood of persons who died violently to cure epilepsy persevered into the nineteenth century. Hans Christian Andersen's autobiography, for example, describes an execution he witnessed in 1823: "I saw a poor sick man, whom his superstitious parents made drink a cup of the blood of an executed person, that he might be healed of epilepsy; after which they ran with him wildly until he sank to the ground."

Blood was used to treat leprosy. An ancient rabbinical commentary on Exodus 2:23—"A long time passed, during which the king of Egypt died"—states that the king was considered dead because he had contracted leprosy and that the Egyptian priests prescribed a grisly cure: the king had to bathe twice daily in the blood of three hundred Israelite children. One legend held that Richard, the king of England from 1189 to 1199, had leprosy. Because nothing seemed to help, he called on a famous Jewish physician, who recommended that Richard bathe in the blood of a newborn child and eat the child's heart. It is interesting to note that great anti-Semitic animosity arose in the thirteenth and fourteenth centuries because of the appearance of red spots on consecrated communion wafers in some churches. These spots were thought to be Jesus's blood, the result of the secret piercing of the wafers by Jews. This belief persisted until the German scientist Ehrenberg presented a paper at the Academy of Sciences at Berlin in 1848, demonstrating that the "blood" was really a bacterial growth that flourished under certain conditions.

Following the crusades, Europe was flooded with relics, such as the bones and body parts of saints, that were objects of veneration and in many cases were used in healing practices. In various European popular beliefs, afflicted persons have been urged to use corpse fragments; for example, pressing a corpse's finger on an aching tooth supposedly cured toothache.

Sadism and Murder

Donatien-Alphonse-François de Sade (1740–1814), better known as the Marquis de Sade, devoted his life and his writings to the glorification of sexual gratification associated with inflicting pain on others (Gillette 1966). He spent sixteen years in prison and eleven more years at the asylum for the criminally insane at Charenton, where he died. His first serious offense occurred when he trapped a woman, whipped her severely, and then superficially sliced the skin of her entire body with a knife. In 1772 he masterminded the "Cantharidic Bonbon Orgy" in which he placed Spanish fly (officially known as cantharides, this chemical was thought to be an aphrodisiac but in reality is a dangerous astringent) in the chocolate dessert served at a ball. According to some accounts the ball turned into a sexual orgy orchestrated by de Sade. Several people supposedly died as a result of esophageal strictures caused by eating the Spanish fly, and de Sade was charged with sodomy and murder.

Certainly de Sade cannot be accused of being a great writer. In his novella *Justine*, for example, a lecher shows Justine the realistic wax effigy of a woman in the same posture as the crucified Christ and then says, "This statue is the representation of my former mistress, who died nailed to this wall. I had it constructed to replace her real body when it began to decompose." *The One Hundred Twenty Days of Sodom* contains a catalog of sexual vices, most of which are silly or improbable. For example, "A man extracts all of a woman's teeth, replacing them with red-hot nails which he secures in place with a hammer. This is done after he forces her to perform fellatio."

Count Leopold von Sacher-Masoch was de Sade's counterpart in that his literary writings depicted sexual pleasure derived from being the object of pain. Both sadism and masochism are, by definition, associated with sexual pleasure, while self-injury is usually not. In my study of 250 chronic self-injurers, only 2 percent said they were often or always sexually aroused when they decided to harm themselves; 3 percent said self-harm often or always aroused sexual feelings in them. Twenty percent said they sometimes used self-harm as a method of ridding themselves of troublesome sexual feelings. There does exist, however, a definite subgroup of self-injurers who are sexually excited by limb amputation, especially of the feet and toes (Wakefield et al. 1977). Additionally, some persons enjoy pain during sexual activity (hot wax dripped on their breasts, use of oversized dildos, pinching), and some like to engage in painful nonsuicidal self-injury (NSSI), such as sticking pins into their skin. While participation in bondage scenarios involving mild flagellation and being tied up with ropes and chains may be considered within the spectrum of normal sexual behavior nowadays, extensive tissue damage is pathological. One patient, whose major sexual outlet was masturbation in front of a full-length mirror, was able to excite himself by whipping himself with wires (the cuts often took seven to fourteen days to heal), lacerating his penis with brush bristles, squeezing his testicles in a door jamb, and burning himself with candle wax. As a child, this patient was forced to engage in sexual acts with both parents in which he was whipped, had rubber probes stuck into his penis, had clamps placed on his testicles, and was given ice-water enemas.

Many murderers who mutilate their victims are psychotic and sadistic. Some, like Jack the Ripper, gained notoriety because of the multiple mutilative murders they committed. The most infamous mentally ill mutilator, however, was Gilles de Rais, a French nobleman born in 1404. He fought against the English with Joan of Arc and was her military instructor.

My suppositions are that he was schizophrenic and that the content of his illness was influenced by the zeitgeist of his era. His was an era of witchcraft, demonology, and Satanism. Persons were accused of such sacrilegious acts as using communion wafers for sodomistic purposes and using children's blood in place of consecrated wine. Gilles de Rais turned to necromancy with a vengeance, abetted by an Italian ex-priest, Francesco Prelati, who taught that contact with Satan could best be achieved by performing the most brutal and sinful acts imaginable.

De Rais began by sodomizing young boys, but Prelati said that this was not enough to entice the devil. De Rais then kidnapped a boy, cut his throat, removed his hands, eyes, and heart, and offered the pieces to Satan in a mock religious ceremony. But still the devil did not materialize.

De Rais supposedly sodomized, mutilated, and murdered more than seven hundred children. At his trial he told of his usual procedure of sexually assaulting boys in the cellar of a tower, cutting open their chests and burying his face in their lungs, and opening their abdomens and handling their intestines. He also confessed to necrophilia with the dismembered bodies and to attempted intercourse with a fetus he cut out of a pregnant woman.

At his trial in 1440, de Rais repented, and the bishop of Nantes was forced to receive him back into the church saying, "Weep, you madman, that thy tears may wash away the pollutions of the charnel-house within you." De Rais and Prelati were then simultaneously hanged and burned to death.

Mutilative Imagery in Religion

Although the next chapter is devoted to religion, here I first focus on three totally different belief systems—Tibetan Tantrism, North American Indian mysticism, and Christianity—that contain exceedingly vivid images of mutilation. These powerful images are not superficial bits of drama but rather are intrinsic to the meaningfulness of the belief systems. Stripped of blood and torn flesh, most religions become no different from fairy tales. The True Cross is not sparkling clean and silver plated.

Tibetan Tantrism

The *Tibetan Book of the Dead,* or *The Great Liberation through Hearing in the Bardo,* describes a series of meditations on death and birth as experienced in six psychological states. During these states the mediator must deal with various deities who appear. "The concept of bardo is based on the period between sanity and insanity, or the period between confusion and . . . wisdom . . . between death and birth. The past situation has just occurred and the future situation has not yet manifested itself so there is a gap between the two. This is basically the bardo experience" (Rinpoche 1975, pp. 10–11).

The bardo retreat, seven weeks in total darkness, is the most rewarding but dangerous form of meditation. The meditator experiences luminosity and visions accompanied by brilliant colors and sounds. The meditator feels detached from the world, like a gigantic head floating in space, and hears the sounds of a thousand claps of thunder, yet there is nothing to vibrate.

The first visions are those of the peaceful divinities, who permit the meditator to experience the eternal peace of the cosmos. But then the terrifying, wrathful deities of mutilation appear as a sign of cosmic passion and aggression. Perfect instantaneous enlightenment occurs when the meditator understands that he is projecting these horrible images from within himself.

> With teeth biting the lower lip, glassy-eyed, their hair tied on top of their heads, with huge bellies and thin necks, holding the records of karma in their hands, chanting "Strike!" and "Kill!" licking up brains, tearing heads from bodies, pulling out internal organs: in this way they will come.
>
> When projections appear like this do not be afraid. You have a mental body of unconscious tendencies, so even if you are killed and cut into pieces, you cannot die.

After death comes rebirth. The reading of the *Bardo* is especially significant to dying persons because, with the insights gained, they can search out an appropriate womb to enter during reincarnation. But even if a person has died, the *Bardo* should be read in the presence of the corpse "until blood and pus come out of the nostrils. . . . This profound instruction leads great sinners on the secret path."

North American Indian Mysticism

The Sun Dance of the Plains Indians is a ritual Alexander (1967) describes as "the index of an entire culture, not merely in a material sense but especially with respect to the whole pattern of life, social and ideal, which guided into its development the particular genius of the hunters and warriors of the prairie. . . . The Sun Dance is essentially an interpretation [and] a philosophy of life" (p. 137). It is an eight-day ritual characteristic of buffalo-hunting tribes, such as the Arapahoe, Cheyenne, and Dakota. Although participants volunteer out of personal initiative, the entire tribe cooperates in its performance, for it is the entire tribe that benefits from the suffering and self-mutilation of the dancers.

The climax of the ceremony is the Gazing-at-the-Sun dance, which portrays the dangers of a warrior's life, namely, Capture, Torture, and Release. The dancers are "captured" by warriors while women sing songs of grief. In earlier times they were then tortured (although bloodletting is currently prohibited by U.S. federal law). Incisions were made on their backs and chests, and pieces of wood with attached leather thongs were inserted under the cut muscles. The thongs of some dancers were attached to buffalo skulls, but others had the thongs attached to the top of the Sacred Pole. They then danced; those who were attached to the Pole were hoisted into the air while they gazed at the sun. They then struggled to break free of their bonds. Some, unable to stand the pain, were cut free. Others successfully struggled until the wooden skewers ripped through their flesh. The pure in heart able to withstand this religious ordeal expected to receive a vision that, when understood, would make clear the meaning and course of their lives.

"Possibly, in a more mystical sense, here is shown the drama of all embodied human life—for more than one religion and philosophy, from the ancients onward, have depicted man as snared in the flesh, there to suffer and endure, and if by the prowess of his spirit enduring to the end, escaped and triumphant in a newer and more spiritual vision. Assuredly there is here an elemental coincidence between the essential elements of Indian and Neo-Platonic or even Christian thinking" (Alexander 1967, p. 169).

Christianity

The most enduring images central to Western cultural tradition are those of the Passion of Christ. The most powerful and intense images were developed during the fourteenth through seventeenth centuries and have been classified by art historians (Ferguson 1954; Schiller 1972). Some are drawn directly from biblical accounts, while others are ahistorical images drawn from the imaginations of the artists. Christ willingly submitted to his Passion. His voluntary suffering, crucifixion, and resurrection both fulfilled and transcended the old prophesies.

The fourteenth century saw the rise of the flagellant cults, and many paintings of that period depict the Flagellation of Christ. He is shown tied to a column while his captors unmercifully whip him. His body is covered with multiple wounds as the surrounding crowd listens to Pilate's unsuccessful pleas for sympathy. In *Ecce Homo* (Behold the Man) scenes, Pilate displays the wounded Christ to the angry crowd in the hope that the pitiful sight will satisfy its lust for blood.

Painters also depicted Christ nailed to the Cross, wearing a crown of thorns while metal spikes are hammered through his outstretched hands and crossed feet. An interesting feminine variation of this theme was inspired by the mystical piety associated with convents. In these images Christ, nailed to the cross, is stuck with a lance by women representing the virtues Ecclesia, Synagogue, and Caritas. Because humanity's salvation was made possible by Christ's, it was considered virtuous to assist Christ by torturing him.

Christ Crucified on the Cross is perhaps the most commonly painted scene in Western art. While some paintings portray Christ free of wounds, many others spare no details. These images echo the vision of Saint Bridget of Sweden (1303–1373): "He was crowned with thorns. Blood trickled over his eyes, his ears, his beard; his mouth was open, his tongue bleeding, his cheeks hollow. His body was so greatly sunk that it seemed he no longer had any entrails."

In Lamentation scenes the body of Christ is mourned. In one of the most famous, by Andrea Mantegna (about 1500), Christ rests on a wooden bed. No spikes are visible, but Christ's hands and feet prominently display the jagged wounds. Pietà scenes portray Mary's grief at her son's death. Particularly gruesome yet touching are German wood carvings of the Pietà in which a sorrowful, adoring Mary holds the emaciated and ravaged body of Christ in her lap. Another related devotional image is the *Man of Sorrows*, in which Christ's suffering is emphasized, although it is not associated with any specific event in his life. Such scenes were invitations for viewers to fulfill themselves by imitating Christ.

Reformation art had its own special focus on the Passion. In Lucas Cranach's *Christ on the Cross, and the Risen Christ Slays Death and the Devil* (1553), for example, John the Baptist, Cranach himself, and Martin Luther stand at the foot of the cross. From a wound in Christ's side a jet of blood—representing the stream of grace—falls on the painter's head, while Luther holds open a Bible, his finger pointing to the words "The Blood of Jesus Christ cleanseth us from all sin."

Arma Christi scenes focus single-mindedly on Christ's suffering. *Arma* refers

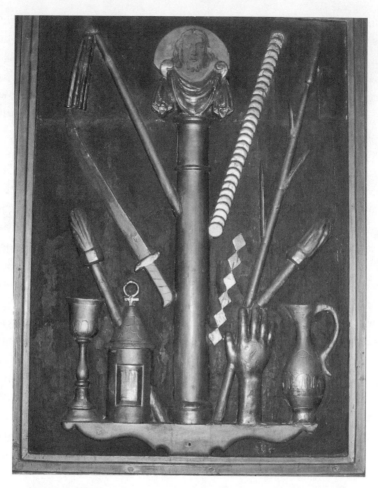

This medieval Arma Christi scene from the French church of Saint-Pierre
de Collonges-la-rouge depicts images from Christ's Passion: the flagellum
used to whip him; the pillar where he was whipped, topped by the veil
that Veronica used to wipe the sweat from his face as he walked on the
Via Dolorosa to Calvary; the hand that slapped his face; the pitcher of gall
and vinegar that was offered to him during his crucifixion; the thirty
pieces of silver paid to Judas for betraying him; the dice used by soldiers
to game for his robe; the torches, lamps, and sword of the arresting
soldiers; and a reed scepter. (Photo courtesy Jean Poussin)

to the weapons with which Christ conquered death and Satan. They symbolized
triumph and were a sort of coat of arms. Typical *Arma Christi* images include the
lance used to pierce Christ, the nails used to fasten him to the cross, instruments
such as whips, pincers, and scourges used to torture him, a crown of thorns, and

even the bloody knife used to circumcise him. The *Arma Christi* image sometimes replaced the crucifixion as the center of Passion scenes. Instead of depicting Christ in his entirety, only his mutilated body parts were shown; sometimes
the central image was a large crown of thorns containing four roses. Each rose
framed either a wounded hand or foot of Christ. In the center of the crown was
Jesus's heart, dripping blood, pierced by a lance. In fact, in the year 1354 the Feast
of the Lance was proclaimed, and a Christian cult arose that venerated the lance
stuck into Christ's side by the Roman soldier Longinus.

Although for twelve centuries Jesus's heart was not especially venerated, it has
become his most revered body part. In the thirteenth century, French and German nuns prone to mysticism declared visions of glory blazing from Christ's
wounded heart. In these visions the heart was still firmly within Jesus's body; the
blazing glory was interpreted as saving grace and, in paintings, became a stream
of blood that gushed from Christ's side onto a person's head or into a chalice.

In 1610, Saint Francis de Sales founded the Order of the Visitation for nuns.
The order's coat of arms featured an image of Jesus's heart with arrows sticking
out of it and with a crown of thorns and a cross at its top. From 1673 to 1675 a
member of that order, Saint Marguerite-Marie Alacoque, had widely publicized
ecstatic visions: "The Heart of Jesus was represented to me as on a throne formed
of fire and flames, surrounded by rays more brilliant than the sun and transpar-
ent as crystal. The wound which He received on the cross was clearly seen there.
Around this Sacred Heart was a crown of thorns, and above it a cross which was
planted in it" (Saint Margaret Mary 1931, p. 64). Her visions climaxed decades of
attempts by a small group of priests to establish the Sacred Heart as an approved
devotional image.

The Council of Trent (1545–63) carefully considered the question of religious
images and had produced a list of acceptable ones. Jesus's heart was not on the
list. Despite this prohibition the Sacred Heart image was commonly used in the
imagery of the Catholic church in Mexico. Kehoe (1979) has demonstrated that
this image diffused from Mexico to Europe. The heart of the Aztec death god, for
example, was often portrayed through a wound in his chest. From this heart a
dynamic "fluid" streamed out while the god held another heart crowned with
flaming leaves in his hand. Thus, the Catholic church appropriated Mexican religious symbols and integrated them into mainstream Christian iconography (Keleman 1967).

Christian art over the centuries has associated human body parts and instruments of torture with biblical figures and saints (Ferguson 1954). A severed head,
depending on the context, might refer to Goliath, or to Holofernes, or to Salome,

or to John the Baptist. Saint Agatha, a third-century martyr, had her breasts cut off with shears; paintings of her show a dish with her mutilated breasts on it. Saint Catherine of Alexandria, another early martyr, was torn to death; her special attribute is the spiked wheel. One of Saint Eustace's attributes is the instrument of his martyrdom, a life-sized, iron brazen bull into whose red-hot body he was placed. Saint Laurence's attribute is the gridiron, on which he was roasted. Saint Lucy is often portrayed holding her self-enucleated eyes in her hand.

Devotional books, such as Gallonio's *De SS Martyrum Cruciatibus*, describe the gruesome fate of the martyrs not only in words but also in vivid drawings; martyrs are shown being flayed alive, dismembered, having their teeth and tongue cut off, being gored by bulls, cooked alive, and eaten by wild animals. Although many of the legends about the early Christian martyrs are clearly embellishments designed to impress the faithful, the torture and suffering they (and later on the Tudor martyrs in England) endured were real and horrible.

From a psychiatric perspective, one of the most interesting and unusual martyrs was Saint Wilgefortis, who was the daughter of a cruel Portuguese king and supposedly lived around A.D. 800. Having made a vow of virginity, she was shocked when her father not only made sexual advances but also betrothed her to a Saracen Sicilian king. She prayed to God to stop the marriage by depriving her of her beauty. She became an ascetic, starved herself, developed an unattractive, hairy body, and even grew a beard! The Sicilian king refused to marry her, and her enraged father had her crucified. While on the cross, she spoke of "the passion that encumbrances all women" and urged women to pray that through her they would be similarly blessed and liberated from worldly care. From A.D. 1200 her cult spread. Lacey (1982) considers her to have had anorexia nervosa, culminating "in Wilgefortis's crucifixion by her father with the support and encouragement of her family, the symbolism of which would not be lost on the anorectic patient of today" (p. 817).

Mutilative Imagery in Secular Art

Although it is beyond the scope of this volume to survey the artistic history of mutilation, the visual images of Hieronymus Bosch's triptych of the *Garden of Delights* (sixteenth century) are among the most famous and incredible in Western art. The theme of the painting is man's fall from grace, his indulgence in sinful pursuits (especially lust), and the hellish punishments for his transgressions. Sinners are grouped together; gamblers, for example, are pictured with dice in their detached hands, while dogs and rodents gnaw at their bodies. Men overly given to delight in music cry in agony because flutes have been shoved up their rectums. Two mutilated ears with a long dagger protruding between them (a bizarre phallic war machine) slash their way among those who have reveled in hearing evil. A central figure is known as the Tree-Man (some critics refer to the figure as Alchemical Man), a strange creature whose legs are lacerated tree trunks and whose egg-shaped torso is cracked open to reveal a tavern full of lost souls. Knights given to anger are ripped apart. A sinner with blackbirds flying out of his anus is devoured by a disgusting bird who, in turn, defecates his human meal into a cesspool full of vomit, feces, and gold coins. Similar themes are portrayed in another of Bosch's famous triptychs, *The Last Judgment.* Here we see some sinners sliced up and placed in a frying pan while others are impaled by spears and still others are ripped apart and tortured.

Bosch remains an enigmatic artist who left no letters, probably never traveled from his hometown, did not date his paintings, and inspired no early biographies. A complete understanding of all his images requires knowledge of the minutiae of medieval symbolism and of Dutch variants. A person who painted such horrifying images today might well be exhibiting schizophrenic pathology, but Bosch's images were well attuned to the cultural climate of his time. Mutilation and torture were regarded as the inevitable "rewards" of leading a sinful life. It was a time in which God's Eye saw every misdeed. Indeed, Bosch's painting *The Seven Deadly Sins* depicts a mutilated Christ as the pupil of God's Eye, which clearly sees humankind's transgressions. "Beware, Beware, God Sees" are the words inscribed around the pupil.

Certainly many of the most highly regarded twentieth-century artistic images reflect a peculiar type of mutilation. One thinks of surrealism, especially Dali's nightmarish figures, and of Picasso and the Cubists, who ripped apart the human body and reassembled it in bizarre ways in an attempt to clarify our perceptions through distortion. And perhaps it would be remiss not to mention two of the most enduring images of classical art—the headless *Winged Victory of Samothrace,* the essence of grace, and that epitome of feminine beauty, the mutilated torso of the Venus de Milo.

Mutilation in Literature

Throughout this book I refer to the famous, classical literary mutilation scenes found in Sophocles' *Oedipus Rex,* in Ovid's *Metamorphoses,* in Catullus's poem about the self-emasculation of Attis, and in Shakespeare's grisly drama *Titus Andronicus.* Although a complete survey of literary depictions of mutilation would constitute an entire large volume in itself, I present several examples that demonstrate mutilation and self-mutilation in differing contexts, namely, mental illness, theatricality, the judicial process, religion, and mob violence.

The oldest, fairly detailed literary example of self-mutilation associated with mental illness that I have found is in book 6 of Herodotus. Cleomenes, a Spartan leader, lost his wits completely and poked his staff into the face of everyone he met. His relatives put him in the stocks. As he was lying there, fast bound, he noticed that all his guards had left him except one. He asked this man, who was a serf, to lend him his knife. At first the fellow refused, but Cleomenes, by threats of what he would do to him when he recovered his liberty, so frightened him that he at last consented. As soon as the knife was in his hands, Cleomenes began to mutilate himself, beginning on his shins. "He sliced his flesh into strips, working upwards to his thighs, hips, and sides until he reached his belly, which he chopped into mincemeat."

Franz Kafka, perhaps more than any other author, has succeeded in developing self-mutilation as a most peculiar and penetrating literary genre. *The Hunger Artist* is about a professional faster, a man who was booked to sit in a cage and starve himself for forty days in full public view. Teams of permanent watchers (usually butchers) watched closely to ensure that the hunger artist did not secretly break his fast. He found himself deserted as people sought other amusements. He was neglected more and more until one day an overseer's eye fell on his cage. He asked why nothing was in it except dirty straw. Workers poked into the straw with sticks and to their surprise found the hunger artist. When the overseer told the hunger artist that he admired his fasting, the reply was, "But you shouldn't admire it because I have to fast. I can't help it because I couldn't find the food I liked. If I had found it, believe me, I should have made no fuss and stuffed myself like you or anyone else." With that the overseer cleaned out the cage and buried the hunger artist, straw and all. And into the cage he placed a wild, young panther whose joy of life was a real crowd pleaser.

Kafka's *In the Penal Colony* begins with the portentous phrase "It's a remarkable piece of apparatus." The apparatus in question is a machine on which persons are mutilated and then executed. It consists of a bed, a control device called a designer, and a harrow or set of needles. A condemned man is strapped naked to the bed, and then, over the course of twelve hours, the harrow carves words into the prisoner's flesh. The prisoner is not told the nature of his crime or the sentence that has been passed on him. In fact, he learns of it only by deciphering the message that is carved on his body. An insubordinate soldier, for example, would have the words "Honor Thy Superiors!" carved on him. After the prisoner deciphers the message and is enlightened through his wounds, the harrow pierces him and casts him into a bloody pit, where he is buried.

A more contemporary depiction of self-mutilation is found in Flannery O'Connor's highly acclaimed novel *Wise Blood*. Amid a setting of rural southern poverty, the protagonist, Hazel Motes, "saw Jesus move from tree to tree in the back of his mind, a wild ragged figure motioning him to turn around and come off into the dark where he was not sure of his footing, where he might be walking on the water and not know it and then suddenly know it and drown." He becomes a bizarre preacher of the Church-of-Christ-without-Christ, a church where the blind don't see, and the lame don't walk, and the dead stay dead, and the blood of Jesus doesn't save. Tortured by his struggles to reject or to accept Jesus, he finally pokes out both his eyes with a pointed stick, stops preaching, and lives in a small boardinghouse, where he puts rocks in his shoes. When asked by his landlady why he walks on rocks, he answers, "To pay." She then discovers that he wears strands of barbed wire under his shirt and says, "It's not normal. It's like one of them gory stories, it's something that people have quit doing—like boiling in oil or being a saint or walling up cats. People have quit doing it. . . . What do you do it for?" "I'm not clean," he replies. Having finally found Christ, he contracts influenza and dies, the winter winds slashing at the boardinghouse, "making a sound like sharp knives swirling in the air."

Germinal (1885), Emile Zola's great novel about social injustice in the French mine pits, vividly demonstrates the theme of mob violence. The story recounts how starved mine workers revolted against management. They cornered Maigrat, the hated shop owner, when he fell, smashed his head on a stone wall, and his brains spouted out.

Then old Mother Brule yelled, "Cut him like a tom-cat!" The other women pulled off his trousers and raised his legs. Mother Brule separated his thighs, grabbed his genitals, and tore them off the corpse. "I've got it! I've got it," she laughed triumphantly. Another woman said, "Swine! You won't fill our daughters anymore! We don't have to offer you our backside in return for a loaf of bread anymore." The women shook with terrible gaiety and spat on the lump of hairy, bleeding flesh. "Mother Brule then planted the whole lump on the end of her stick, and holding it in the air, bore it about like a banner, rushing along the road, followed, helter-skelter, by the yelling troop of women. Drops of blood rained down, and that pitiful flesh hung like a waste piece of meat on a butcher's stall."

Zola's likening of the mutilation of a man to the mutilation of a cat was an accurate reflection of European folk beliefs. Darnton (1984) shed light on this curious aspect of mutilation by examining ways of thinking in eighteenth-century France. One theme he developed is the mutilation and torture of animals, especially cats. In fact, his lead essay begins, "The funniest thing that ever happened in the printing shop of Jacques Vincent, according to a worker who witnessed it, was a riotous massacre of cats." The episode he examined is a revolt by printer's apprentices in Paris during the 1730s. The apprentices led a miserable existence, and even at night they were unable to sleep in their dingy bedroom because the wife of the printing shop's owner allowed her cats to sit on the roof and howl. When the howling became too much for even the shop owner, he asked the apprentices to get rid of the cats, except for the one favorite feline of his wife. The apprentices gleefully collected all of the cats, beginning with the one they were asked to save, and proceeded to massacre them by placing them in sacks and smashing them with iron bars. They then gathered the cats, some still barely alive, and held a mock trial. The cats were pronounced guilty, given last holy rites, and hanged on a small gallows. The shop owner and his wife, aroused by the men's laughter, flew into a rage, but the apprentices were delirious with "joy, disorder, and laughter." During the following days, the apprentices joked about the event and reenacted the scene in mime at least twenty times. Years later one of the participants noted that it was the most hilarious event of his life.

What was so special about cats? As Darnton points out, cats have long fascinated humankind in general, and artists and poets in particular. Their night howling sometimes sounds like a human scream. And cats are well suited for staging ceremonies: "You cannot make a charivari with a cow. You do it with cats: you decide to *faire le chat*, to make *Katzenmusik*." Torturing cats was a popular form of amusement in Europe. In France, during the *dimanches des brandons* in Samur, children attached cats to poles and roasted them over bonfires. In Aix-en-Provence cats were smashed on the ground. People were described as being "patient as a cat whose claws are being grilled." Hogarth's drawings *The Stages of Cruelty* vividly depict the joyousness obtained from animal mutilation.

Cats were popularly associated with witchcraft in Europe. The devil himself was depicted often as a huge tomcat who presided over sexual orgies. The standard method of protecting oneself from sorcery was to maim a cat by smashing its legs, cutting its tail, or burning its fur, thus stripping it of its evil powers. Cats also had occult powers (e.g., a person could hasten recovery from a bad fall by sucking the blood from a cat's freshly amputated tail). Also, when a new house was built the French often placed a live cat in the walls. Finally, cats were, and are, connected with sex. The slang word *pussy* means the same in French as in English, and the shrieks of copulating cats sometimes refer to cuckoldry. Thus, the printer's apprentices "could hear a great deal in the wail of a cat . . . witchcraft, orgy, cuckoldry, charivari, and massacre."

CHAPTER TWO

Self-mutilation in Myths of Creation, Shamanism, and Religion

Et nos servasti . . . sanguine fuso
[And you saved us by shedding blood]
— Mithraic inscription in the Roman church of Santa Prisca

Self-mutilation is a violent act associated with suffering, either immediate or delayed. However, there are many culturally sanctioned instances when persons willingly mutilate themselves or allow others to mutilate them in the belief that their behavior serves a higher purpose beneficial to themselves or their community. Michael and Aubine Kirtley (1982), for example, photographed and described the New Year festival of the Abidji tribe (Ivory Coast). On the eve of the festival, tribal members attend meetings devoted to reconciling divisive personal and communal issues. On the day of the festival, bad spirits are driven away, and some individuals enter a trance state to the accompaniment of rhythmic drumming. Guided by *sekes*, beneficent spirits that possess their bodies, they plunge a knife into their abdomen. The serious wounds that result are treated with poultices of kaolin, herbs, and raw eggs. Healing occurs, and the entranced mutilators say that their *seke* prescribes both the wound and the cure. Although the Abidji cannot explain clearly the reasons for this ritual, it probably serves as a physical demonstration of the social healing that has occurred within the entire community.

Most mentally ill persons are nonviolent and suffer because of their illness. Why should they wreak violence on themselves and endure even more suffering through the act of self-injury? The simplest answer provided by patients is that self-injury provides relief, at least temporarily, from pathological symptoms such as anxiety, guilt, and hallucinations and from aversive social situations. The psychiatric theories that attempt to explain this process are discussed later in this book. Here, however, I examine the process from a different perspective, namely, that of religion and its offspring, shamanism.

The decision to examine self-injury in the context of religion stems from several

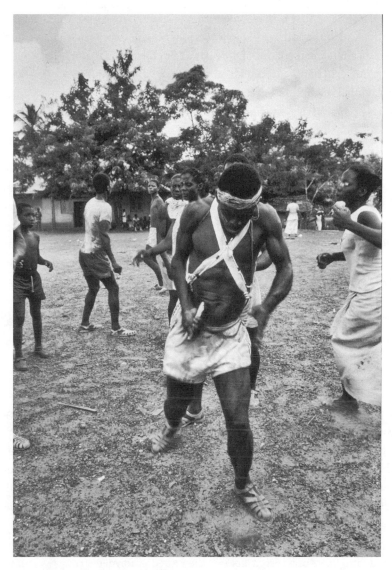

An African native from the Ivory Coast (Abidji tribe) mutilates himself while in a trance during the New Year festival. The wounds, although often severe, typically heal without difficulty. On the eve of the festival, tribal members meet to reconcile divisive personal and communal issues. The self-mutilation probably symbolizes the social healing that has occurred within the entire community. (Photo by Michael and Aubine Kirtley, courtesy of National Geographic Society)

observations. The first is that some forms of mental illness are characterized by symptoms such as shifting levels of consciousness, auditory and visual hallucinations, and altered perceptions of the body and of the environment that are similar to religious experiences; indeed, some mentally ill self-injurers experience and articulate their condition in religious terms, for example, they claim to be a god or to have a special relationship with the spirit world. A second observation is that many religions have extolled the practice of bodily mortification. A third is that violence, according to some scholars, is at the core of religion; as stated by Girard (1977, p. 24), "Violence is the heart and secret soul of the sacred. . . . Religion shelters us from violence just as violence seeks shelter in religion." A fourth is that religion functions in great part to help individuals deal with the suffering inherent in life.

Religious sentiments, albeit in varying degrees, are present among many mentally ill self-mutilators, especially those who experience psychosis, and an understanding of religion helps us understand why such persons injure themselves. In this context, self-injury may be regarded not only as a destructive act but also as a creative one. Let us, therefore, begin at the beginning when the world itself was created.

Myths of Creation

The primary Indo-European cosmogonic myth is that the world was created as the result of the sacrifice and mutilation of the primordial hermaphroditic being. Lincoln (1975) noted that cosmogonic myths establish the order of the world. He reconstructed the basic Proto-Indo-European myth of the creation of the world from the dismembered body of a primordial being by examining three classic texts, the *Rigveda* (India), the *Greater Bundahisn* (Iran), and the *Prose Edda* (Scandinavia).

The *Rigveda* states that the gods tied up Purusa, sacrificed him, and divided his body into portions. From his eye the sun was formed, from his mind the moon, from his navel the midair, and from his head the sky. Earth came from his feet, and from his ear came the regions of the earth. From the dripping fat were formed the creatures of the air and animals both wild and tame. His mouth became the Brahman, his arms the Rajanya, his thighs the Vaisya, his feet the Sudra.

The *Greater Bundahisn* tells how Ahriman, the Evil Spirit, dismembered both an ox and Gayomart. From the semen of the dead ox were created corn, medicinal herbs, and a pair of every species of animal. From Gayomart's head lead was fashioned; his blood became tin, his marrow silver, his feet iron, his bones copper, his fat glass, his arms steel, his life's departure (breath?) gold. As he lay dying, Gayomart's sperm spilled to the earth and from it came the ten species of humanity.

In the Scandinavian *Prose Edda*, both a cow and the giant Ymir are mutilated by the gods. From Ymir's body the world was made. His blood became the sea and lakes; his flesh became the earth; his bones became mountains; his teeth and jaw became rocks and pebbles; his skull became the sky.

Despite minor variation, the three primordial victims are structurally similar. From semantic and phonological studies it is also apparent that they are all derived from a Proto-Indo-European mythic figure.

Even in China, the giant figure of P'an-ku can be traced to the Indian Purusa. When P'an-ku was sliced up, his breath became the wind and clouds, his voice the thunder, his eyes the sun and moon, his limbs and fingers the earth and mountains, his blood the rivers, his sweat the rain, his skin and hair the plants and trees, his teeth and bones the metal and stones, and the parasites on his body became human beings.

The first sacrifice of the Primordial Being was the origin of the world, and from his mutilation society and social order were established. Over the millennia, this myth in its various elaborations has been and continues to be reenacted in countless religious rituals. With each reenactment, the world and social order are recreated. Participants in these rituals experience the suffering and terror that come with sacrifice and mutilation, but they are rewarded for their participation by feelings of security, solace, well-being, and personal order.

The self-mutilative acts of some mentally ill persons may be understood in the light of this mythic process. Their bodies become a microcosm of the vaster cosmos, and the irresistible urge to self-mutilation becomes an unconscious reenactment of the cosmogonic myth in which chaos is averted and a new order established. Self-mutilation offers a temporary respite from illness rather than a permanent cure because the sacrificial death of the Primordial Being is not emulated; the mentally ill person sacrifices only a body part or a portion of blood to achieve a modicum of well-being. A partial sacrifice achieves only a partial peace.

Shamanism

From the earliest days of human history, special men and women have devoted their lives to healing the illnesses and reversing the misfortunes of the members of their community. One such group, known as shamans, attends to these difficult tasks through personal contact with the spirit world. Revered for their wisdom and granted a lofty status by their social groups, shamans hold special interest for us because they voluntarily participate in their own bodily mutilation to become healers.

Persons who receive a calling to shamanism enter into a crisis and endure an initiatory sickness. They must endure a traditional sequence of mystical events, resolve their crisis, and emerge "resurrected" as new persons able to travel to the spirit world to protect and to heal the members of their tribe. According to Eliade (1975), shamanic initiation has five important moments: (1) torture and dismemberment of the body; (2) reduction of the body to a skeleton by scraping away the flesh; (3) substitution of the viscera and renewal of the blood; (4) time spent in Hell, during which the future shaman learns from demons and from the souls of dead shamans; and (5) an ascent to Heaven in order to be consecrated by God.

"The sufferings of the elected man are exactly like the tortures of initiation; just as in puberty rites or rites for entrance into a secret society, the novice is 'killed' by semi-divine or demonic Beings, so the future shaman sees in dreams his own body dismembered by demons; he watches them, for example, cutting off his head and tearing out his tongue" (Eliade 1975, p. 89). In the shamanic world, these experiences of suffering and mutilation are intense and are perceived as real and dangerous (Eliade 1960; 1974).

Would-be Yakut (Siberia) shamans "die" and lie silently for several days in a secluded place during their initiatory sickness. Demons scrape the flesh off their bones, remove the fluids from their bodies, and tear out their eyeballs. In this condition they are transported to Hell for three years, where their heads are cut off and their bodies are finely chopped and distributed to diseased spirits. In this process the would-be shamans endure great suffering and learn the secrets of healing. When their bones are covered with new flesh and their bodies given new blood, they emerge from the underworld with a new personality, that of a true shaman.

Similar stories are told by Australian aboriginal shamans. A medicine man of the Unmatjera tribe stated that he was killed when an old tribal doctor threw stones at him that went through his head. The doctor then removed his internal organs, packed his body cavity with stones, and sang over him. He was given a new set of internal organs and brought back to life.

Dyak (Borneo) shamans assert that their heads are cut open. To achieve insight into healing, their brains are washed and restored into their heads. Gold dust is inserted into their eyes to empower them to see souls that might wander off. Their hearts are pierced with arrows to enhance their ability to sympathize with the sick and suffering.

These examples from disparate, ancient traditions point to bodily mutilation as a stepping-stone to wisdom, special capacities for healing oneself and others, and a higher level of existence. Shamans allow their bodies to be dismembered painfully and then reconstructed so that they emerge as wiser and healthier persons. Shamans have discovered the therapeutic value of self-mutilation. Is it not possible that some mentally ill persons faced with suffering and misfortune have unwittingly made the same discovery?

Religion

- A 46-year-old woman cut out her tongue with a razor. She said that she had "received a message from God to cut out my tongue. . . . Duty demanded it."
- A 26-year-old man believed that he possessed some of Jesus's features and that God had talked with him. He blinded himself by scratching out his eyes, stating that "God told me to prevent people suffering."
- A 32-year-old man had sought to purify his spirit for six years. Burdened by guilt over episodes of drunkenness, aggression, and sexual transgressions, he cut off both his testicles "as a freewill offering to God." He entered into a brief homosexual relationship. Disgusted by this, he turned to the New Testament and read that "there be eunuchs who have made themselves eunuchs for the Kingdom of Heaven's sake." When he felt sexual desire two weeks later, he cut off his penis with a razor and burned it in a fire, stating, "Even if I do get certified [as legally insane] and in the eyes of the world I am mad, it is far better for me to have cleansed myself."

In each of these clinical cases, the diagnosis of schizophrenia was made. However, in certain historical and cultural contexts, these incidents of self-mutilation might have been regarded as socially meaningful or even inspired. In most religious traditions, gods, prophets, martyrs, saints, and sinners in search of redemption have mortified, mutilated, and sacrificed themselves. That some people who are mentally ill model their behavior on that of these spiritual heroes is clear and, at least on a superficial level, understandable. Identification with a conquering hero may permit psychotic persons to feel in control of a world that appears to be crumbling around them (the consolation of illusion). For self-mutilators, however, not any hero will do. Napoleon is never chosen, but Jesus frequently is. Even in non-Christian cultures, self-mutilators tend to identify with religious heroes. Is there, then, some special connection between self-mutilation and religion?

Religion means many things to many people and can be appreciated on various levels. Surely religion is love, compassion, purity, joy, and tranquility. Yet at the core of religion one finds violence, sacrifice, blood, suffering, martyrdom, and self-mutilation. Two of the most revered symbols, for example, are the cross of Christianity and the Siva lingam of Hinduism.[1] Others before me have reached the same conclusion (Bowker 1970; Burkert 1983; Girard 1977). This bloody violence has from the earliest times served to establish and to preserve cosmological and personal order. Likewise, some modern-day people who are mentally ill mutilate themselves to establish and to preserve order in their lives. I do not believe that they consciously understand the significance of their actions, however. Although the "religious" self-mutilations of people who are mentally ill are idiosyncratic and, unlike truly "sacred" mutilations, devoid of meaning for the community, they touch on a profound, mythic process. The following lyrical scenario attempts to reveal the essence of the Sacred.

Let us imagine a group of travelers in search of the Sacred. They pass through consecrated grounds and enter the Holy Temple. As they penetrate the gilded antechambers sweet music fills their ears. Through the disorienting mist of incense they see the object of their quest, the True Altar. A blinding yet strangely peaceful light reflects off the altar's gold and pure-white marble sides. Bedazzled, most of the travelers feel no need to go further. They are satisfied with their sense of awe and refresh themselves with a little bread and wine given to them by the priests. But those brave souls who truly wish to experience the terror, bliss, and recognition of supreme authority (*mysterium temendum, fascinans, et augustum*) of the Holy go on bended knees to the True Altar's edge. The sound of hymns has disappeared, replaced by groans and muffled shrieks of agony from the Altar's center. Fearful, they peer over the top of the Holy Altar into the Well of Eternal Life. What they see disgusts them momentarily, but they are powerless to avert their eyes. The well is deep, so deep that it reaches the very center of the earth, and it is apparent it is the source of all the streams and rivers of the world. Should this well dry up, no crops would grow. It is apparent, too, that this well supplies humankind with a special type of sustenance called the Sacred. Without it Chaos

---

1. According to Hindu belief, Brahma the Creator was unsuccessful in creating human beings and so commanded Siva to do it. Siva initially refused to create imperfect beings and in anger responded to his father's command by castrating himself. Siva's severed penis or lingam sunk into the ground, penetrated the netherworld, and then shot up into the sky as a burning pillar of flames. His lingam is a most sacred object. Naturally formed stone representations of the pillar, some of them ten feet tall, often include carvings of Siva's face, indicating the relationship between procreation and creative thought. According to Kramrisch (1981): "In the world of Siva, the significance of the *linga* is comparable to that of the Cross in the Christian world, and that of Siva with the *linga*, or the faces of Siva together with the shape of the *linga*, to the figure of the Savior on the Cross."

would control the universe and people would exist in hopeless lawlessness, devouring one another like wolves.

There is no water in the Well of the One True Altar, only blood and bits of flesh and bone that pop to the surface. Look! There is Odin's eye, and Jesus's heart with a lance tip in it. Now Osiris's lost phallus floats by, and Attis's private parts. Now the breasts of Saint Agatha appear, and slices of Buddha's limbs. Here is the marrow of P'an-ku, the chest muscles of some courageous Sioux braves, and the charred skins of the Tudor martyrs. Although the violent commotion has comingled all of the blood, one can discern different textures and colors. The blood from blessed bulls and rams and oxen swirls to the top but is displaced by Dionysus's claret-colored blood and the crimson blood of Mithra.

Here, in the presence of the Sacred, the voyagers understand that everything in the universe—the crops, the forests, the rivers, the animals, the ordering of human groups, the moon, the sun, the stars—is dependent on the continued beneficence of the Holy Well. And they understand that the blood and flesh in the Well must be periodically replenished, especially during those times when the forces of chaos and evil let loose the dogs of war and set locusts on the fields, when pestilence and plague run rampant, and the sun darkens the sky. But whose blood shall be shed, whose flesh shall be picked apart to save us all?

Sacrifice and Suffering

During several manic episodes over the course of twelve years, a woman bit off a large piece of her tongue, wounded her arms, badly lacerated her vagina with her hand, burned her skin, and blinded herself while trying to gouge out her eyes. She claimed that God had ordered her to purify herself by sacrificing parts of her body.

A 48-year-old widow accused herself of being a great sinner. She went naked into the street and felt that her eyes were sinful. Having read Matthew's (5:28–29) claim that those who have lustful thoughts should remove their eyes, she quietly took out both of her eyes and asked the doctors to cut off her legs and feet, stating that because Christ had sacrificed his blood, she too must sacrifice her blood to become saintly.

A 25-year-old man removed both testicles with a razor blade. He said he did this because he heard the voice of his mother, who told him that he would be denied entry into the kingdom of heaven unless he sacrificed his penis and testicles.

In these cases as well as in many others described in this book, it is clear that the self-mutilations of some mentally ill persons occur in a context of religious sacrifice. Throughout history, persons who have endured suffering and death willingly out of devotion to their god have been revered as martyrs. Few religious followers become martyrs, but many choose to emulate their suffering and may inflict suffering on themselves deliberately. They are, in effect, engaging in a partial sacrifice.

Why are sacrifice and a focus on suffering so important to religion? What purposes do they serve? Why do some mentally ill persons perceive their acts of self-mutilation as sacrificial? What do they gain by inflicting suffering on themselves?[2]

The concept of sacrifice was an important concern of the founders of modern anthropology at the end of the nineteenth century (Bourdillon and Fortes 1980). Tylor's theory is that a person who offers a valuable sacrificial gift to a deity anticipates that the deity will respond with a special favor, such as recovery from illness, or general beneficence. Frazer's theory holds that the blood and flesh of sacrificial victims serve to rejuvenate the gods and to keep them from dying. Smith's theory focuses on the communion that is established between a group and its deity as a result of eating the flesh of the sacrificial animal or human victim. Hubert and Mauss's (1899) theory defines a sacrificial rite as "a procedure to establish a communion between a sacred world and the profane world through the intermediary of a victim." Some of these early anthropologists also noted that a powerful "energy" is released at the moment of sacrifice.

Perhaps the most astute modern student of sacred sacrifice is René Girard (1977). According to him, sacrifice is a religious act that protects a group from its own violence, restores harmony to a community, and reinforces the social fabric by focusing communal dissension onto a sacrificial victim. Sacrificial victims have been primarily such persons as prisoners of war, slaves, small children, and the handicapped, persons who are not fully integrated into communal life and who do not share close social bonds with a broad cross section of citizens.

Religious sacrifice entails suffering, whether it be the suffering of an animal whose throat is slit, a person whose heart is ripped out, or a god who is crucified; certainly in Christianity Jesus's suffering is an integral component of his self-sacrifice. In addition to this linkage with sacrifice, suffering is the raison d'être of the widespread religious practice of self-mortification.

Hinduism, perhaps the most complex of all religious systems, presents fertile grounds for self-mortification and self-mutilation. As recounted in the holy Vedas, the world "is just food and the eater of food," an endless cycle of devouring and

2. Among the best sources for a theoretical understanding of sacrifice and suffering are the books by Money-Kryle (1930), James (1962), Girard (1977), and Bourdillon and Fortes (1980).

being devoured. Through sacrifice one identifies with this cycle of creation and destruction and attempts to gain some measure of control over it.

In the Hindu pantheon of gods, Siva personifies the forces of destruction and evil in the universe. Bowker (1970) noted that Siva must be propitiated and "on the basis of the threefold relationship of devourer, devoured, and devouring, the propitiation of the devourer sometimes took on frightening and awe-inspiring forms" (p. 204). Kali, the Dark Goddess, is a ferocious and bloodthirsty aspect of Siva. Her teeth are fangs, and she wears a necklace of skulls and a belt of amputated limbs. In her four hands she carries a sword and a decapitated head dripping blood. Campbell (1962) noted that "in the temples of the Black Goddess Kali, the terrible one of many names, whose stomach is a void and so can never be filled and whose womb is giving birth forever to all things, a river of blood has been pouring continuously for millenniums, from beheaded offerings, through channels carved to return it, still living, to its divine source" (p. 5). Human sacrifices to Kali were abundant until forbidden by law in 1835. Today her temples in India and Nepal are still the scene of animal sacrifices.

The Hindu gods represent opposite and complementary qualities. Siva is the force of destruction as well as the force of creation. These qualities represent different aspects of a unitary process.

In Hinduism, suffering is inherent to the tensions of the cosmos. Again, according to Bowker, "Basically suffering is a part of the universe of being. It may be extremely beneficial, particularly if it is the foundation of better things, or if it is the knife which cuts humans off from their attachment to unworthy objects. . . . That explains why asceticism, privation voluntarily accepted, is so important in Hinduism. It is a part of the process of getting suffering in perspective. . . . Suffering is the process of being devoured, and as such it is the relationship between the two conflicting principles of the universe, the urge to life and the urge to death" (1970, p. 207).

Indeed, travelers to India cannot help but be impressed by the numbers of ascetic holy men, some of whom appear wasted and who twist their bodies into odd positions to free themselves from the bondage of attachment to worldly objects; also seen are numerous beggars, some of whom have deliberately mutilated their bodies. Ronald Simons produced an exceptional film called *Floating in the Air, Followed by the Wind*, which depicts a yearly Tamil festival in which devotees go into trance, pierce their tongues and cheeks with thick pins, and carry heavy religious objects that are anchored to their bodies by hundreds of fish hooks.

Within the mystical Islamic tradition of Sufism, asceticism and self-mortification are prominent. In Morocco, a Sufic brotherhood called the Hamadsha engage in head slashing during healing rituals. In describing this and similar brotherhoods, Crapanzano (1973) noted their extreme behavior: "wild dances, including ecstatic, frenetic trances; drinking boiling water; eating spiny cactus and other defilements; charming poisonous snakes; and innumerable acts of self-mutilation. All of them attempt to produce some sort of extraordinary psychic state which may be interpreted as union with God or possession by a demon" (p. 3). Indeed, al-Halla j (A.D. 858–922), the most revered Sufi martyr, advocated suffering as an important pathway to salvation, in emulation of Jesus's crucifixion, and many Sufic traditions are derived more from the Christian Desert Fathers than from mainstream Islam.

In Shia Islam (the Shiites are the second largest sect, the first being the Sunnis) great attention is given to the martyrdoms of the religious heroes Ali, Hasan, and especially Husain. During yearly passion festivals the deaths of these martyrs are reenacted so fervently that both the actors and spectators inflict wounds on their bodies. During the festival of Husain thousands of Shiites flagellate themselves frenetically while recalling his words: "Trial, afflictions, and pains, the thicker they fall on man, the better do they prepare him for his journey heavenward."

Is self-mutilation encountered among mentally ill Muslims? Several British psychiatrists with experience in Arabic countries have told me that the prevalence of self-mutilation there is somewhat higher than in Europe. In questioning several leading Islamic psychiatrists from the Middle East, however, I was assured that self-mutilation is *never* encountered because suffering is forbidden by the Koran. Indeed, I vividly recall a conversation with an elderly and stately Muslim psychiatrist who became a bit irritated by my questions. He stated that no Muslim would ever mutilate himself and added, while pointing a finger at me and twisting it, "Remember that the Prophet said that even when you kill an infidel you should twist the knife rapidly so as to cause him no pain."

Buddhism is the religion that most focuses on suffering. The essence of Buddha's wisdom, presented in his First Sermon at Benares, is that most everything in life—birth, death, aging, sickness, sorrow, association with the unpleasant, not getting what one desires—is suffering. Suffering is inevitable and should not be taken personally. Mortification of one's body is painful, unworthy, and unprofitable. Self-mutilation has a low incidence in Buddhist culture areas but Buddhism has many differing traditions. In Chinese monasteries, for example, burning off one's fingers as offerings to Buddha was practiced through the nineteenth century (Williams 1989; also see Benn 2007; Conze et al. 1995). Self-burning, including immolation, also has been practiced to achieve practical and political goals such as the ending of droughts and persecution. Bigot (1938) reported ten cases of self-castration by Vietnamese monks who had succumbed to sexual desires.

The Judaic tradition and Christian traditions cannot be comprehended accurately without reference to bloodshed, sacrifice, and suffering. Indeed, the sacred text of the Bible, a book that has greatly influenced human behavior and the course of events for millennia, devotes many pages to these topics. And from the New Testament has come the most famous example of sacrifice and suffering in all history and the most potent of all religious symbols—the bloody cross of the crucifixion.

The ancient notion that suffering is a just punishment for sins is found in the Old Testament, but some of its writers were well aware that this is not invariably the case. Thus, Jeremiah (12:1) pleaded with God to answer, "Why is it that the wicked live so prosperously? Why do scoundrels enjoy peace?" The answer that emerged is described by Bowker as "perhaps the supreme contribution of Israel to a human response to suffering, that suffering can be made redemptive, that it can become the foundation of better things, collectively, if not individually" (1970, p. 51). Nowhere is this more poignantly expressed than in Isaiah's description of the Servant (a metaphor for the people of Israel): "Ours were the sufferings he bore, ours the sorrows he carried. But we thought of him as someone punished, struck by God, and afflicted. Yet he was wounded for our transgressions, crushed for our sin. On him lies a punishment that brings us peace, and through his wounds we are healed. . . . Yahweh burdened him with the sins of us all" (53:4–6).

Traditionally for the Jews, the messiah that would come to rule in justice and in peace was an idealized version of King David. But then, according to James (1962), "The tribulation of the Jews during and after the fall of Jerusalem in A.D. 70 led to the Rabbinic interpretation of self-inflicted suffering as an atoning sacrifice in expiation of the national guilt, in preparation for the coming of the Messiah and the establishment of his righteous reign" (p. 116).

Enter Jesus, a man-god whose life assumed both unique meanings and linkages with older deities such as Mithra, Attis, and Dionysus.[3] Within the new Christian tradition, Jesus is both the glorious King David and the Suffering Servant. Indeed, 1 Peter 2 states: "Christ also suffered for you, leaving you an example,

---

3. Sinless Mithra was born on 25 December, the old date of the winter solstice. His sacrifice of the primal bull was repeated by thousands of his initiates over the ages. From the bull's spinal cord grew wheat and from his blood grew grape vines—the prototypical bread and wine of the communion meal. Attis castrated himself and was resurrected. His love was Cybele, the great mother goddess whose shrines were converted into shrines to the Virgin Mary. Dionysus, born of a virgin, was mutilated as a child and eventually resurrected.

that you should follow in his steps. . . . He himself bore our sins in his body on the tree, that we might die to sin and live to righteousness. By his wounds you have been healed."

In the Bible enormous emphasis was placed on Christ's suffering, on the metaphor of the Christian congregation as the body of Christ, on the literal need for individuals to present their bodies to God, and on the redemptive value of suffering.

— It is now my happiness to suffer for you. This is my way of helping to complete, in my poor human flesh, the full tale of Christ's afflictions still to be endured; for the sake of his body which is the church. (Col. 1:24)

— My dear friends, do not be bewildered by the fiery ordeal that is upon you, as though it were something extraordinary. It gives you a share in Christ's sufferings, and that is cause for joy. (1 Pet. 4)

— According to the law almost everything is purified by the blood, and without the shedding of blood there is no forgiveness. . . . So Christ was offered up once to take away the sins of many. (Heb. 9:22, 28)

— All men have sinned and are deprived of the glory of God. All men are now undeservedly justified by the gift of God, through the redemption wrought in Jesus Christ. Through his blood, God made him the means of expiation for all who believe. (Rom. 3:24–25)

Thus, Christ's suffering and crucifixion were a true sacrifice involving consecration of the victim, spilling of blood, death, expiation of sins, and establishment of a sacramental meal in which believers could partake of a portion of divinity by eating the victim's flesh and blood. Christ was both priest and victim whose self-sacrifice, an act of redeeming love, was followed by his victorious resurrection, and it afforded humankind the opportunity to reestablish a right relationship with God. To enter into this relationship, humankind had to participate in certain rituals, hold certain beliefs, and follow certain rules of conduct. For our study of self-mutilation, the one rule of conduct that has proven most portentous is stated in Matthew 18:7–9 (almost identical words are used in Mark 9:43–48):

What terrible things will come on the world through scandal! It is inevitable that scandal should occur. Nonetheless, woe to that man through whom scandal comes! If your hand or foot is your undoing, cut it off and throw it from you! Better to enter life maimed or crippled than be thrown with two hands or two feet into endless fire. If your eye is your downfall, gouge it out and cast it from you! Better to enter life with one eye than be thrown with both into Gehenna.

Martyrs and the Company of Saints

The early Christian church was distinguished by numerous martyrs who willingly died for their faith and endured incredible tortures. These men, women, and children epitomized the formation of a collective social body out of their individual bodies. Martyrs aggressively sought a passive death—the bloodier the better. Their model was Christ crucified. "In dying, the martyr's victory over Satan, instinct, and the world was confirmed; in suffering, his power was demonstrated" (Bradford 1990). The theologian Tertullian, at the end of the second century A.D., wrote his impassioned tracts *On Flight in Persecution* and *The Antidote for the Scorpion*: "At this present moment, it is the very middle of the heat, the very dog-days of persecution. Some Christians have been tested by the fire, some by the sword, some by the beasts; some, lashed and torn with hooks, have just tasted martyrdom, and lie hungering for it in prison. . . . We say, and we say it openly while you are torturing us, torn and bleeding, we cry aloud, 'We worship God through Christ!' . . . Nothing whatever is achieved by each more exquisite cruelty you invent; on the contrary, it wins men for our school. We are made more as often as you mow us down. The blood of Christians is seed [*semen est sanguis Christianorum*]."

The *Acts of the Martyrs* by the Bollandists comprises fifty folio tomes in which the lives of the martyrs are recorded to serve as models for all believers. The life of Saint Potitus, an example, tells how he was persecuted by his father because of his Christian beliefs. His father asked, "My child, do you not fear the punishments to be inflicted on Christians? If you are brought before the Emperor Antoninus, what will become of you? Those strange doctrines of yours will cause your flesh to be torn to pieces by hooks, and you will be eaten by the lions." Potitus responded, "Father, you can never frighten me with these things. In the name of the Father, and of the Son, and of the Holy Ghost, I am prepared to suffer everything for Jesus Christ."

Potitus cured a rich woman of leprosy by invoking Christ's help. At that time Antoninus's daughter was possessed by a devil who caused her to scream. Sacrifices to the Roman gods did not help. Potitus was asked by the emperor to cure the girl. "If I cure your daughter, will you believe in the God I believe in?" asked Potitus. The emperor said, "I will." Potitus succeeded, in Christ's name, in exorcising the demon from the girl leaving behind the stench of fire and brimstone. The emperor reneged on his promise, however, and tried to force Potitus to sacrifice to the Roman gods. When he refused, Antoninus brought him to the Colosseum, where, before a large crowd, he ordered the tortures to begin.

Although Potitus was stretched on the rack, for him it was like lying on a bed of roses. Starved and ferocious beasts were let loose, but they merely licked Potitus's feet. Four gladiators entered the arena, but their weapons fell harmlessly to the ground. Pincers with two large spikes were set on Potitus's head; when the pincers closed the spikes would pass through his brain. But, in response to Potitus's prayers, the pincers were lifted and were set by an invisible hand on the emperor's head. He shrieked in agony; Potitus agreed to remove them only if the emperor agreed to allow his daughter to become a Christian. After Antoninus assented, Potitus announced that he, a servant of Christ, was victorious and that now he desired to be united with Christ, whereupon Roman troops cut off his head.

Obviously the stories were embellished, but they were widely read (e.g., Voragine's *Legenda Aurea*) and served to inspire countless sermons over the centuries. More true to fact are the accounts in John Foxe's *Acts and Monuments* of the three hundred Protestant martyrs who were burned at the stake in Tudor England between 1531 and 1558. Especially interesting is an episode on the eve of the martyrdom of Thomas Bilney, the first Tudor martyr, in which he burned off a finger by placing it over the flame of a candle. Asked what he was doing Bilney replied, "Nothing but frying my flesh by God's grace, and burning one joint, when tomorrow God's rods shall burn the whole body in the fire."[4]

The ascendency of the Desert Fathers, holy men and women who sought salvation in the solitude of the Egyptian desert, in the fourth century A.D. made an enormous impact on Christianity. Large monasteries, some with ten thousand inhabitants, were established. In their small cells these seekers of religion practiced severe asceticism, desiring to rid themselves of all passions of the flesh. Their lives represented the concepts found in Socrates' *Phaedo* and echoed the saying of Dorotheus the Theban: "I kill my body, for it kills me." Their ideal was *solus ad solum*, alone to the alone, and as Waddell (1957) points out, they gave the intellectual concept of eternity to Europe: "These men, by the very exaggeration of their lives, stamped infinity on the imagination of the West" (p. 23).

The first Desert Father was Saint Anthony (A.D. 251–356). The widely circulated book *Vita S. Antonii* was highly influential in the spread of the ascetic movement. Anthony opted for a life of celibacy and lived in empty tombs where he had

---

4. Byman (1978) interpreted Bilney's action as one of many counterphobic devices utilized by the martyrs to overcome their fears and the pain of the fire. Other examples include those of martyrs embracing the stake upon which they were to be burned, lifting their hands to heaven while their bodies were being burned, and praying. In fact, ritualistic acts and compulsive behaviors are performed by some self-injurers, especially chronic self-cutters.

visions of demons who whipped him. He then lived alone in a deep pit for twenty years. His disciples lowered bread to him every six months. During this time he neither washed nor removed his only garment, a coarse animal skin. His fame spread, and his behavior served to inspire others (although centuries later the historian Gibbon described him as "a hideous, distorted emaciated maniac, without knowledge, without patriotism, without natural affection, spending his life in a long routine of useless and atrocious self-torture, and quailing before the phantoms of his deluded brain").

The most fantastic desert hermit was Saint Simeon Stylites, whose odd behavior inspired a cult of imitators. He devoted himself to celibacy and to self-starvation and went to a deserted mountaintop and had his foot chained to a large rock. The chain sunk into his flesh, creating a large ulcer. The ulcer became infested with worms, and as the worms fell to the ground Simeon placed them back into the wound, saying, "Eat what God has given you." He is best known for climbing onto a small platform at the top of a sixty-foot pillar and living there for the last thirty years of his life. Sparse amounts of food were passed up to him in a basket.

With the development of the great monastic orders in Europe during the eleventh century, the spirit of asceticism and self-mortification once again became prominent, and in this spirit self-flagellation as a voluntary act of penance became widespread. Heinrich Suso, a German mystic, wrote the following famous third-person account of his flagellatory experience: "He shut himself in his cell and stripped himself naked, and took his scourge with the sharp spikes, and beat himself on the body and on the arms and on the legs, till blood poured off him as from a man who had been cupped. One of the spikes on the scourge was bent like a hook, and whatever flesh it caught tore off. He beat himself so hard that the scourge broke into three pieces and the points flew against the wall. He stood there bleeding and gazed at himself. It was such a wretched sight that he was reminded in many ways of the appearance of the beloved Christ, when he was fearfully beaten. Out of pity for himself, he began to weep bitterly. And he knelt down, naked and covered in blood, in the frosty air, and prayed to God to wipe out his sins from before his gentle eyes" (Cohn 1958, p. 124). Self-flagellation was not a Christian invention, but rather was widely practiced in many circum-Mediterranean religions; for example, the priests of the cult of Attis scandalized the Romans because of such odd practices as self-flagellation, the hearing of confessions, and self-castration.

The first followers of Saint Francis were passionate flagellators, as were Saint Dominic and Peter Damian (who taught that one thousand lashes equaled the recitation of ten penitential psalms). Joachim of Fiore preached that the year 1260 would usher in the age of "the Eternal Gospel," a time of peace and happiness. Public expectations were high and reached a fever pitch as the year progressed. Then, in November 1260, an epidemic of self-flagellation began.

Thousands of Perugians spontaneously beat themselves with small leather whips. The Italian historian Salimbene wrote an eyewitness account: "All men, both great and small, noble knights and men of the people, scourged themselves naked, in procession through the cities, with the Bishops and men of religion at their head; and peace was made in many places, and men restored what they had unlawfully taken away; and they confessed their sins so earnestly that the priests had scarce leisure to eat" (Jones 1961, p. 50).

The epidemic spread and took hold in Germany, where flagellant leaders produced a Heavenly Letter, supposedly dictated by Christ, which stated that God was angry because people neglected religion and practiced usury and adultery. God decided to punish humankind by sending disease, famine, and pagan invasions. Because people still did not change their evil ways, God decided to destroy them all. But the Virgin Mary begged God to give humankind one last chance, and an angel ordered mass flagellation if humanity was to save itself.

In the face of prolonged drought and poverty, the masses responded to the warning of the Heavenly Letter. In 1348, the bubonic plague spread from Hungary. The high death rate and fears associated with the plague gave renewed impetus to the cause of the flagellants. Itinerant bands organized into disciplined groups of from fifty to several hundred men, with uniforms reminiscent of those worn by the crusaders and with lay leaders, who, contrary to the church's orders, heard confessions and granted absolution from sins. These groups flagellated themselves twice a day for thirty-three and a half days (a number corresponding with the years of Jesus's life) and were received enthusiastically. They would march up to a church, take off their clothes, don a special skirt, and pray and sing while they whipped themselves before an admiring public who believed that the flagellants would protect them from the plague and from death. "It became a privilege to welcome and assist such people. . . . People not only brought the sick to be healed by these holy men, they dipped clothes in the flowing blood and treasured them as sacred relics" (Cohn 1958, p. 134).

The influence of the flagellant cults, whose emphasis on self-prescribed penance threatened the authority of the church and whose popularity threatened the social order, led to suppression highlighted by actions taken at the Council of Constance in 1417. Many flagellants violently attacked the church, killed priests, and massacred Jews, who, they claimed, spread the plague by poisoning wells. It took the church and state authorities about fifteen years to control fully the flagellant movement everywhere except in central Germany. There, the cult remained secretly organized and adopted new practices, such as whipping babies and baptizing them in their own blood. The last German flagellators were burned at the stake as heretics in the 1480s.

Although the movement waned, individual devotees continue to flagellate themselves. Public self-flagellation, particularly during Eastertide, still takes place in the Philippine Islands, Mexico, and the southwestern United States.

A goodly number of the saints, holy persons whose lives serve as models for the faithful, engaged in self-mutilative practices. Pope Benedict XIV (1675–1758) wrote in *Heroic Virtue* that "with the exception of the martyrs, the Church venerates and gives the sanction of her authority to the sanctity of those only whom she finds to have been zealous in the mortification of the flesh and senses."

An extreme example of a saint who was zealous in the mortification of her flesh and senses is Saint Mary Magdalene de'Pazzi. Born in Florence in 1566 of an aristocratic family, Caterina de'Pazzi was religiously precocious. At age 10 she made a vow of perpetual chastity, secretly whipped herself, and wore a crown of thorns. Although unhappy with her behavior, her parents allowed her to enter a Carmelite convent, where she chose the name of the holy harlot, Mary Magdalene, and gained a reputation for outstanding virtue. She reportedly was able to cure diseases; one procedure she followed was to lick the skin lesions of afflicted nuns, including one who was a leper, and to suck the maggots out of skin ulcers.

At age 20, she declared that God had ordered her to eat only bread and water. With swollen feet she crawled around the convent and kissed the feet of the bewildered nuns. Hounded by devils, she frenetically whipped her body to chase them away and threw herself naked on thorn bushes until she was covered with blood. She burned her skin with hot wax and cajoled the novices in the convent to whip her and to step on her mouth.

At about age 37, emaciated and racked with coughing and pain, she took to her bed until she died four years later. Her painful gums were so badly infected that her teeth fell out, one by one. Her body was covered with putrefying bed sores, but when the sisters offered to move her she warned them off for fear that by touching her body they might experience sexual desires.

Because of her virtuous life, her miraculous healing, her clairvoyance, and the presence of a perfumed fragrance that emanated from her corpse, she was made a saint in 1668. A large statue of her holding a flagellant whip can be seen in her church in Florence, where people from around the world still come to pay her tribute.

Stigmatics

When Saint Paul attempted to win converts for his yet unnamed religion, he was badly beaten. He said that the stigmata (marks) on his body were those of Jesus (Gal. 6:17), and he called for church members to share in Christ's suffering. For more than a thousand years, this call was generally heeded, and then a miraculous event occurred in 1224 on the mountain called La Verna, near the Italian town of Assisi.

As a young man, Francis di Bernadone enjoyed the good life provided by his prosperous father. However, after he joined a military group on a raid against nearby Perugia, he was imprisoned for a year, during which he contracted malaria. Upon his release, he began to hear voices and to behave oddly; for example, he kissed the infected hands of lepers.

Francis visited a dilapidated country church and while praying heard Jesus tell him to restore the church. He sold his father's possessions and gave the money to the priest in charge of the church. Enraged, his father demanded restitution and even asked the local bishop to hold a church court. Francis appeared at the hearing, returned the money, stripped off all his clothes, and said that god in heaven was his only father.

He devoted his life to praising god, winning souls, and renouncing worldly pleasures. He fasted and wore only a coarse tunic, even on the coldest days. The malaria stayed with him and he developed a serious disease. Saint Bonaventure's biography states that by 1224 Francis "began to suffer from diverse ailments so grievously that scarce one of his limbs was free from pain and sore suffering. At length, by diverse sickness, prolonged and continuous, he was brought to such a point that his flesh was wasted away and only as it were the skin clove to his bone."

According to the *Fioretti* (Little Flowers), a book about Francis written a century later, he contemplated Christ's Passion, "and his fervour grew so strong in him that he became wholly transformed into Jesus through love and compassion." He saw a vision of Christ crucified, and "in the hands and feet of St. Francis began to appear the marks of the nails in the same manner as he had seen them in the body of Jesus." Until his death two years later, his body carried the five wounds of Christ, which often trickled blood.

News of Francis's stigmatization spread rapidly throughout Europe. Thirty-one cases of the stigmata appeared in the next twenty-five years (for accounts of these and other cases see Jacobi 1923; Thurston 1952; Whitlock and Hynes 1978; Wilson 1992). About three hundred cases of the stigmata have been reported since the time of Saint Francis. Most of these (271) have been women. Many are clearly the result of deliberately self-inflicted wounds, some are readily explained by psychological processes, and a few are problematic.

In 1869 Louise Lateau was seriously ill with throat abscesses and experienced mystical visions. A year later, at age 19, she developed the stigmata. Her wounds bled every Friday until her death at age 33 (Jesus's age at death). She was studied by Dr. Warlomont (1875) under the auspices of the Belgian Royal Academy of Medicine. He noted that every Thursday morning one-inch oval spots on her hands, feet, and chest turned pink and after several hours turned into vesicles. In the middle of the night, the vesicles would rupture, and blood would flow for a day. The lesions did not appear to be deliberately induced. When the blood was present, Lateau was "in an ecstatic state of deep contemplation," changing often to sadness, terror, and contrition, and claimed that she saw Christ in person and all the scenes of his Passion.

The stigmatic wounds of Theresa Neumann (1898–1962), a Bavarian peasant and member of the Third Order of Saint Francis, persevered for thirty-six years, and blood also dripped from her eyes (Hyneck 1932). She was examined for two weeks by the professor of psychiatry at Erlangen, Dr. G. Ewald. He noted that her medical history included episodes of blindness, deafness, and paralysis that suddenly remitted. She was amenorrheic, and her conviction that she was medically ill was strengthened by her parish priest, who continually pointed out the sufferings of Christ and the virtue of emulating the suffering of the martyrs. Neumann developed stigmata on her hands, feet, chest (over her heart), and scalp, as well as bloody tears. Some lesions bled continuously for a while, but then only on Fridays. She claimed to be in an ecstasy when blood came from her lesions, during which she lived through the scenes of Christ's Passion. When she experienced his crucifixion, she extended her arms, stared blankly, spoke in an Aramaic dialect, and fell into a swoon. Ewald concluded that the stigmata were genuine (in the sense that they were not deliberately caused), although he considered her a hysteric. Her diet supposedly consisted of only water and a daily communion wafer. She was ridiculed by the authorities for her anti-Nazi sentiments.

An American physician, Joseph Klauder (1938), examined her several years later. Neumann impressed him as being "emotionally normal, plain, and humble. She did not exploit or talk about herself or the stigmas; on the contrary she was reticent and showed them reluctantly." He concluded that her stigmata were genuine and noted that even among some Muslims there are reported cases of stigmata appearing during periods of contemplation on the battle wounds of Muhammad. Klauder believed that cases of genuine stigmata should be classified as

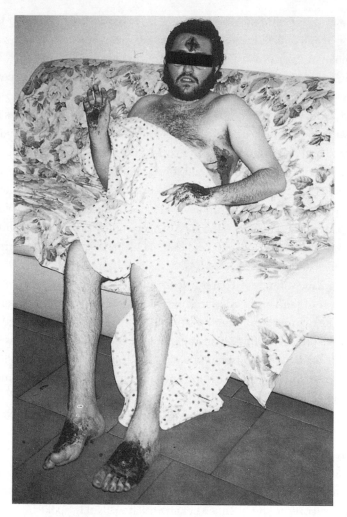

A man who claimed that the stigmata appeared on his body
whenever he meditated intensely on Christ's crucifixion.
(Photo by Armando Favazza)

an "exotic dermatosis," and he favored a psychological explanation for their patho-
physiology (for example, autosuggestion, vasomotor lability, and "latent powers"
associated with mysticism).[5]

5. Newspapers and magazines covered the case extensively, often showing gruesome photographs
of Neumann's bloody face. In 1928 a German psychiatrist, Alfred Lechler, encountered a 26-year-old
patient known as Elizabeth K (Lechler 1933; Wilson 1992). Her long list of symptoms included severe
trembling, episodes of paralysis, bouts of anorexia, and urinary and fecal incontinence. Lechler treated
her with hypnotherapy and hired her to serve as a maid in his home. She heard a sermon about Christ's

Wilson (1992) listed nineteen stigmatics in the twentieth century, although the actual number is probably much greater. The most famous is Padre Pio, an Italian monk whose wounds stayed open from 1918 until his death in 1978. An 11-year-old African American Baptist girl, Cloretta Robinson, in Oakland, California, bled from the palm while in a school classroom. She had just read a book about the crucifixion of Jesus. Stigmatic wounds on her hands, feet, and forehead, appeared during the period of Lent. Jane Hunt, a bus driver's wife in England, developed the stigmata in 1985 while shopping for groceries. The wounds disappeared two years later after she received a hysterectomy.

Most literary portrayals of stigmatics are forgettable. The one exception is Ron Hansen's *Mariette in Ecstasy* (1992), the story of a 17-year-old postulant at a priory of the Sisters of the Crucifixion. When Mariette develops the stigmata, life in the convent is turned topsy-turvy. One nun licks Mariette's wounds, while others accuse her of seeking attention, of fabricating everything, of contaminating everyone with her wiles. Mariette herself wonders if she hasn't made it all up in some way. She gets caught reading medical and religious books about the stigmata. She writes to a priest not to believe anything she says. When her father cleans the blood off her skin, he finds no lesions. Mariette declares that "Christ took back the wounds." Her father smirks and tells the nuns, "You have all been duped." But have they?

The Religious Context of Self-mutilation in People Who Are Mentally Ill

Self-mutilation—the hacking off of a hand or the gouging out of an eye or the slicing off of a penis—by a person who is mentally ill is a dramatically awesome act reminiscent of a sacrificial rite.[6]

The bodies of some mentally ill self-mutilators can be thought of as a stage on which is enacted a personal drama that reflects, in varying proportions, personal psychopathology, social stresses, and cultural myths, especially those of a religious nature. The themes of these myths are suffering, dismemberment, blood

---

crucifixion on Good Friday and told Lechler that she could literally feel nails being driven into her extremities. Lechler, cognizant of the Neumann case, made a hypnotic suggestion that Elizabeth concentrate on nails being hammered into her hands and feet. On the next day, wounds appeared. He then suggested that she concentrate on pictures of Neumann with bloody tears. Within hours, Elizabeth bled from inside her eyelids. When Lechler suggested that the blood cease from flowing, quite quickly it stopped.

6. In his classic study of Nuer (African) sacrifice, Evans-Pritchard (1956) noted that the sacrificer is "acting a part in a drama" and that "we seem indeed to be watching a play or to be listening to someone's account of what he had dreamt" (p. 322).

sacrifice, resurrection, rebirth, and the establishment (or reestablishment) of a new, prosperous, healthy, and amicable order. Although an audience might regard the self-mutilative act as the tension-heightening conclusion of a tragedy, the actors—at least at the moment of their self-mutilation—might regard it as a tension-reducing, cathartic moment, or a moment of clarification, or a moment that harbingers a new, more joyous conclusion to the drama. For some, pain and blood are associated with death, but for others they are associated with birth.

Religious ritual and some acts of self-mutilation share an interesting interplay with time and reality. During religious rituals, the continuing flow of normal, secular time is interrupted by intervals of sacred nontime (Leach 1976). Turner (1968) noted that "in the life of most communities, ancient and modern, there appear to be interludes in historical time, periods of timeless time, that are devoted to the celebration of certain basic postulates of human existence, biological and cultural . . . the moment when ritual is being performed" (p. 5). Some mentally ill persons have frightening episodes of depersonalization, during which time and reality are distorted. The act of self-mutilation often serves to terminate these episodes. It allows self-mutilators to reexperience their biological existence and place in society.

While some mentally ill self-mutilators consciously believe and publicly declare themselves to be gods or members of the company of saints, others seem to tap unconsciously into such beliefs. In this context acts of self-mutilation and mortification may take on a sacrificial quality. At a personal level these sacrifices often have profound consequences. By gouging out an eye, for example, the self-selected victim may avert suicide (martyrdom) and may cause group members to reevaluate their relationships. The power of drama to influence the lives of both the actors and the audience cannot be underestimated.

The acts of mentally ill self-mutilators, however, have no transcendency. They have little meaning for the universe or the world or the community at large but rather affect only the self-mutilators and occasionally the members of their small social networks. Deviant self-mutilators are not liminal objects (Turner 1977), and the flow of their blood opens no significant channels between God and Man. Their use of religious symbolism is based on private rather than public delusions. Although therapists should try to use powerful religious and shamanic symbols in selected cases, the fact remains that self-mutilators are neither gods nor saints but rather frightened prophets manqué.

CHAPTER THREE

Self-injury and Eating Disorders

Lillian Malcove (1933), a psychoanalyst, wrote that the experience of learning to eat is the prototype of the fear of being dismembered or mutilated. A child sees food cut into pieces and mashed by special instruments (knives, forks, and spoons) and finally eats it. "Since the child's thinking is at this stage animistic, that food that he cuts and eats is endowed with attributes of human life, and can therefore easily be identified with himself or other persons. . . . The identification of the child's self with his food . . . is facilitated by fairy tales, or oral caresses and endearments, and by games improvised to expedite the feeding procedure. For the child, eating is literally a cannibalistic procedure which includes the antemortem tortures of cutting and crushing, and in which the table silver supplements the teeth and the hands."

Much evidence points to a relationship between nonsuicidal self injury (NSSI) and eating disorders (see Favazza et al. 1989 and especially Levitt et al. 2004). Typing "eating disorders and self-injury" into any computer search engine reveals hundreds of programs—inpatient, outpatient, individual and group therapy, Internet meeting sites, support groups, message boards, and so on—as well as brief informational articles on the topic.

Brenda and William Parry-Jones (1993) traced the earliest literary reference of an eating disorder connected with self-harm to a story in Ovid's *Metamorphoses*. Because he scorned the gods and violated the sacred groves of Ceres, Erysichthon was punished with an insatiable craving for food: "At last when . . . his grievous malady needed more food, the wretched man began to tear his limbs and rend them apart with his teeth and, by consuming his own body, fed himself." The authors also examine the case of the famous eighteenth-century author Dr. Samuel Johnson, who was a lifelong bulimic and ruminator given to melancholy, tormenting scruples, obsessive-compulsive rituals, and hypochondriasis: "His eating pattern was characterised by excesses of uncontrolled consumption, interspersed by attempts at abstinence or reduced intake. . . . His table manners were crude, his ingestion rapid like a cormorant, and mastication was perfunctory." His companion and biographer James Boswell wrote: "Such was the heat and insatiability of his blood that not only did he pare his nails to the quick; but scraped the joints of his fingers with a pen-knife, till they seemed quite red and raw" (quoted in Parry-Jones 1993). He also reportedly bit and rubbed his lips continually. It is likely that Johnson's NSSI was a form of punishment for indulging his impulses as well as a way to relieve tension, perhaps in association with his intense fear of giving in to masturbation. Recent medical historians make a good case for Tourette's syndrome, a neuropsychiatric disorder characterized by many of the behaviors, including minor self-mutilation, demonstrated by Dr. Johnson (McHenry 1985; Murray 1979).

Parry-Jones (1993) also describes three other historical cases from England of self-mutilation associated with bulimia. The first, reported in 1745, was of a 10-year-old boy who ate fifty-five to seventy-eight pounds of food daily and immediately vomited. If not fed on demand, "he would gnaw the very flesh off his own bones." The boy was described as cheerful and with a healthy-looking face. He died of emaciation within two years of the onset of his "extraordinary Boulimia." The second case (1786–1828) was of a girl with a voracious appetite; for example, she ate ten pounds of bread daily at age 6. A year later her menses began, she was sexually attacked by her father, and she developed epilepsy. As an adult she had attacks of great hunger; it was reported that "if her wants are not satisfied . . . [she] bites her own flesh." She was thought to be normal mentally except during her paroxysms of hunger. The last case, reported in 1815, was of a 16-year-old boy who developed such an insatiable appetite during the course of typhus fever that he tried to eat his fingers.

In modern times the association between eating disorders and self-mutilation was noted in three articles that stressed female genital self-injury. French and Nelson (1972) reported on a 38-year-old housewife hospitalized for intractable binge eating and self-induced vomiting. After a marital argument, she slashed her genital area with a razor blade. Simpson (1973) discussed a 22-year-old patient with such problems as severe dieting, compulsive overeating, self-induced vomiting, wrist cutting, breast slashing, and the cutting of her vagina with a butcher knife. On the basis of three cases, Goldney and Simpson (1975) described a syndrome of female genital self-mutilation, eating disorders, and hysterical personality disorder.

Several studies of patients identified as self-mutilators note the presence of eating disorders. Of fifteen adolescent female self-mutilators, "12 were moderately overweight to obese and 2 were extremely thin and exhibited some anorexic behavior in the hospital. . . . Several reported extreme and rapid fluctuations in weight" (Simpson and Porter 1981). Another study reported that fifteen of twenty-three self-cutters described compulsive overeating or severe anorexia or periods of each (Rosenthal et al. 1972). A study of twelve female self-mutilators who had slashed themselves an average of thirty-eight times found that, in "an early pubertal phase," six had had anorexia nervosa and three both anorexia nervosa and bulimia (Yaryura-Tobias and Neziroglu 1978). Coid et al. (1983) reported that four of seven hospitalized female habitual self-mutilators demonstrated either anorexia or anorexia/bulimia and noted that "severely disturbed patients who habitually mutilate themselves show profound disturbances of appetite characterized by both bulimic and anorexic episodes."

Another body of literature describes NSSI in patients identified as having anorexia nervosa and/or bulimia nervosa. Pierloot et al. (1975) associated NSSI with poor outcome in thirty-two anorexic women. Garfinkel et al. (1980) reported a 9.2 percent NSSI rate among sixty-eight bulimics. Yellowlees (1985) found that four of fifteen bulimics had deliberately injured themselves. Jacobs and Isaacs (1986) reported a 35 percent self-injury/suicide attempt rate in forty subjects with pre- and postpubertal anorexia nervosa. A comparison of eighty-four laxative-abusing bulimics with 101 non-laxative-abusing bulimics recorded NSSI in 40.5 percent of the former group and 25.7 percent of the latter (Mitchell et al. 1986). Claes (2004) compared eating disorder patients with (twenty-seven subjects) and without (thirty-eight subjects) NSSI. The former scored much higher on measures of impulsivity (drug abuse, shoplifting, suicide attempts), of personality disorders (borderline and histrionic), of dissociative experiences (identify fragmentation and amnesia), and of traumatic experiences (most endured a combination of sexual, physical, and emotional abuse, and 100 percent of subjects who were sexually abused before the age of 11 years engaged in NSSI). In 2005 the National Eating Disorders Association issued a warning about Web sites that foster anorexic and bulimic lifestyles. Persons can now purchase beaded bracelets that identify themselves as anorectic (red) or bulimic (purple), and can add black and blue beaded bracelets if they also cut themselves.

Favazza and Conterio (1989) gathered data on 290 female self-mutilators. The typical subject was a 28-year-old single Caucasian female who had cut herself on more than fifty occasions. Half of the women reported the history of an eating disorder. Of the total sample, 22 percent listed bulimia nervosa, 15 percent listed anorexia nervosa, and 13 percent listed both. The same survey data were gathered on a large group of female undergraduate students enrolled in a basic psychology course; 14.5 percent had an eating disorder and 38 percent of this group also had a history of NSSI.

A typical and instructive case history demonstrating the self-mutilation and eating disorder linkage is the following.

Ms. C, aged 24 years, first cut herself at age 13 because she was angry with her alcoholic father, who had sexually abused her for many years: "I couldn't get back at him, so I cut myself and I felt better." From the ages of 17 to 19, she repeatedly cut herself because, "It made me feel less depressed." During the next four years, Ms. C did not cut herself but became a severe alcoholic and abuser of street drugs ("Drinking and drugs took the place of cutting for me"). She was hospitalized for anorexia nervosa at age 23 after a fifty-pound weight loss. This hospitalization occurred several months after she had markedly decreased her alcohol and drug use. Upon discharge, her weight slowly but steadily ballooned to the point of moderate obesity. She then resumed heavy alcohol use and was hospitalized. She was placed on a diet and was denied access to alcohol on a locked ward, so she "had to start cutting again." On one occasion she escaped from the ward, went to a bus stop, and proceeded to scream wildly and slash herself many times with a razor blade in front of a group of frightened onlookers. Ms. C stated that cutting herself, drinking alcohol, and not eating were "interchangeable ways of hurting myself." However, she felt that cutting herself was the best method because it prevented people from getting too close to her, helped her to get back at her father, let her feel that she was "in control" (although she admitted that most times she could not control her desire to cut herself), and brought her back to reality when she had "no feelings, like I'm hypnotized."

Ms. C's symptoms shifted over time. I met her when NSSI was the major symptom. Had I encountered her at another time during the course of her illness, the primary diagnosis might have been anorexia nervosa or substance abuse. German psychiatrists studied thirty-two females whom they termed "multi-impulsive bulimics"; a history of NSSI was found in twenty-four (75%) of the women, while eleven (34%) reported alcohol abuse and seven (22%) drug abuse (Fichter et al. 1994). This shifting of impulsive symptomatology is characteristic of what I and Richard Rosenthal (1993) term the syndrome of repetitive NSSI.

Parkin and Eagles (1993) described an odd form of NSSI, namely, deliberate bloodletting by venipuncture, in three women who had lengthy histories of bulimia preceded by anorexia. All three had some medical training and proficiency in venipuncture that, like binging and purging, relieved their anxiety, tension, and anger. One woman developed anorexia nervosa at age 17. This was followed by six years of bulimia nervosa during which she overdosed once, burned herself several times, and cut herself three times. She began self-bloodletting in her senior year of medical school and claimed that it reduced tension and gave her a sense of control and satisfaction. She also believed that it helped her to lose weight (she removed a liter of blood each time). Other cases have been reported by Margo and Newman (1989) and by Brown (1993).

Food for Thought

Cross (1993) related the finding that skin-cutting and eating disorders are present more often in females than in males to women's perceptions of their bodies as functionally mysterious and prone to abrupt, profound transformations. The female genitalia, for example, are partially internal; menstruation cannot be controlled; changes in body contours at puberty may be dramatic; during pregnancy the fetus is experienced as the "other within;" the lactating breast belongs both to the child and to the mother. Thus, there are elements of ambiguity, paradox, and discontinuity in females' experiences of their bodies. Cross states that self-cutting and eating disorders are "attempts to own the body, to perceive it as self (not other), known (not uncharted and unpredictable), and impenetrable (not invaded or controlled from the outside)." She theorized that certain girls reared in an environment of severe physical pain, sexual abuse, or extremely unempathetic parenting develop a developmental deficit. A "psychological chasm between body and self" is erected. As adolescents, those girls try to overcontrol their unruly emotions, sexual feelings, and bodily changes by the seemingly simple and efficient maneuver of transforming "in a kind of internal projection" their psychological problems into concrete, physical ones. Their body becomes both their whipping boy and their solace. "The metaphorical destruction between body and self collapses: thinness is self-sufficiency, bleeding emotional catharsis, bingeing is the assuaging of loneliness, and purging is the moral purification of the self." The process ultimately fails because "the body comes to resent its task master . . . escapes control and inflicts its own persecution . . . as body and self constantly shift roles of victim and victimizer, master and slave."

The sympathetic conjectures of Cross do not explain the basic relationship between self-mutilation and eating disorders. Malcove (1933) notes children's identification with food. If true, then the act of eating during the early stages of life serves to make self-mutilation a palatable behavior because it is inherent in the human condition. The child's act of eating is rewarded by a primary gain because hunger is temporarily satisfied. In later life, NSSI also offers a primary gain, namely, temporary respite from unpleasant experiences such as anxiety, tension, depersonalization, and racing thoughts. Food, like NSSI, is a source of solace.

Children can express willful anger toward their parents either by refusing to eat or by spitting out their food. This behavior may be the prototype of NSSI as a retaliation against an abusive adult. By eating what their parents offer, children also are able to please their parents and win affection. This form of secondary gain may be the prototype of NSSI as manipulation of others.

Malcove's final point is that eating is a "cannibalistic procedure" to a child. The horrible truth of this insight is seen in repressed, psychotic persons who amputate a body part and then consume it (Betts 1964). A mild derivative of this behavior is commonly encountered in nonpsychotic self-cutters who drink their own blood. Certainly, in Western societies cannibalism is thought of as the ultimate ghastly antisocial act of aggression (Sagan 1974). And the anthropologist W. Arens (1979) notes that Westerners have used ritual cannibalism in primitive groups as a justification both for colonization and for a sense of righteousness. For evidence of "friendly" ritual cannibalism usually associated with mortuary rituals and of "aggressive" cannibalism when enemy flesh is eaten, see Berndt (1962), Dupeyrat (1954), and Brown and Tuzin (1983). Poole (1983), for example, has reported that when a leading Bimin-Kuskumin (Papua New Guinea) male elder dies, parts of his raw heart tissue are eaten by other male elders in order to perpetuate his great ritual power and knowledge. When a leading female elder dies, parts of her uterus and vagina are eaten by her female relatives and by other female elders to perpetuate her ritual power and to diffuse her reproductive power.

Western culture includes outstanding examples of groups defaming others through accusations of cannibalism and blood sacrifice. The Romans accused the early Christians, who in turn accused competing sects. Epiphanius (305–403) wrote that the Gnostics' Passover meal consisted of an aborted human fetus. Saint Augustine charged the Manicheans with eating sperm and menstrual blood in their communion rituals. He also dealt with pagan attacks on the concept of the resurrection of the body in which, according to Luke 21, not one hair from the head of believers would be harmed. Scoffers asked if bodies would be resurrected with all the hair that barbers had cut from their heads or if fingernail clippings would rejoin their bodies. The question that most stymied Saint Augustine was, "Whose flesh shall that man's be in the resurrection, which is eaten by another man through compulsion of hunger? For it is turned into the flesh of the person who eats it and fills that part that famine had made hungry and lean." For details of charges of cannibalism against Jews dating from the eleventh century see Strack's *The Jew and Human Sacrifice* (1909).

Cannibalism and Psychosis

Individual acts of cannibalism have certainly occurred throughout human history in times of extreme famine. Starved inmates in Nazi concentration camps resorted to cannibalism (Russell 1954), and Roheim (1932) reported that famished Australian aborigines induced abortions to provide food for the rest of the family. Cannibalism within the context of starvation was even the topic of a famous literary essay. Jonathan Swift's political parody and censure of Irish helplessness and English voraciousness was titled *A Modest Proposal for preventing the Children of Poor People from being a Burthen to their Parents, or the Country, and for making them Beneficial to the Publick* (1729). Swift's modest proposal was that the impoverished and starving Irish sell their children at age 12 months to the rich of England, who would then eat them, thus improving the diet of one group and the wealth of the other.

Individual acts of cannibalism rarely have occurred among psychotic persons, usually with a religious overlay. A psychiatrist in Papua New Guinea, for example, reported the case of a 30-year-old psychotic native who killed and ate his son (Burton-Bradley 1976). The patient had a family history of mental disorder, was a heavy betel nut chewer (the chemical arecoline in betel nuts induces a euphoria known as arecolinism) and spree drinker of alcohol, and was an avid reader of Christian literature provided by missionaries. He had read about the Apostles, about Jesus's fast of forty days, and about Abraham and the sacrifice of Isaac. He then decided on a course of action.

I decided to kill my child. After I made up my mind, I fasted for 5 days. I then took my little boy into the bush and came to the place where I had decided to kill him. I struck him twice on the forehead with my axe. I then took my knife and cut him in the stomach and upward toward the chest through the bone. I then took his heart out. I chopped it up and ate some of it. I also made some cuts in my own body and mixed some of my son's blood with this. Then I put the body in the grave. I had brought some glue and petrol with me which I mixed with the remaining slices of my son's heart. I tried to boil it but was not successful. I had hoped that the steam and the rest of the mixture would go up to God and he would then send me the power in my dreams to do the right things for my people. The people's heads would also become clear, and they would then do the necessary things to bring about the white man's way of life. God would send many goods to the people and we would find money. Then I lay down in the grave and slept with my dead son. I dreamed that I saw a light go up to heaven. I then covered the grave and returned to my village.

Burton-Bradley noted that native informants considered the man's act to be pathological. The official diagnosis was an acute schizophrenic reaction; a year later "the autism and ambitendencies of nuclear schizophrenia were well in evidence." The patient's bizarre act was probably also influenced by the effect of starvation-induced chemical changes as well as by the euphoria of arecolinism. Cannibalism has a tradition in Papua New Guinea (e.g., as a method of revenge or of absorbing a victim's life principle or of facilitating conception, as part of warfare, and as an act of justice). Indeed, a Supreme Court judge in Melanesia had ruled that cannibalism per se was neither improper nor indecent but rather must be understood within a cultural context (Griffin 1971). In this case, however, the cultural context was overshadowed by the presence of mental illness.

A psychiatric report of idiosyncratic cannibalism (Benezech et al. 1981) deals with a 41-year-old paranoid schizophrenic man. He traveled across Europe because God's voice told him to undertake religious missions. These auditory hallucinations controlled much of his subsequent behavior. His wife died of an apparent drowning, but he later confessed to killing her. His attempt to rape a young girl and drink her blood was subverted when the girl's mother appeared. He then murdered an elderly person, ate large pieces of the victim's thigh, and tried to suck the blood from his victim's femoral artery. The following day, the man killed a farmer and his wife with a pitchfork and beat their maid severely. He stated that God had told him to kill everyone. The killings proved that he was bad and, therefore, he ate the victim's flesh to be united with God. "I ate his flesh and drank his blood to obey the sentence: who will eat my body and drink my blood will live." His reference was to Jesus's words in John 6:54–56, "He who feeds on my flesh and drinks my blood has life eternal, and I will raise him up on the last day. For my flesh is real food, and my blood real drink. The man who feeds on my flesh and drinks my blood remains in me, and I in him."

Totem, Taboo, and Depression

There is something morbidly enticing about cannibalism. Ever since the 1930s, anthropological and psychiatric literature has made numerous references to a mental illness termed *windigo psychosis* among Algonkian Indians, such as the Ojibwa and Cree, in northwestern Canada. The disorder is frequently classified as a "culture-bound psychosis" characterized by a compulsive desire to eat human flesh. However, as pointed out by Marano (1982), windigo psychosis has never existed. In fact, Marano concluded that the situation is an example of mass suggestibility among anthropologists who, enticed by the exotic notion of cannibalism, fabricated the disorder in an attempt to explain certain events.

The notion that cannibalism is inherent in the human condition was set forth by Sir Thomas Browne in his lyrical *Religio Medici* (1634): "We are what we all abhor, Anthropophagi and Cannibals, devourers not onely of men, but of our selves; and that not in an allegory, but a positive truth; for all this mass of flesh which we behold, came in at our mouths; this frame we look upon, hath been upon our trenchers; in brief, we have devour'd our selves."

A modern version of this idea was developed by Freud in *Totem and Taboo* (1950). Freud theorized the existence of a primal horde in the earliest stage of the development of humankind. The leader of the horde was a powerful father who, in order to maintain his authority, drove out his rebellious sons:

> One day, the brothers who had been driven out came together, killed, and devoured their father and so made an end of the patriarchal horde. United, they had the courage to do and succeeded in doing what would have been impossible for them individually. . . . Cannibal savages as they were, it goes without saying that they devoured their victim as well as killing him . . . and in the act of devouring him they accompanied their identification with him, and each one of them acquired a portion of his strength. The totem meal, which is perhaps mankind's earliest festival, would thus be a repetition and a commemoration of this memorable and criminal deed, which was the beginning of so many things—of social organization, or moral restrictions, and of religion. (p. 142)

Freud's scenario is based on his reading of anthropological reports and on his observations during the psychoanalyses of neurotic patients (he reckoned that the psychological regression experienced by these patients sheds light on the primitive mentality of early humans.) He asserted that the events in his scenario might have existed in fact or might have existed only in the imaginations of primitive people, who nonetheless experienced them as real. Although the validity of Freud's scenario has been strongly challenged by many modern scholars, it contains a certain elegance and heuristic value. Freud contended that a cannibal feast gave rise to three elements of human life—namely, social organization, moral restrictions, and religion—that we know to be significant in both culturally sanctioned and pathological self-injury.

According to Freud's formulation, social organization in society arose because the brothers planned and carried out their act of murder and cannibalism and then established clan solidarity. Many culturally sanctioned mutilative rites serve this same purpose, for example, initiation rites often include mutilations (such as skin cutting, tooth removal, and circumcision) that serve to bind group members together and validate membership in the tribe and cults. The brothers' deeds also demonstrated acts of independence from authority and proof of masculinity. These same motives underlie some instances of NSSI, especially in institutionalized mental patients and prisoners. Not infrequently, for example, prison gang members cover their bodies with visible, grotesque, and often obscene tattoos to prove their masculinity, to assert their dislike of authority, and to enhance a sense of belonging among group members.

The origins of moral restrictions in society in Freud's scenario derive from the brothers' desire not to share the same fate as their father. Thus, they prohibited the killing and eating of each other. In time, these prohibitions were generalized to other clan members and eventually evolved into the simple injunction "Thou shalt not kill." Many mutilative rites are linked to moral restrictions; for example, the vaginas of young African girls are sewn closed to prevent sexual intercourse until marriage. Among people who are mentally ill, self-mutilation rarely may serve as an alternative to suicide—a depressed patient begged staff to kill him, and then he plucked out both his eyes, stating that he did it so that he could continue living.

The link between cannibalism and religion is complicated but significant for our understanding of self-injury among some patients. For Freud, the talion law— an eye for an eye, a tooth for a tooth—is deeply rooted in human nature. Thus, when Christ redeemed humankind from the burden of original sin by sacrificing his own life, he was expiating the original murder of the primal father by the sons. Christ was the incarnation of the sons who displaced their father just as the son-religion of Christianity displaced the father-religion of Judaism. The original cannibalistic meal evolved into the sacrament of communion, in which god's flesh and blood are eaten.

Many anthropologists have attempted to account for *ritual* cannibalism in an evolutionary format. Thus, primitive humans ate human flesh simply because it was available as a food source. As humankind developed, cannibalism became part of religious rituals, especially in the complex non-Western civilizations, while it was replaced by animal sacrifice, especially in Western (Judeo-Christian) cultures. With further cultural evolution, cannibalism and animal sacrifice were superseded when the religious belief in transubstantiation was developed. According to this belief, cereals and other substances could be transformed into flesh by the recitation of certain prayers and the performance of ritualistic acts.

In Christian practice, for example, a priest is thought to be able to convert bread and wine either symbolically or in fact into the flesh and blood of Jesus, which is then eaten by the communicants.

The transubstantiation of bread into the flesh of a god is popularly associated with Christianity, where it was ecclesiastically established at the fourth Lateran synod in 1215, but a chapter entitled "Eating the God" in Frazer's *Golden Bough* (1958; original 1890) provides examples of the practice both in pre-Christian and non-Christian cultures. The Aryans of ancient India, for example, believed in the transubstantiation of rice cakes into flesh during holy sacrificial rites. Thus, "When it (the rice cake) still consists of rice-meal it is the hair. When he (the Brahman priest) pours water on it, it becomes skin. When he mixes it, it becomes flesh; for then it becomes consistent; and consistent also in the flesh. When it is baked, it becomes bone. . . . And when he is about to take it off (the fire) and sprinkles it with butter, he changes it into marrow" (vol. 2, p. 81). Spanish priests who came to Mexico with the conquistadors discovered that the Aztecs practiced a transubstantiation ritual twice a year. At the festival of the winter solstice in December, for example, the Aztecs made an image of the god Huitzilopochtli out of dough mixed with the blood of children. The image was venerated and then cut into pieces by a priest. This ritual was called "killing the God Huitzilopochtli so that his body might be eaten." The Aztec king was given a piece of dough cut out from the heart area of the image while all the males attending the ceremony were given a crumb from the image. The ceremony was called *teoquado*, which means "god is eaten."

Cannibals are persons who traditionally live on the fringes of Western civilization (Arens 1979). When the boundaries of this civilization greatly expanded during the fifteenth century cannibals were supposedly encountered. Thus, Christopher Columbus's journal notes that the Arawak Indians described their enemies, the Caribs, as "men with one eye, and others with dogs' noses, who ate men, and when they took a man, they cut off his head and drank his blood, and castrated him." A papal representative at the Spanish court, Peter d'Anghera, embellished Columbus's account and wrote fantastic dispatches that had great popularity. He described cannibals, mermaids, giants, and Amazon women.[1]

1. The Amazons were a tribe of warrior women whose name derives from the Greek words meaning "without a breast"; in some Latin manuscripts the word *Amazon* is written *unimamma* (Schecter 1962). Homer's *Iliad* contains many references to these fierce women. In his *Judgements Derived from Heaven*, Ptolemy states, "Such are the Amazons, who avoid having contact with men, and who apply themselves to weapons, and who made their daughters hardy from childhood, cutting off their right breast in order that they may be better fitted to military exercises, and who uncover this portion of their bosom in exploits of war and in combats, so as to reveal their natural vigor and male courage." According to Hippocrates, the Amazons cauterized the right breast of their daughters with a hot copper instrument.

People who have severe depression are at high risk for self-mutilation (many cases are included in this book). On one level, this association may be understood as a derivative of cannibalism. As Freud first showed in *Mourning and Melancholia* (1917), the psychological processes of mourning and of severe depression are qualitatively similar and are modeled on the earliest infantile interaction with reality, namely, taking in food. As expressed by Cameron (1963), in the mourning process "the mourner tends to take over some of the characteristics of the lost one and to act like him, speak as he did, even to look like him and live as he did. It is as though the mourner were saying to the world, 'He lives again in me!' . . . It seems to be a normal defense against crushing loss, a process of taking onto oneself parts of the behavior and appearance of the lost persons, in that they are in a sense preserved alive." In psychodynamic terms, the mourner *identifies* with, or feels like, the deceased. This process is based on the mechanism of *introjection* (the internalization of the deceased).

The vast majority of cannibalistic acts occur during mortuary rites. In fact, Sagan (1974) defines "affectionate" cannibalism as the eating of body parts of kinsmen who have died a natural death and notes that the emotions associated with this form of cannibalism "are very similar to our own feelings toward dead relatives—affection, sorrow, and the desire to preserve and remember the virtues of the deceased." I have already noted the aboriginal Bimin-Kuskumin, who practice affectionate cannibalism in order to assume the generative and ritual strength of a deceased kinsman, believing that by eating a dead person's flesh, some characteristics of the deceased will be kept alive and recycled. One wonders during the course of human development whether such cannibalistic mortuary rites developed as a concrete expression of the emotions associated with the mourning process or whether the psychological process of mourning that we now experience (often associated in many cultures with a feast or special meal) evolved from primitive cannibalism.

The relationship between mourning and cannibalism is clearly demonstrated by the Wari tribe of western Brazil, which practiced cannibalism until the 1960s. When enemy flesh was eaten, obvious hostility was demonstrated, and the body parts were abused and treated disrespectfully; but when the flesh of a Wari was

---

By burning the breast, its development was arrested. Without this impediment, the Amazons were better able to handle weapons and to draw their bows when shooting arrows. According to several ancient commentators, the Amazons maimed male children by dislocating their knee and hip joints so that they would not try to conspire against the women when they grew up. Over the centuries, the term *Amazon* came to mean female warrior, without any reference to breast mutilation, and it was in this sense that Columbus used the term. In fact, the Amazon River in South America was named after a group of female warriors of the Tapuya tribe encountered by one of Pizarro's officers in 1541.

eaten at funerals, great honor and respect was demonstrated. Unlike the Bimin-Kuskumin, the Wari did not believe that eating human flesh recycles the characteristics of the dead person. Instead, they ate the flesh of tribal members to help the mourners' "gradual detachment from thinking about and remembering the dead . . . for prolonged sadness is believed to endanger individual health and productivity" (Conklin 1995). By devouring the corpse instead of putting it in the ground to rot, the dead person's spirit was free to become a Water Spirit and then to return as a peccary (a piglike, hoofed animal), which could be hunted and eaten. For the Wari, mourning lasted about ten months. At that time the mourners went on an extended hunt and killed as many animals as possible. A successful hunt signified that the spirit of the deceased was prospering in the afterworld. Amid feasting and singing, the Wari said, "Sadness has ended; now happiness begins."

Many people who are depressed overuse the psychological mechanism of introjection and enter into dependent relationships. In Cameron's (1963) words, "The depressive adult is a person who has had to meet implacable demands for compliance during infancy by the overuse of introjection. Introjection is a symbolic engulfing, a perceptual taking in, the primitive forerunner of social role organization. The infant incorporates his mother symbolically, as he has previously incorporated his food, and sets her up inside as a regulating image. Instead of internalizing merely the role . . . he internalizes the whole frightening image, which then controls what he does" (p. 553). Depressive persons typically have much repressed anger over their situation and regard the controlling maternal image with ambivalence. Because they overuse introjection, the anger they experience at the loss of a loved one or a prize possession is turned inward, thus potentiating the repressed anger. The result may be psychotic decompensation, replete with feelings of great guilt and sometimes with self-injury. The cultural prototype of this process is apparent in cannibalistic and self-mutilative mortuary rites. The eating of a dead person's flesh, with no matter how much affection, contains elements of aggression and of ambivalence. Anthropophagy during mourning satisfies at some level the feeling of anger at the deceased for having abandoned the mourner, and it is common in many cultural groups for mourners to mutilate themselves, especially by chopping off a finger. In some cultures this activity has become symbolic. Mourners, for example, may wear black clothing, cut off their hair, and put ashes on their body. Among patients we find some who mutilate themselves upon the death of a loved one. For example, a 24-year-old man became depressed after his father died; he then attempted to circumcise himself with a pair of scissors, saying that this might lift him out of his depression.

The conquering cannibal literally tastes the fruits of his victory, but victory can also be achieved by exactly the opposite action, namely, self-starvation. In many religious traditions, enlightenment and victory over the forces of evil come after a period of prolonged fasting. Cannibalism and self-starvation appear to be linked poles representing the opposite sides of revenge-victory. Political activists in India and more recently in Northern Ireland attempted to overthrow British rule by starving themselves. The metaphor for their actions is clear: the British have devoured our country and now we will demonstrate vividly how this devouring leads to weakness and to total destruction.

In like manner, anorexia nervosa is an object lesson. It is a form of indirect self-injury in which the patient achieves victory over real and fantastic enemies through fasting. To eat is to accept the status quo. To eat is to partake of a regenerative cannibalistic ritual. To eat is to open one's self to the possibility of being devoured and to participate in the cycle of life. The episodic gorging often accompanying anorexia is a sign of weakness, a dent in the anorectic person's armor, and must be undone by self-induced vomiting. Anorexia is tragic because it overshoots the mark. Once a certain point is reached, the catabolic process relentlessly feeds on itself until the anorectic person's body and will to live are shrunken. The therapist's task is to reverse the process of decay and to convince the patient that victory may be won short of fasting unto death.

CHAPTER FOUR

Animals and Automutilation

Much of what we know about the cause and treatment of human diseases derives from studies of animals. In psychiatry, for example, basic knowledge of brain physiology has come from experiments done with squids and snails; many basic psychological principles have resulted from laboratory work with dogs, rats, and mice; an illness much like major depression in humans can be induced in monkeys. In this chapter, reports of animal automutilation (I use the prefix *auto* instead of *self* because no one knows whether an animal has a true sense of self) are examined in an attempt to better understand human self-mutilation.

Through experiments with automutilation in animals, scientists hope to explain the pathophysiological mechanisms underlying the self-mutilation found in certain human diseases with a strong biological component. Such experiments involve strategically placed surgical lesions and the administration of drugs that alter brain chemistry. To learn about social factors influencing human self-mutilation, scientists are experimenting with restrictive environments that cause automutilation in animals. Some theorists believe that self- and automutilation derive from an innate aggressive drive and that an understanding of human self-mutilative behavior is enhanced by ethological observations.

The earliest medical reference is contained in the 13 February 1855 "Proceedings of the Pathological Section of the Irish College of Surgeons." Discussion focused on a case of automutilation in a 12-year-old lioness that lived in the Dublin Zoological Gardens. The animal had been in good health and had given birth to four litters of cubs. She had a history of regular menstrual periods except for the year previous when she had not been "in season." One morning she was discovered to have bitten off six inches of her tail. Shortly, she bit off another large piece and finally demolished the remainder. After a brief interval, she began to eat one of her paws. Despite attempts to treat her by changing her diet, applying topical medicines, and other means, she continued to mutilate herself. She presented such a pitiful sight that the staff decided to destroy her. The only finding on autopsy was some ovarian degeneration.

The secretary of the Zoological Gardens found it necessary to drown animals that incessantly bit their tails, and he linked tail biting with the tendency of female animals to destroy their offspring.[1] The surgeons noted that animal automutilators were almost always females who appeared to have some interruption or disturbance of their sexual functioning, and they suggested that automutilation was due "to something akin to mental derangement, or as one of the manifestations in the lower animals of the protean hysteria" (p. 211). Back then, hysteria in females, both animal and human, was thought to result from ovarian pathology.

Although the Irish surgeons' comment likening animal automutilation to hysteria in humans seems far-fetched, people (predominantly women) who have hysterical personality disorder are, in fact, prone to nonsuicidal self-injury (NSSI). Additionally, people who have this disorder typically are attentive to their physical appearance and grooming. Interestingly, the majority of automutilative lesions in monkeys, such as hair pulling and scratching, are "aberrations of normal grooming behavior" (Jones et al. 1979).

Biochemical Lesions

From the study of neural tissue in animals much as been learned about how human brains function. Nerve cells (neurons) in the brain generate measurable impulses that transfer information to other neurons by chemical "transmitters" released at one side of a synapse that affect the receptor neuron. It is thought that imbalances of chemical transmitters such as dopamine, norepinephrine, serotonin, opiates, glutamate, and GABA (gamma-amino-butyric acid) may increase or decrease impulses and play a significant role in various psychiatric and neurological disorders. Among the many human disorders in which neurotransmitter imbalances have been implicated are three possibly related syndromes characterized by self-mutilation, namely, the Lesch-Nyhan syndrome (severe mutilation), and the de Lange and Tourette's syndromes (moderate mutilation). These syndromes are discussed in later chapters. Scientists are developing models in which animals are given drugs that cause chemical and neurotransmitter changes that

---

1. Konrad Lorenz (1954) reported on the instinctive reactions of female animals who have just given birth. Normally, the mother sucks, lifts, bites, removes, and eats the fetal membranes, placenta, and umbilical cord from her offspring. Sometimes, however, the impulse to devour the fetal wrappings goes awry, and the mother will rip open the abdomen of, and even eat, her offspring. Lorenz stated that this occurs in domestic mammals, such as pigs and rabbits. If the offspring are removed immediately from their mother and are returned to her, cleaned and dried, several hours later when her devouring impulses have passed, they are in no further danger. Among feral animals, however, mothers destroy their young only if they are diseased. He recounted the story of a 2-month-old sickly jaguar at an Austrian zoo. Its mother was seen licking it nervously and shoving her mouth under its belly near the umbilicus. Spectators at the zoo interpreted the action as maternal solicitude for a sick baby, but Lorenz noted the "beginning of conflict between brood-tending reaction and impulse to devour dead young." The next morning the young jaguar had disappeared, having been eaten by its mother.

lead to automutilation. The obvious value of producing an animal model is that it might then be possible to develop medications that would eliminate mutilative behaviors. It is important to note that drugs cause changes in many neurotransmitters at the same time, even though studies may emphasize only one or two transmitters. An understanding of the complexity of neurotransmitter responses that occur simultaneously is an ongoing work in progress.

A classic observation of animal automutilation was made by Peters (1967) when testing the response of rats to caffeine. After administering high doses of caffeine he observed that 90 percent of semistarved rats demonstrated a sequence of behaviors that progressed to stereotyped acts, such as running backward or in circles and tail chasing, and culminated in biting of their legs and tails. The mutilation was so intense that some rats died from hemorrhage. "A ball of wire put in the cage served as a temporary substitute for self-aggression but ultimately the animal would turn upon itself. . . . Attacks came intermittently. When biting itself, the animal would shriek and then stop biting" (pp. 141–42). Interestingly, when the rats were aggregated, the amount of automutilation declined because the rats' "aggressive behavior appeared to be satisfied to a large extent by chasing and biting neighbor rats which usually ran away before they had become severely mutilated."

The finding that high doses of caffeine often produce automutilation in rats has been often duplicated and partially explained by increases in brain dopamine. Persons who ingest large amounts of caffeine—especially in "energy" drinks that may contain as much caffeine as fourteen cans of a cola drink—can experience heightened anxiety, restlessness, and irritability. Some turn to NSSI to decrease these unpleasant symptoms.

A second proposed model is based on the administration of the drug pemoline to rats. Pemoline is an amphetaminelike central nervous system stimulant that selectively increases levels of the neurotransmitter dopamine. In humans it is a second tier medication for attention deficit disorder. When given to rats, it causes hyperactivity, highly repetitive behaviors (stereotypes), avoidance of physical contact with others, abnormal social behavior, and automutilation such as foot biting (sometimes to the point of amputation) that appears to be a fragmented, exaggerated grooming response. The behavioral similarities between pemoline-treated rats and humans with the de Lange syndrome (who often indulge in acts suggestive of exaggerated grooming behavior such as hand licking, hair stroking, and eye picking) have led researchers to speculate that the two conditions also share neurochemical similarities (Mueller and Hsiao 1980). A comparison of caffeine- and pemoline-treated rats demonstrated that the latter engaged in

self-injurious behaviors more quickly and more severely in a dose-orderly manner across the pemoline doses. The substantial individual variability seen in the
induction of self-injury with moderate/high doses of pemoline is akin to the situation in human beings with neurobiological disorders, where some engage in
self-injury while others do not (Kies and Devine 2004).

Pemoline-induced automutilation in rats can be blocked by coadministration
of naltrexone (an opiate blocker) and dopamine blocker antipsychotics such as
haloperidol and pimozide, drugs that are sometimes used, albeit with scant success, in treating NSSI in human beings (King et al. 1993; Mueller and Nyhan
1982). A more recent study demonstrated that three other medications used,
again with scant success, in treating human NSSI-attenuated pemoline-induced
automutilation in rats (Muehlmann et al. 2008). The most effective was risperi-
done (an antipsychotic dopamine blocker) followed by valproate (a mood stabilizer and antiepileptic GABA enhancer) and then by topiramate (an antiepileptic
drug that interacts with multiple systems that affect neurotransmission). In the
rare human Prader-Willi syndrome topiramate has been shown to decrease severe skin-picking, although this effect may be due to the drug's ability to promote
healing of skin wounds (Shapira et al. 2002).

Another animal model is based on the observation that very high doses of
amphetamine in rats cause occasional automutilation as well as marked stereotypic behavior. These same reactions may be seen in some human beings. Researchers are now able to induce automutilation without stereotypy in rats by
implanting silicone pellets that continuously release small doses of amphetamine
(Mueller et al. 1982). This new model is superior to the caffeine and pemoline
models in that it produces more specific behavior effects at lower doses and also
appears to affect selectively dopamine transmitter levels in a specific area of the
brain (the caudate nucleus).

Clonidine is a drug that affects self-injurious behavior differently in humans
and animals. It works on certain (alpha 2 adrenergic and imidazoline) receptors
in the brain. In human beings, it primarily reduces high blood pressure but is
also used to treat withdrawal symptoms from opiates and alcohol, to reduce anxiety and aggression, and occasionally to reduce stereotypic self-injurious behaviors such as eye gouging and finger biting as well as NSSI. Clonidine, however,
produces severe autobiting in isolated and food-deprived mice (Bhattacharya et al.
1988). The larger the dose, the greater the biting and gnawing off of forelimb
digits. It also worsens rat automutilation induced by caffeine and amphetamine
(Mueller and Nyhan 1983).

Nifedipine, like clonidine, is primarily used to reduce high blood pressure, but its mechanism of action is to block calcium ions from causing neuronal transmission in various organs including both the heart and the brain. In an interesting study Blake et al. (2007) induced automutilation in rats using four different models: administration of a calcium channel enhancer (Bay K 8644), pemoline, amphetamine, and a dopamine enhancer in rats with lesions in their dopamine pathways. In all four situations, nifedipine successfully suppressed self-injurious behaviors. This effect does not seem to be caused by nonspecific factors, such as sedation, because other types of behaviors remain stable. To date, there are no reports of nifedipine treatment for human NSSI.

The most significant biochemical finding regarding self-injurious behavior in human beings is a direct result of animal studies implicating serotonin. For decades, numerous studies have shown that decreased brain serotonin results in increased aggression in both rats and nonhuman primates. In a classic study (Weld et al. 1998), rhesus monkeys who engaged in spontaneous self-biting requiring suturing were given L-tryptophan, a dietary supplement that is a chemical precursor of serotonin. After one week, the marked reduction in self-biting to below baseline measures was correlated with increased brain serotonin levels as measured by the amount of a serotonin metabolite (5-hydroxyindolacetic acid) in the monkeys' cerebrospinal fluid. The same doses of L-tryptophan did not affect the behavior or serotonin metabolism in monkeys without a history of self-biting. Diminished serotonin levels are consistently seen in persons who engage in repetitive NSSI.

Studies of human self-mutilation have primarily emphasized the role of lowered brain serotonin activity, but it is becoming more apparent that other neurotransmitters (dopamine as well as norepinephrine) also are significant. They may well play a permissive or mediating role, and might be responsible for irritability and hyperarousal, which are traits that facilitate self-mutilative and impulsively aggressive behaviors (Markowitz and Coccaro 1995). The importance of dopamine, for example, was demonstrated in an important study of very young rats whose levels of brain dopamine were reduced by administration of a lesion-producing drug (Breece et al. 2005). These rats engaged in self-biting when, as adults, they were give a drug that increased their dopamine levels (as well as decreasing their serotonin levels). Adult rats who had not been brain lesioned did not self-bite when their dopamine levels were increased. The timing of the lesions in early life with the resulting reduction of brain dopamine was thought by the authors to be a possible model for understanding not only the severe self-injurious behavior associated with Lesch-Nyhan syndrome but also the hyper-activity seen in attention deficit disorder as well as functional changes seen in schizophrenia.

The dopaminergic mediation of self-biting in mice was also shown in an elegant study (Kasim and Jinnah 2003). The mice were given drugs that depleted their brain dopamine. When challenged by administration of another drug, a calcium channel enhancer that causes self-biting to increase (Jinnah et al. 1999), the mice markedly reduced their automutilation.

Although most of the animal automutilation studies have focused on neu-rotransmitters, other biochemical factors also are involved. Hormones secreted by the interconnected glandular hypothalamic-pituitary-adrenal (HPA) axis play a role. Cortisol, for example, a hormone produced by the adrenal gland in response to stress, has many actions. Several studies have found disregulation of the HPA axis with low cortisol levels in stressed monkeys who engage in self-biting (Novak 2003; Tiefenbacher et al. 2004). The automutilation rapidly lowered the monkeys' escalating heart rates and positively affected HPA disregulation. NSSI, such as skin-cutting, serves the same function in human beings. High cortisol levels that result from acute stress may trigger self-injurious behavior as seen in monkeys with a history of past self-biting who are relocated to a new facility (Davenport et al. 2008). Acute stress similarly may result in NSSI in human skin-cutters.

A study by Mori et al. (2007) implicates oxidative stress in self-injurious behavior. Oxidative stress refers to the body's constant process of reducing the harmful chemicals that result from the cellular metabolism of oxygen. Rats with methamphetamine-induced self-biting significantly reduced this behavior when given a drug that decreased oxidative stress in brain neurons.

Localized Biological Lesions

Some animals will gnaw off a trapped limb to free themselves. Foxes are especially known for such behavior; in fact, a fox will bite off an injured limb even when the injury is less serious than that sustained by being caught in a trap. Of more interest is the observation that animals will lick, gnaw, and scratch parts of their bodies that are abnormally sensitive, for example, as a result of infections, skin irritations, vitamin deficiencies, parasite and flea infestation, and poor blood supply. This pathological "cleaning behavior" may cause severe tissue damage. Opossums, long-tailed monkeys, small South American monkeys, and carnivorous mammals are especially prone to such automutilation. Meyer-Holzapfel (1968) provided examples from zoos of an opossum that gnawed away its hind leg, of a hyena that gnawed away both hind paws, of a Moor macaque monkey that ate its penis, scrotum, and testes, and of lions that gnawed their paws and tails.

A study of a large mouse production colony found that 8.5 percent of the males mutilated themselves by biting off their penises. Evidently the vigorous sexual activity of the mice resulted in spontaneous incomplete ejaculations and consequent formation of acellular, mucuslike plugs that blocked the urethra. Urinary retention ensued, causing such pain that the mice bit off their penises (Hong and Ediger 1978).

Although it seems unlikely that localized lesions play a role in most human self-mutilation, two observations come to mind. First, some people who are mentally ill excoriate their skin severely, often under the delusion that insects or parasites are present. As noted in chapter 7, these people may seriously gouge their skin with knives and needles in an attempt to dig out these imaginary invaders. They may even bring bags with pieces of skin, dried blood, and dirt to the physician for inspection. Second, some people mutilate body parts that are abnormal, for example, some self-castrators have a history of testicular pathology, such as undescended testicles or mumps orchitis. In these cases, it seems likely that both psychological and biological factors operate to focus the person's attention on the abnormal body part and make it a target for destruction. The memory of pain in a body part may persist even though the original lesion is no longer "really" painful, especially if the body part—such as the testicles—is heavily associated with symbolic meanings. The importance of pain memory to mutilation has been demonstrated in experiments with rats (Dennis and Melzack 1979). If the sensory fibers from a rat's forelimb are surgically cut, the rat will mutilate the organ. If the forelimb is painfully irritated before the destruction of the sensory fibers, the automutilation of the organ is accelerated, often to the point of amputation by chewing. Because the surgical cut makes it impossible for the rat to receive sensations from its forelimb, it is thought that the memory of the pain operates through brain mechanisms to accelerate an automutilative chewing response. Administration of the antiepileptic drug phenytoin (Dilantin) prevents the automutilative response, presumably by affecting the neural circuits that process pain memory.

Several hereditary automutilating disorders result from the loss of sensation due to lesions of spinal cord fibers and cells (e.g., rats and dogs who bite their feet) (Cummings et al. 1981; Jacobs et al. 1981). Similar hereditary neuropathies affect human beings who mutilate their limbs.

Mutilation in Captive Animals

In an attempt to better understand the role of environmental and social factors in human self-mutilation, researchers have performed many experiments using animals, namely monkeys, that are high on the evolutionary scale. It is clear that animals placed in artificial environments, such as zoos or laboratories, are predisposed to automutilation, that social isolation increases this predisposition, and that stressful events, such as a frustrated sex act, threatening stimuli, or thwarted aggression, may precipitate this behavior (Jones and Barraclough 1978).

Tinklepaugh's complicated case of a male monkey named Cupid is the best-known early report on automutilation (1928). Cupid established a relationship with a female monkey named Psyche. He reacted violently and attacked two other female monkeys, Topsy and Eva, when they replaced Psyche in his cage. Through various experimental manipulations, Cupid developed a relationship with Topsy. When Topsy was then replaced by Psyche, Cupid seemed fine. After two weeks, Topsy replaced Psyche. Just as Cupid was about to copulate with Topsy, "he jumped away and began biting his hind feet." For three days, he repeated this behavior, never completing copulation, so his hind feet became badly torn. As he was being attended to medically, Psyche shrieked from her nearby cage and threatened Topsy, who was in Cupid's cage. Without warning, Cupid viciously bit his feet, jumped down, ripped open his scrotum, mutilated the end of his tail, and tore a three-inch gash in his hip. During the following four months, he appeared to be in a "state comparable to the depression of some psychoses." He eventually was able to interact normally with both Psyche and Topsy, but whenever Tinklepaugh approached the cage Cupid began to bite his own paws and scrotum.

Although Tinklepaugh did not draw any firm conclusions from this case, he suggested that the automutilation may have resulted from the frustrations of disturbed sexual bonding. Similar behavior in monkeys frustrated by incomplete copulation has been reported by Sackett (1968). Time and again, it has been shown that automutilation in adult laboratory monkeys is highly associated with social isolation during the first year of life; other behaviors associated with early social isolation include social withdrawal, rocking, huddling, clasping, excessive fearfulness or arousal, stereotyped actions, and inappropriate heterosexual and maternal reactions. These behaviors are most severe and persistent when the isolation is total, begins at birth, and continues for at least six months. In general, automutilation increases in isolation-reared monkeys under conditions of frustration, such as when a human experimenter interferes with a monkey's

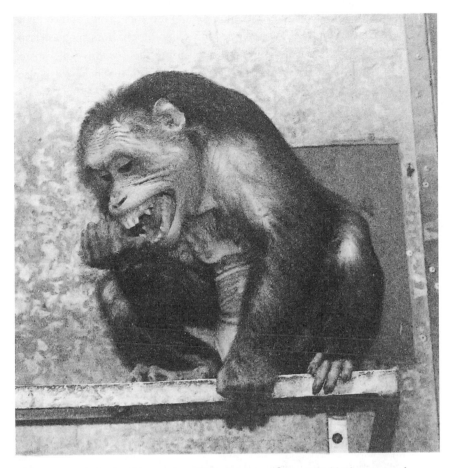

Autoinjurious behavior in a monkey. (Photo courtesy of Drs. Arnold Chamove and J. R. Anderson)

cage, although it may occur even without human interference (Cross and Harlow 1965).

All captive monkeys during their second year of life demonstrate social aggression (biting, grabbing, threatening, and chasing other monkeys) three times more frequently than autoaggression. During autoaggression, a monkey may bite its arm, knee, or foot, slap itself in the face, attempt to "surprise" itself, and threaten or attack the limb that "surprised" it. On reaching maturity (the fifth year of life), however, monkeys raised with social contacts no longer engage in autoaggression while monkeys raised in isolation demonstrate increasing levels of autoaggression (see the appendix to this chapter).

It appears that inadequate social input leads to the appearance and continuance of autoaggression in monkeys raised in isolation. Behaviors such as clasping, sucking, and brief vigorous biting begin during the first three months of isolation and may be a prècursor of autoaggression. The normal behavior of play-fighting among monkey peers is subverted during isolation. The socially deprived monkeys may learn to use themselves as targets for aggression as a means of stimulating themselves. The monkeys may also learn that autoaggression is more controllable and safer than social aggression; for example, a dominant male will not interfere with a monkey that is hurting itself but will threaten or attack socially aggressive monkeys. This tendency to autoaggression is established during the first two months of isolation and can be decreased or eliminated if soon after the first two months the monkey is placed in consistent contact with peers or, better still, with a receptive adult female monkey.

Comparisons between Animal Automutilation and Human Self-mutilation

In considering the comparability of automutilation in animals with self-mutilation in humans, we need to address the question of similarities in the behavior itself. Clearly, some mutilative behaviors appear identically in animals and humans. Mild acts such as hair pulling, head hitting, and skin scratching, for example, are seen in confined monkeys as well as in about 17 percent of normal children. More severe acts such as head banging, face slapping, eye and ear digging, and self-biting are seen in laboratory monkeys as well as in humans who have severe mental retardation. Both humans and animals scratch, gouge, and bite accessible body tissue. Animals use their claws and large incisor teeth for automutilation; during the course of evolution humans have substituted tools, such as knives and razor blades. Thus, the behaviors appear to be comparable.[2]

Automutilation seems to be a device to increase or decrease levels of arousal. Monkeys that are highly aroused as manifested by agitation and rage become calm following an act of automutilation. This sequence of events also occurs in

---

2. Although no animal models have been developed for schizophrenia or manic-depressive disorder, claims have been made that animals may develop severe depression although many authors are careful to use very precise language. Thus, Moran and McKinney (1975) state that "assorted techniques have been developed by various researchers in an attempt to reproduce in non-human primates that state of despair and withdrawal that is labeled depression in human primates." One such technique is to confine monkeys in a steel vertical chamber designed to induce feelings of helplessness and hopelessness.

many cases of human NSSI—persons report mounting tension and anger before the act and lowering of tension, even calmness, after it.

Monkeys, especially in isolation settings, automutilate. This behavior has been interpreted as autostimulation used to counteract low levels of arousal. As will be discussed in greater detail in subsequent chapters, human self-mutilation often serves to increase low arousal levels; for example, head banging in people who have mental retardation and in sensory-deprived children may serve this purpose. Sociopaths may engage in stimulus-seeking behavior, including NSSI, in an attempt to counteract low cortical arousal levels. Human prisoners are especially prone to NSSI, although the social isolation of a prison cannot fully compare with the total isolation of experimental monkeys. Convicts frequently experience loneliness, alienation, and frustration in social relationships while living in overcrowded prisons. The notion that people can feel isolated even while in the company of other persons has been popularized in the concept of "the lonely crowd."

The automutilation resulting from early social isolation is probably due to a variety of mechanisms that include impaired learning of social skills, impaired ability to adapt to change (a consequence of perceptual-motor deficits resulting from a lack of critical experiences in early life), increased frustration, a tendency toward depression, and general developmental lag (Jones 1982; McKinney 1974). A large number of human self-mutilators report pathological childhood experiences, including physical and psychological abuse by parents and inadequate supplies of parental love, nurturance, and comforting physical contact. As children, self-mutilators often experience a sense of abandonment, of loneliness, and of unlovability, and they may carry these traits into adolescence and adult life. Loneliness is a common complaint among psychiatric patients, and relative social isolation during childhood along with a current inability to form close relationships is often reported by persons who deliberately injure themselves. According to Jones (1982), "This series of events—developmental isolation, bonding disturbance, and later predominant feelings of social isolation, loneliness, and anomie, with consequent frustration in interpersonal situations—is the sort of sequence that might be predicted from the animal model" (p. 146).

Many of the inferences we make about animal behavior indicate that it often may be identical to or similar to human behavior, but the human capacity to use symbols and to communicate information about thoughts, emotions, and perceptions bespeaks a major problem in comparing human and animal behaviors. Thus, comparative environmental and social studies, while instructive, are handicapped by the complexity of the human situation.

APPENDIX

A number of publicly acclaimed books, such as Konrad Lorenz's *On Aggression* (1966), Desmond Morris's *The Naked Ape* (1967) and *The Human Zoo* (1969), and Eibl-Eibelsfeldt's *On Love and Hate* (1972), address animal aggression and its relationship to human aggression. As neatly summarized by Fromm (1973), these books draw similar conclusions, namely, that "man's aggressive behavior as manifested in war, crime, personal quarrels, and all kinds of destructive and sadistic behavior is due to a phylogenetically programmed, innate instinct which seeks for discharge and waits for the proper occasion to be expressed" (p. 23). Presumably, self-mutilation can be added to this list of humanity's aggressive behaviors.

Lorenz's work is of interest because so many subsequent ethological studies derive from his observations. Lorenz holds that animals are innately aggressive but not destructive, that an animal's aggression is predominantly directed toward competitive members of its own species, and that aggression is a positive force. The aggressive drive has important value for survival in that it functions to balance the distribution of animals of the same species over the environment and thus ensures an adequate food supply. Therefore, animals will claim a territory sufficient to meet their nutritional and other needs and will aggressively protect this territory from competitive animals. The aggressive drive also affects sexual selection; the strongest and fittest males will chase away their weaker rivals during the breeding season, gain access to females, and protect their offspring from predators. Another function of the aggressive drive is the development of a ranking order, "a principle of organization without which a more advanced social life cannot develop in high vertebrates. . . . Under this rule every individual in the society knows which one is stronger and which weaker than itself, so that everyone can retreat from the stronger and expect submission from the weaker if they should get in each other's way" (p. 40). The establishment of a ranking order provides peace and order within a group in that the dominant animals use their force to control intragroup fighting, to provide leadership against attacks by predators, to diminish group tensions by ensuring some sort of consistency, and even to serve as role models.

For Lorenz, the aggressive drive is a species-preserving instinct, but the spontaneity of the instinct is what makes it dangerous, especially in humans. Aggression sometimes is a reaction to external factors, but it also may explode without demonstrable external stimulation; for example, when the central nervous system lowers the aggression threshold, or when the stimuli that normally release aggression fail to operate for an appreciable period of time, then an organism will search actively for a "missing stimulus" against which aggression can be unleashed. Lorenz holds that this process of unleashing dammed-up aggression becomes especially dangerous in situations where group members know each other well. He provides an example: a person sneezes in the presence of a close friend with dammed-up aggression. The friend may overreact to this trivial stimulus. In rare instances the friend may kill the person who sneezed; usually, however, the overreaction takes the form of a redirected activity in which the aggression is expressed by smashing some object. Likewise, one could develop a scenario in which a mentally ill person who has dammed-up aggression responds to an irritating stimulus by redirecting aggression through the process of NSSI. Redirection of aggression is an evolutionary expedient for neutralizing aggression. A related mechanism is the display of an appeasing attitude; for example, a strong attacking animal will stop its attack if a weaker animal adopts a submissive, vulnerable posture. The ritualization of appeasement attitudes results in social bonding among animals. Lorenz notes that the personal bond of an individual friendship is formed only in animals with highly developed intraspecific aggression, that in many cases love develops through ritualization of a redirected attack, and that these rituals eventually assume an autonomous existence in which an aggressive animal's partner becomes highly valued. In the case of an imaginary stimulus such as a threatening auditory hallucination, the redirection of aggression onto the self (certainly the aggression cannot be directed physically against a hallucination) through NSSI may also be a type of appeasement attitude. By demonstrating their wounds and vulnerability, self-injurers may hope to forestall further attacks against themselves. In some cases repetitive NSSI may represent an attempt to form a social bond with a perceived attacker such as a vicious cell mate in a prison. On an unconscious level, it may even represent an attempt to obtain a loving relationship with a parent.

While most scientists would agree that animals possess an aggressive instinct, a great many would not agree that irrational behavior in humans has phylogenetic origins or that behavioral principles derived from the study of animal instincts have any application to humans. Ashley Montagu's *Man and Aggression* (1973) contains twenty chapters by noted scholars, each of whom debunks the ethological concept of aggression as applied to humans. In Montagu's words, "There is, in fact, not the slightest evidence or ground for assuming that the alleged 'phylogenetically adapted instinctive' behavior of other animals is in any way relevant to the discussion of the motive-forces of human behavior. The fact is, that with the exception of the instinctoid reactions in infants to sudden withdrawals of support and to sudden loud noises, the human being is entirely instinctless. . . . That is not to say that man is born a *tabula rasa*. Clearly, the reason why man is not an ape is that he possesses genetic capacities, the result of a long and unique evolutionary history, which, under the appropriate environmental stimulation, enable him to function as a human being. The most important of these genetic capacities is that for learning, educability, literally the species trait of *Homo sapiens*. Man is capable of learning virtually anything" (p. 11). These critics go on to attack the concept of innate human depravity and aggressiveness and put forth the concept that human aggression is learned behavior. In Leon Eisenberg's eloquent words, "To believe that man's aggressiveness or territoriality is in the nature of the beast is to mistake all men for some men, contemporary societies for all societies, and, by a remarkable transformation, to justify what is as what needs must be; social repression becomes a response to, rather than a cause of, human violence" (p. 56).

The concept of a human aggressive instinct and, indeed, of aggression in general has been extremely problematic for psychiatrists. Alfred Adler first mentioned *Aggressionstrieb* (aggressive instinct) in 1908 in "The Aggressive Instinct in Life and in Neurosis." For a full explication of the Freudian concept of aggression, I refer the reader to Fromm's *The Anatomy of Human Destructiveness* (1973). Suffice it to say that Freud adopted the term *Aggressionstrieb* and, in fact, used it as well as the terms *Destruktionstrieb* (destructive instinct) and *Todestrieb* (death instinct). In *Civilization and Its Discontents* (1930) he wrote, "Starting with speculations on the beginning of life and from biological parallels I drew the conclusion that, besides the instinct to preserve living substance, there must exist another, contrary instinct seeking to dissolve those units and to bring them back to their primaeval, inorganic state. That is to say, as well as Eros there was an instinct of death." Freud placed the source of the death instinct within the individual constitution; that is, aggression is not reactive but innate. Thus, life itself is a conflict and a compromise between the continuance of life and a striving toward death, between metabolism and catabolism. Although both Lorenz and Freud have proposed an innate aggressive (destructive) instinct, Fromm is correct in pointing out that the former's aggressive drive serves life, while the latter's death instinct serves death. Both Lorenz and Freud believed that failure to express aggression in action may result in psychopathology.

Most contemporary psychiatrists have discounted the Freudian notion of a death instinct, and the few that have written about ethology are cautious about drawing parallels with human behavior. One psychiatrist who has attempted to explain human aggressiveness on the basis of ethological concepts is Anthony Storr (1968). He notes that we now tend to "accept the idea that sex is an internal force which has to be satisfied." Satisfaction—the release of sexual tension—may be achieved best with the help of a partner but may also be obtained through masturbation. Because the physiological state of the body in both sexual and aggressive arousal is similar and because the sexual and aggressive instincts share certain components, Storr proposes the notion that, like sex, aggression is an internal force that has to be satisfied. The reduction of aggressive tension may be obtained through activities such as war, hunting, sports competition, initiation rites, and religious sacrifice. This argument could be extended to include NSSI. In fact, many persons describe themselves as filled with unbearable tension; an act of NSSI may lead to dissipation of this tension and to a feeling of relief. Thus, as a tension-relieving device, self-mutilation may be analogous to masturbation.

PART TWO

MUTILATION AND SELF-INJURY
OF BODY PARTS
Cultural and Clinical Cases

In this section, data on culturally sanctioned and deviant self-injury are presented according to the various body parts that are affected: the head and its subdivisions, the limbs, the skin and body, and the genitals. Using an anatomical model is more than a device that allows us to make sense of a wide array of mutilative practices. In fact, most culturally sanctioned self-mutilation focuses on a specific body area such as the skull or genitals. Similarly, mentally ill persons tend to damage one body part such as the eye or the skin.

From a cultural perspective, rituals and practices involving the sanctioned destruction or alteration of specific body parts are examined. In some instances the body modification is self-inflicted, while in others individuals voluntarily allow themselves to be mutilated. In the case of infants and young children, parental consent is given in accord with social expectations. Relevant folkloric, literary, and mythological references to body parts are presented in addition to native and scientific explanations for the mutilative behavior. As will be seen, the selection of a specific anatomical part for mutilation is often intertwined with cultural concerns such as beauty and social status.

From a psychiatric perspective, cases are described in which self-injury is the product of mental illness. Whenever possible the self-injurers' own statements about their behavior are presented, as well as psychiatric understandings of the behavior. The word *self-injury* has a broad meaning that refers to all types of direct, deliberate, self-inflicted bodily harm. Self-mutilation refers to self-injury involving a major, significant body part such as enucleation of an eye or limb amputation. NSSI refers to nonsuicidal self-injury such as skin-cutting, head banging, and pulling out body hair. People who engage in NSSI most commonly refer to themselves as self-injurers. It should be noted that all self-injury, with rare exceptions such as some cases of eye enucleation and self-castration, does not involve conscious suicidal intent.

Deviant self-injury can be understood most fully by examining the cultural context (historical and contemporary) in which it occurs. This section presents the data on which the conclusions of the third section of this book are based.

CHAPTER FIVE

The Head and Its Parts

The head is importantly associated with two major facets of human life: aesthetics and control. Although our perception of physical beauty involves the total human body, the head holds a preeminent place. A minor anatomical rearrangement, such as the crossing of an eye or elongation of a nose can turn beauty into ugliness. Cultural practices (head molding, ear piercing, lip stretching, etc.) are often linked with aesthetics, and facial plastic surgery for reasons of vanity is a common practice in many cultures.

The notion of the head as the locus of control of the body is related both to the presence of the brain within the skull and to the head's position atop the body. In a common social metaphor a king, president, or chief is the head of his or her people and controls them just as the human head controls its body. The power to control others emanates from the mouth and eyes. From the mouth come words that can entreat, cajole, flatter, deceive, persuade, bless, and curse. From the eyes, according to a widespread folk belief, comes a potent evil force. When propelled by a glance, it can cause sickness and misfortune in the person it strikes.

The mouth, nose, eyes, and brain are head parts that play a special role in the prevention and treatment of illnesses and in the remediation of sin. The mouth can confess sins and pathogenic secrets, pray for forgiveness and deliverance, invoke the healing intercession of beneficent spirits, name and cast out harmful spirits, and engage in a talk cure with a therapist. Nose bleeding can be induced, often in imitation of female menstruation, to rid the body of poisons. Self-inflicted destruction of the eyes—a highly prized body part—is a method of obtaining relief from the guilt associated with a terrible thought or deed. In modern thought, mental illness is, to a great extent, linked with chemical and structural defects in the brain. Among the procedures used to correct such defects are the administration of drugs, the use of electrical and magnetic devices, and, more rarely, the surgical destruction of brain tissue. In past centuries, mental illness was sometimes thought to result from pathological forces, such as evil spirits or humors, in the cranial cavity. One method of treatment was to drill holes into the skull to allow these forces to exit.

The Skull and Head

This section presents three examples of culturally sanctioned mutilative practices involving the skull and head: head molding, trephination, and head slashing. This is followed by a discussion of the most common form of deviant head self-mutilative behavior, head banging.

Deviant self-mutilation of the skull is rare. Sinclair (1886–87) describes a 25-year-old delusional man who had self-mutilative tendencies. While in the hospital, he cut out his testicle with a nail, claiming that it belonged to another patient. Five months later, he excised his remaining testicle and ate it "to prevent anyone else getting it." Whenever possible, he scratched himself with pieces of wood, stone, or glass. He placed a nail against his forehead, hit it in with his hand, and drove it all the way into his skull by banging his head against the wall. Hospital staff noticed only a superficial scratch, which he said was caused by a belt buckle. Two months later, he became very ill and told the staff about the nail. It was surgically removed, but the patient died the next day. An autopsy showed that the nail had reached the frontal lobe, resulting in a large cavity filled with blood, pus, and broken-down brain tissue.

Head Molding

In ancient Egypt, a powerful king, probably Akhenaton, was born with a distinctive head shape. In imitation, the Egyptian aristocracy placed constricting bandages around the heads of their infants to produce a head shape similar to that of the king. In fact, an infant's skull is soft and can be molded by techniques such as massage and the application of pressure with bandages, boards, and stones. Head shaping was a prerogative of the upper classes in Egypt, and it created an ideal of beauty and a mark of social status that was imitated for thousands of years. The skull shape of the beautiful Queen Nefertiti was clearly the product of molding. Head molding spread from Egypt throughout much of the world. In modern times the Nazis encouraged German parents to massage their children's heads to produce an "Aryan"-type skull.

References to head molding are found in classical Greek literature. Zenobius described a group, the Syrakoi, who chose as their leader the man with the longest head. This group may have been the same as the Macrocephali, who were described by Hippocrates in *On Air, Land, and Water*. Hippocrates wrote, "There is no other race of men which have heads in the least resembling theirs. They think those the most noble who have the longest heads. . . . Immediately after the child is born, and while its head is still tender, they fashion it with their hands, and constrain it to assume a lengthened shape by applying bandages and other suitable contrivances whereby the spherical form of the head is destroyed, and it is made to increase in length."

Head molding was practiced throughout much of Europe, especially in Holland and France, until the middle of the nineteenth century. It was greatly influenced by phrenology. To increase desired mental functioning, parents reshaped infants' heads. Although primarily a rural practice, it affected the urban population as well because of the custom of sending city children to the country to be reared.

In Normandy, handkerchiefs were tightly and painfully wound around the heads of children. These constricting bandages were rarely removed and served as breeding grounds for lice. Many of the children developed skin ulcers. In Limousin and Languedoc, the molded heads of women were distinctive; the molding was caused by tight-fitting bonnets that produced a pleasing head shape and supposedly enhanced intelligence and memory.

Achille Foville, a nineteenth-century French physician who worked in mental asylums, found that 247 out of 431 patients had deformed heads as a result of being forced to wear a constricting bandeau that flattened the upper part of the skull and deformed ear tissue. He correlated the severity of head deformation with the severity and intractability of mental symptoms. Many French physicians regarded head molding as medically dangerous and thought it could result in epilepsy, mental retardation, and chronic insanity (Dingwall 1931).

In Africa, head molding has been influenced most directly by the Egyptian concept of beauty and social status. Many African statues of elongated heads are not the result of artistic conceits but rather reflect the actual shape (albeit somewhat stylized) of admired models. Head molding is still carried out in some areas of Africa, especially on female infants.

Many reports of head shaping have come from the Pacific Islands. The natives of Malekula developed a most peculiar circular, small head shape with a double depression in the upper part of the skull. The British explorer Captain James Cook described them as "the most ugly, ill proportioned people I ever saw, and in every respect different from any we had met within this sea." Some anthropologists, unaware that the natives deliberately created the head shapes by applying constricting bands, initially thought the Malekula skulls represented a special racial type. The Samoans wrapped stones in cloth to flatten the foreheads and noses of children; for them, Western noses were ugly and were referred to as "canoes."

The Maya Indians in Central America applied a board to the forehead that caused the frontal bone to slant backward so far that the nose and forehead formed a straight line. Head deformation was also found in Peru, where myth has it that the custom of forming tapering, elongated heads arose from a native desire to resemble a holy volcano from which the tribes supposedly originated.

In North America, the Chinook, or Flathead, Indians were the leading practitioners of head shaping. Immediately after birth infants were strapped on a board; a flat piece of wood was placed on their foreheads and tied tightly to the plank for a year, thus flattening the forehead and forcing the head to rise at the top. A European observer described a child on such a contraption: "Its little black eyes, forced out by tightness of the bandages, resembled those of a mouse choked in a trap" (Dingwall 1931, p. 166). Another observer described a child whose head had just been removed from the apparatus as the most frightful and disgusting object he had ever seen. The frontal part of the skull was completely flattened, and the child's inflamed eyes protruded half an inch from the sockets. As the children grew up, their heads did not appear to be grotesquely abnormal, except for a broad face. The Chinooks bought and captured many slaves who were readily distinguishable by their "ugly," round, natural heads.

Trephination

Trephination, the deliberate removal of bone from the skull, is an ancient surgical procedure that has persisted to current times. Over one thousand trephined skulls have been found in South America, especially in Bolivia and Peru. Trephined skulls have been found in Oceania, France, Russia, Sweden, North Africa, the Balkans, and ancient Egypt (Hrdlicka 1939; Wehrli 1939).

The most common procedure was for a surgeon to cut through the scalp and scrape the skull with a sharp tool. This is relatively safe as long as the dura, the covering of the brain, is not damaged. More dangerous procedures included sawing, cutting, or drilling directly into the skull and then breaking off the bone to remove a plug. From evidence of healing in the area of the trephination, various estimates have been made about the mortality rate of the procedure. Two studies involving 214 and 400 Peruvian skulls demonstrated healing in 55.6 percent and 62.5 percent, respectively. One skull showed healing from seven distinct operations. It is not uncommon today for persons in eastern Africa to survive several trephinations.

In sixteenth-century Europe, Paracelsus advocated surgical opening of the head as a last resort to cure mania; the procedure allowed an exit for hot humors that caused insanity by touching the brain. Itinerant charlatans known as stonecutters flourished in Holland and Belgium in the fifteenth and sixteenth centuries. They made small incisions in the heads of the mentally ill and by sleight of hand pretended to remove "stones of folly," as demonstrated in paintings by Bosch and Breughel (Grabman 1975).

How and why humans first thought of putting holes in their heads is unknown. One theory is that the practice arose from an ancient method of treating sheep for the disease called "staggers," namely, opening the sheep's skull and removing worm larvae from its brain. In Yugoslavian folklore, beetles are removed from the human brain, and in Tibet, centipedes. A simpler explanation is that trephination was devised to cure headaches by allowing evil spirits to exit.

Coxon (1962) reported on trephination among the Kisii, a small, remote African tribe of cattle farmers. A clear history of head trauma must be present, with or without subsequent severe headaches. The "surgeons" use chisels and saws and are careful neither to cross cranial suture lines nor to cut into the dura. Anesthesia consists of diverting patients' attention by poking their ears with thorns while relatives hold them down during the six-hour ordeal. Some patients have multiple operations. "The Kisii must have set a record in one man who has survived thirty-five trephinings. Although he has little cranium left, with a tin hat and an unlimited supply of aspirins he is free from headache and a successful farmer." By carefully selecting their patients and by adhering closely to empirically derived surgical techniques, the surgeons rarely have any complications. In fact, should the patient die or become seriously ill, the surgeon faces imprisonment and even capital punishment because it is presupposed that he acted out of carelessness or stupidity.

A number of trephined skulls show evidence of fracture lines, thus indicating that the procedure was also used to relieve pressure on the brain. In the mining districts of Cornwall, in England, surgeons continued to trephine until the late nineteenth century. Many miners sustained head injuries in the narrow shafts (the caps they wore did not offer sufficient protection, and blasting devices to loosen the earth were crude), and surgeons there considered it good practice to drill holes in the skull even before symptoms of compression were present. Other therapeutic indications for trephination throughout the world include epilepsy, mental illness, vertigo, coma, and delirium. It reportedly was done in Melanesia to promote longevity.

John Mitchell (1984) recounts the story of a Dutchman, Dr. Bart Hughes, who developed a small following. In 1962, Hughes advocated trephination to achieve a transcendent state. He theorized that a consequence of the evolutionary process of adopting an upright stance was a reduction in the flow of blood to the brain because of gravity; as a result humans have reduced the range of their consciousness and lost touch with the dreams and intense perceptions of childhood (a child's skull does not enclose the brain as tightly as an adult's). Hughes's solution was to drill a small hole in his head to allow for increased blood flow. Although he claimed a satisfying state of consciousness as a result of the procedure, he was involuntarily committed to a Dutch mental institution. His cause was taken up by Joseph Mellen and his girlfriend, Amanda Fielding, who ran for Parliament in London; her political plank called for free trephination for everyone under the National Health Service plan. They both put holes in their heads, but Amanda had the foresight to make a movie, called *Heartbeat in the Brain*, of her self-operation. In it she calmly applies an electric drill to her skull to remove a plug of bone. According to Mitchell, the couple lived and worked together in harmony thereafter. They bought an art gallery, and "there is nothing apparently abnormal about them." They frequently lectured about the benefits of trephination and showed the film of Amanda's self-operation to the accompaniment of a soothing musical soundtrack.

Head Slashing

As reported by Crapanzano (1973), the Hamadsha is a lower-social-class, religious, Sufi, healing brotherhood in Morocco whose rituals are considered extreme by most other Muslim mystic groups. Their healing ritual includes drinking boiling water, eating spiny cactus, charming poisonous snakes, and head slashing with razors and knives during ecstatic trances induced by wild dancing.

The Hamadsha are curers of persons who are struck or possessed by jinn spirits. The jinn are capricious, quick-tempered, and dangerous spirits who sometimes assume human or animal forms. When insulted or injured, they may retaliate by striking a person blind, deaf, mute, or paralyzed. They may enter and possess a person as manifested by symptoms such as unconsciousness, fainting, convulsions, tremors, talking in tongues, flights of thought, and abrupt, meaningless changes in activity or talk. Aisha Qandisha is a libidinous, quick-tempered jinn who is extremely important to the Hamadsha. She strangles and scratches anyone who disobeys her; because of her fondness for blood she compels her followers to cut themselves.

The *hadra*, or healing ceremony, is designed to cure jinn illness and to promote health through the acquisition of a miraculous saintly force called *baraka*. *Baraka* enables the Hamadsha to enter a trance and to slash their heads to please the spirits. The saint's healing *baraka* is acquired when a patient eats or is smeared with the blood of an adept.

The ceremony lasts from four to twelve hours and may be attended by forty-five to eighty men, women, and children. After invoking Allah, several musicians play loud, fast, violent music, and the men form a dance line. They jump up and down, hyperventilate, and punch themselves until a trance state is achieved. Occasionally, a woman will enter a frenetic trance, screaming and charging around the dance area. She may convulse, scratch or slash her head with a knife, or even try to cut off a breast. Severe head mutilation, however, is more common among the men who enter a frenetic trance. With a pocketknife a man will slash his head until his face and shoulders are drenched with blood. Sometimes the gashes reach the skull, although usually the cuts are superficial. On some occasions, the Hamadsha slash their heads with axes and hit their heads with heavy iron balls and nail-studded clubs. They may see a vision of Aisha Qandisha slashing at her head, compelling the dancers to slash theirs and to calm her by making their blood flow. They smear the blood from their head wounds on the ailing parts of a patient's body, or they may dip sugar cubes or bread in their blood and give it to the sick to eat. The dancers claim to feel no pain and to be unaware of their wounds until they have emerged from the trance.

Crapanzano's explication of how patients are cured by the Hamadsha details such factors as group support and cult membership, which afford the patient explanations of illness, new social status, an increased social network, and changed self-image and social identity. Achievement of a trance state increases suggestibility, allows partial erasure of old, learned behavior, and facilitates catharsis. The author interprets the mutilation as a symbolic castration. The men, he claims, conceive of illness at some level of consciousness as an inability to live up to the standards of male conduct. To be cured, a man becomes a woman through symbolic castration. Thanks to the *baraka* of the saint, he passes through a feminization stage, is revitalized, revirilized, and able to become a man again. In the process, Aisha Qandisha is transformed from a socially and morally disruptive force into one that preserves order and morality. That most Hamadsha patients periodically continue to participate in *hadras* suggests that cures are temporary and that there is no personality change of long standing.

Head Banging

Although head banging is the most common form of nonsuicidal self-injury (NSSI) involving the skull, mild, limited head banging is found in up to 6 percent of normal children, especially boys. It is often preceded by transient crib rocking or head-body rolling, behaviors that provide some reassurance to the frustrated child attempting to master a new stage of development. This "normal" head banging coincides with tooth eruption and with the change from sitting to crawling (ages 8 to 12 months). It may last for one to three years. Head banging past age 4 is almost always pathological, is primarily found in children who have autism or mental retardation, and may be associated with head punching and slapping, recurrent vomiting, self-induced seizures, detached retinas, and eye hemorrhage (Noel and Clarke 1982).

Many reasons have been proposed to explain head banging, the most fanciful being that it is done to reexperience the comfort of hearing mother's heartbeat when being held in her arms. Other theories regard it as a means of obtaining adult attention, a response to fatigue, a response to understimulation, and an expression of frustration and anger. A traditional psychoanalytic concept holds that head banging is a form of aggression turned inward that is channeled and directed by the superego. Many children, however, engage in head banging at an age before the development of the superego. Freud and Burlingham (1944) described a 14-month-old child who knocked her head violently when isolated in the empty sickroom. At 15 months, "when put into her crib for a nap against her wishes, she threw herself against the bars and banged her whole body as well as her head repeatedly. When other children took her toys or attacked her, she always banged her head in despair. At 16 months she threw herself on the floor and banged her head over and over again when not allowed to take another child's toy" (p. 74).

Collins (1965) described a 26-year-old man with severe mental retardation whose head banging had persisted since the age of 4. By the age of 22, he was confined to bed, where he wore a thick rubber collar and was fully restrained. When the restraints were removed, he would immediately attempt to smash his head on any available object or to hit it with his fist or knee. Even when wearing a football helmet with a face guard, he contused and lacerated his head. The author interpreted the head banging as "an effort to maintain a self-identity through constant reinforcement of the perception of the extent of his body—a most primitive and basic level of existence" (p. 209). Thus, the patient's perceptual world may have been diffuse, not integrated with reality, and meaningless. He was able to experience himself as a separate entity by banging his head. A treatment program was devised in which he was exposed to many stimuli, such as sound from a bedside radio, mobiles hung over his bed, perfumed soaps and lotions, spiced candy and gum, and scheduled trips to the toilet. Attendants spent time with him on walks and played and spoke with him. Within weeks, his intense head banging subsided, and in a year he no longer required restraints. After four years, he was able to participate in simple group games, to follow simple instructions, to withdraw from painful stimuli, and to show obvious joy and affection when visited by his mother.

Bates and Smeltzer (1982) reported a 25-year-old man with severe mental retardation whose intense head banging began at age 2. He had prolonged episodes of insomnia, weight loss, hyperactivity, and terrible head banging. For unknown reasons, he would fling aside his protective helmet and suddenly bang his head against a wall in a staccato frenzy (once measured at three hundred blows in five minutes); often he bloodied his head before he could be restrained, and twice he knocked himself unconscious. Medications including sedatives, major tranquilizers, and lithium were ineffective, as were behavioral extinction programs. At age 21, his behavior and other symptoms were life threatening. He flung himself against walls and floors, butted staff with his head, bit his lips, lacerated himself with his fingernails, and beat his knees together until they bled. Because nothing seemed to help and because he had a family history of manic-depressive illness, electroconvulsive therapy was performed. After six treatments over a two-week period, the patient's symptoms came under control, as did his attempts at self-mutilation. Maximum benefits were achieved after six more treatments, and the patient did well. When symptoms returned in several months, they were then controlled by lithium and a major tranquilizer. At the time of the report, the patient had been under control for three years, although his symptoms reemerged whenever attempts were made to lower the dose of either medication.

Baroff and Tate (1968) described a 9-year-old psychotic boy with a five-year history of head hitting so severe that he had a detached retina and blindness. Treatment consisted of jolting him with an aversive stimulus—an electric cattle prod—whenever he banged his head. The results were dramatic: "In short, a pattern of self-injurious behavior which had existed for more than five years, had resulted in blindness in one eye, and had been completely refractory to standard forms of treatment, was interrupted literally in minutes, reduced to non-injurious minimum within days, and all but disappeared in five months" (p. 464).

Although these cases had successful long-term therapeutic outcomes, most reported cases of severe head banging record limited therapeutic successes. A discussion of behavioral treatment approaches for head banging and other behaviors is presented in chapter 11.

Head banging has become a cultural phenomenon in association with hard rock and heavy metal music. It began in 1968 at a Led Zeppelin concert when people in the front rows reportedly banged their heads on the stage floor in time to the music. The term *headbanger* was born, and it is used today in reference to people at rock concerts who frantically swing their head up and down, side to side, or in a circle, or who bang heads with others, or who bang their heads on the stage. When the movements pass a threshold (more than 146 beats a minute and a range of movement more than 75 degrees), headaches and dizziness are common. Rare injuries include bleeding into the brain and traumatic aneurysm of the cervical vertebral artery (Patton and McIntosh 2008).

The Eyes

The only organs of the human body that have not been subjected to voluntary, ritual mutilation are the anus and the eyes. The anus probably has been spared because it responds to wounds angrily, and its refusal to heal often results in chronic inanition. The eye probably has been spared because it is the most intellectually valuable and magically endowed human organ. Anatomically the eye is unique in that it grows out from the brain, and thus it is the only portion of the central nervous system directly in contact with the outside world.

In mythology, folklore, and literature a host of often contradictory attributes are linked to the eyes. Thus, the eyes may be associated with creativity or with destruction, with purity or with shame and guilt, with love or with sexual transgression. These attributes of the eyes often are significant factors in deviant self-mutilation.

The eye was a potent force in Egyptian mythology. From the eyes of Ptah, the gods were created. Ra, the supreme sun god, rested with his eyes shut in the primordial ocean. He then arose, opened his eyes, and created the universe. When he grew old and senile, ambitious men plotted against him. In anger he sent his Divine Eye to slaughter them.

Horus was the name given to more than twenty Egyptian gods. The earliest Horus was a falcon-headed god whose eyes were the sun and the moon (the hieroglyph for *god* is a falcon). Horus the Elder was the god of the sky. He was the son of Ra and brother of the evil Set. In the horrible battles between Horus and Set, between the forces of good and those of evil, Set plucked out Horus's eye and plunged humankind into chaos. Horus retaliated by emasculating Set. Horus the Younger was a god who eventually took over all the attributes of the previous Horuses. As the final conqueror of Set, Horus the Younger, with his powerful eye in place, restored order to the universe and brought peace to the world.

Hindu mythology contains one of the most bizarre stories about the eye. The god Indra desired the beautiful wife of Gotama. He obtained the help of Chandra, the moon, who took the form of a cock and crowed at midnight. Gotama thought it was time for his morning devotions and went to the riverside, leaving his wife alone. Indra sneaked into her bedroom and had intercourse with her. Upon discovering the deception, Gotama cursed Indra, and Indra's body was covered with a thousand openings like the female vulva to remind him of her sinful deed. Later, these openings were changed into eyes. Indra's eye-covered body is frequently depicted in drawings.

I am indebted to B. B. Sethi, professor at King George's Medical College, in Lucknow, India, for providing two more examples from Hindu mythology in which religious figures enucleated an eye to please a god. In the first story, Lord Rama wishes to offer one hundred lotus flowers to the goddess Durga. He has only ninety-nine flowers, however, so he removes one of his eyes and offers it in place of the missing flower. Another story involves Soordas, a devotee of Lord Krishna. Once he sees Lord Krishna, and to preserve that wonderful sight in his mind, he enucleates both his eyes. Soordas, in fact, literally means "blind disciple."

The myth of Oedipus, especially as told by Sophocles, is the most famous of all self-mutilation stories. Oedipus unwittingly kills his father and marries and sires children by his mother, Jocasta. When the truth becomes known, Jocasta hangs herself, and Oedipus blinds himself by sticking her golden brooches through his eyes:

"Wicked, wicked eyes!" he gasps,
"You shall not see me nor my shame—
Not see my present crime.
Go dark, for all time blind
To what you should have never seen. . . ."
And the bleeding eyeballs gushed and stained his beard.

In the Old Testament, the king of the Ammonites would spare his enemies only if they agreed to let him bore out their right eyes (1 Sam. 11:2); their blindness served as a badge of slavery and prevented them from fighting effectively. Eye mutilation within the Christian tradition has been granted legitimacy by several New Testament admonitions. Mark 9:47–48 notes: "If your eye is your downfall, tear it out! Better for you to enter the kingdom of God with one eye than to be thrown with both eyes into Gehenna, where the worm dies not and the fire is never extinguished." Matthew 5:28–29 states the same theme: "What I say to you is: anyone who looks lustfully at a woman has already committed adultery with her in his thoughts. If your right eye is your trouble, gouge it out and throw it away! Better to lose part of your body than to have it all cast into Gehenna." Matthew continues, in 6:22–23: "The eye is the body's lamp. If your eyes are good, your body will be filled with light: if your eyes are bad, your body will be in darkness. And if your light is darkness, how deep will the darkness be."

The oldest story of a person who removed an eye in accordance with biblical admonitions is told in book 1, chapter 9, of Marco Polo's *Travels* (circa A.D. 1300). The Calif of Baghdad threatened Christians. Unless they could literally move a certain mountain by virtue of their faith, they could choose either to be put to death or to convert to Islam. A one-eyed Christian cobbler saved their lives by moving the mountain. Years earlier he had scooped out his eye in obedience to Matthew's injunction (5:28–29) because he experienced lustful thoughts when he accidentally viewed the leg of a beautiful woman who had come to his shop. Marco Polo commented: "By this act you can judge the excellence of his Faith."

In Christian tradition the lives of the saints, often embellished by regional folklore, were presented as models of comportment. Saints with special characteristics were selected as patrons for specific diseases. Saint Lucy became the patron saint of eyes. She was born in Sicily in about A.D. 283. She consecrated her chastity to God, much to the displeasure of her mother. Her mother finally accepted Lucy's wishes but unfortunately had already betrothed Lucy to a pagan youth. He was angered and reported Lucy as a Christian to the governor of Sicily. She was found guilty and sentenced to a life of prostitution. When she refused to comply, she was tortured, possibly blinded, and finally killed. Several centuries later, a legend about her eyes became popular: A young man had fallen deeply in love with her and was especially attracted by her beautiful eyes. Mindful of her vow of chastity, she cooled the young man's ardor by cutting out her eyes and sending them to him on a plate, a scene depicted by many artists. Her suitor was converted to Christianity, and Lucy's eyes were restored to her, more beautiful than ever.

The evil eye belief is that a harmful force may be projected from the eye of a person or an animal (Maloney 1976). The origins of the belief in the evil eye, however, are prebiblical and widespread throughout Europe, the Near East, and the Indian subcontinent. Among the disorders attributed to the evil eye are disrupted social relationships, diarrhea, vomiting, anorexia, insomnia, impotence, sudden death, hypochondriasis, depression, headaches, malformed fetuses, colic, cataracts, nystagmus, failure to thrive in children, persistent yawning and hiccups, inflammation of the eye, ophthalmia in newborn children, fevers, and epidemic diseases such as plague, smallpox, and cholera. Additionally, the evil eye supposedly can cause spoilage of crops, accidental injuries, and illness in animals. In fact, the fourth century Council of Elvira in Spain prohibited Jews from staring at Christian crops for fear the crops would wither (a German word for evil eye is *Judenblick*, or Jew's glance).

Particularly susceptible to injury by the evil eye are pregnant women, children, nursing mothers, the wealthy, and anyone who is admired. Persons most likely to possess the evil eye are strangers, hunchbacks and others with physical deformities, eccentrics, and anyone who is envious of others. A literary portrayal of a *jettatore* (a person who possesses the lifelong ability to inflict the evil eye) can be found in *Le Corricole*, a minor novel by Alexander Dumas fils. Protection against the evil eye often takes the form of amulets, such as the red chili horn and red ribbons. In some groups, children have dirt rubbed on their faces to detract from their beauty, thus making them less likely targets of the evil eye. A person afflicted by the evil eye may remove it by participating in rituals, for example, dropping oil in water and reciting, "Who has fascinated you? The eye, the thought, and the evil desire. Who will remove the fascination? The Father, the Son, and the Holy Ghost." A most unneighborly type of treatment is to throw the oil-water mixture onto a path in the hope that the evil eye will be removed from the afflicted person by attaching itself to the next person who walks along the path.

For thousands of years, the concept of the evil eye was thought to be based on scientific fact. The Greeks believed that vision flowed out from the eyes just as light flows out from a candle. Plutarch drew an analogy between the voice that emanates from the mouth and the rays that emanate from the eyes; just as words can influence others for better or worse, so too can the eyes' rays. Montaigne's essay "The Power of Imagination" contains the following statement: "Imagination not only acts on one's own body but on the bodies of others, and thus one body may inflict injuries on his neighbor, as is apparent from the plague, smallpox, and the evil eye, which are sent from one to another." The "scientific" theory that one can emit poison from one's eyes and cause it to enter another's eyes by uttering words of praise was proposed in 1550 by Hieronymus Fracastorius: "For praise creates a peculiar pleasure and pleasure in turn opens the heart, the face and especially the eyes so that the closed doors are opened to receive the poison. . . . Therefore, it is most proper whenever we intend to praise a person, we add, 'May it be of no injury to you!' "

The English story of Lady Godiva and Peeping Tom is paradigmatic of stories in which lust is punished by blindness. Lady Godiva of Coventry begged her husband to lower the high taxes that caused the townspeople to suffer. He agreed but only if his wife rode naked on her horse through the town. To his surprise, she accepted his condition. She then ordered the populace to shutter their windows and not look on her during the ride. Tom the tailor, however, peeped at her and was immediately struck blind.

Clinical Cases of Eye Mutilation

> Quoi qu'il en soit, l'automutilation oculaire, si l'on en croit les
> confidences des aliénistes, est moins rares qu'elle ne le parait.
> [Whatever has been said before, self-mutilation of the eyes, if one
> believes the reports of psychiatrists, is less rare than it appears.]
> —A. Terson, 1911

Deliberate eye mutilation is not a common event, but neither is it rare. The actual number of cases is much greater than the number of published cases. I estimate that about five hundred cases of eye enucleation occur each year in the United States and that the incidence of milder forms of eye mutilation, such as the deliberate placing of noxious substances into an eye, greatly exceeds that of self-enucleation.

In case reports from 1846 to the present, eye mutilation is associated with many psychiatric conditions. What follows is a presentation of published and unpublished cases associated with "organic mental" disorders, and schizophrenic, affective, anxiety, somatoform, factitious, and personality disorders. In these cases I have tried to deduce the most appropriate diagnosis, a task complicated by changing symptomatology and methods of reporting over the years. Also, I have categorized cases with multiple diagnoses under what the author of the original article or I considered to be the principal one.

The term *organic mental disorder* has been replaced in psychiatry by the more specific diagnoses of delirium (rapid onset changes in consciousness and cognition [e.g., reasoning, awareness, perception, and judgment]), dementia (defective cognition with memory loss), and amnestic disorder (impaired memory without significant cognitive impairment). Symptoms that may be present include hallucinations, delusions, mood disturbances, impulsivity, and personality changes. These disorders have many causes such as Alzheimer's disease, brain infections, tertiary syphilis, cerebrovascular strokes, ingestion of various drugs (alcohol, amphetamines, cocaine, LSD, etc.), or general medical conditions such as liver failure, hypothyroidism, brain tumor, traumatic brain injury, and vitamin deficiency.

The following are illustrative cases (also see Bergua et al. 2002; Gerhard 1968; Rosen 1972; Soebo 1948; Tuwir et al. 2005).

A 52-year-old man went to a convent and refused to leave. He demonstrated delusions of grandeur, religious exaltation, irritability, and excited behavior. He stuck his fingers in his eyes and displaced them out of their sockets. He said the voice of God told him that he had sinned and demanded that he tear out his eyes because he had seen the nakedness of his daughter. The rapid onset of dementia ensued (Goffin 1887).

A 16-year-old girl who had an eight-year history of chronic encephalitis was found holding her right eye in her hand and said that it had spontaneously fallen out of her head while she was sleeping. She seemed indifferent to the incident and did not complain of pain. Two hours later, she shouted and said that her left eye, which was found on her bed, had also fallen out. She initially denied gouging out her eyes, but several months later she said she felt "hypnotized" at the time and that an irresistible urge made her do it. She also admitted that some peculiar force had caused her to extract some of her teeth over the years and to bite her tongue (Goodhart and Savitsky 1933).

A 34-year-old chronic alcoholic man felt sick from drinking too heavily and demanded that his mother get some medicine for him. When she left to go to the store, the patient was alone for fifteen minutes with his 8-year-old niece. He sexually assaulted the girl, killed her, and then shot himself in the eye with a pistol. He developed total amnesia for his actions. The author concluded that "his own right eye was shot out as a self-castration punishment for his sexual and homicidal crime" (Lewis 1928, p. 180).

A 21-year-old woman with agitation, auditory hallucinations, and ideas of reference—beliefs that external stimuli, such as newspaper articles or the honking of a car horn, pertained to her—gashed her left cornea with a piece of glass and burned her right cornea with a cigarette. She repeatedly said, "I'm evil because my eyes can hurt you." In the years before hospitalization, she changed her lifestyle from that of an "all-American girl" to one of macrobiotics, illicit drug use, and Eastern philosophies. In the week before her eye mutilation, she used amphetamines and marijuana heavily (Westermeyer and Serposs 1972).

An 18-year-old youth with no previous psychiatric history was found wandering in the street nude with his right eyeball in his hand. He had taken LSD for four consecutive days, during which he was forced into a homosexual episode. He then felt that he was going to die, that the devil controlled his mind, and that he should obey the Bible and pluck out his eye because he had offended God. He said, "My mind was so weak because of the LSD that the devil possessed me. Now I've got the devil out of my mind since I plucked my right eye out" (Rosen 1972, p. 1109).

A 35-year-old man blinded himself during a cocaine-induced psychotic episode to rid himself of terrifying visual hallucinations (Wurfler 1956).

A 16-year-old boy with a two-year history of heavy, mixed drug abuse was in an automobile with his mother on his way to admission at a psychiatric hospital. During the lengthy trip, the boy purchased a number of nasal inhalers and swallowed the medication in them to feel "high." They stopped at a restaurant, but the boy remained in the car, where he masturbated while his mother went to eat. When she returned ten minutes later, he screamed, "I did it, I did it! I have to get my balls out." A few seconds later, he gouged out his eyeball, shouting, "I have to get my eyeball out." At the hospital, he was judged psychotic. Although amnesiac for the event, the boy remembered a voice telling him, "If thy right eye offend thee, pluck it out." The hospital staff thought that the boy had a symbiotic relationship with his mother and assumed that he had sexual fantasies about her while in the close confines of the car. Because these fantasies were unacceptable to him, he displaced them to his eyeball. By removing his eye, he was able to remove his fantasy (Carson and Lewis 1971).

A 20-year-old man became preoccupied with lustful thoughts and with the Bible. He ingested phencyclidine and experienced dysphoria, hallucinations, altered perception and judgment, and loss of motor control for several hours. Early the next morning, he decided that the text of Matthew 5:28–29 applied to him, and he proceeded to rupture the globe and severely damage the ocular tissue and optic nerve of his right eye with his fingers. He assumed a Christlike physical appearance and maintained that since losing his eye he had improved his self-control and no longer had lustful thoughts (Moskovitz and Byrd 1983).

A 56-year-old man with severe diabetic renal damage and retinopathy experienced severe pain in his left eye. As a result of marked uremia, his mental capacity was impaired, and he slashed his left eye with a knife in an attempt to control the pain (Brown 1970).

An 85-year-old woman who had dementia and was hospitalized for gastritis and anemia suddenly gouged out her eyes. In response to questions, she simply replied, "Why are you bothering me?" (Malavitis et al. 1967).

Schizophrenic disorders are characterized by deterioration in functioning and by symptoms such as delusions, illogical thinking, loosening of associations between one thought and another, hallucinations, blunted or inappropriate affect, disturbed sense of self, impairment in goal-directed activity, decreased involvement with the external world, and unusual behaviors including stupor, rigid posture, purposeless excited movements, and grimacing. No single symptom is invariably present or seen only in schizophrenia. The following is a sample of cases of eye mutilation in schizophrenic patients, many of whom were inspired by the Bible and preoccupied with the supernatural and with sexuality. (For additional cases, see Arons 1981; Brown 1970; Fan and Fink 2007; Gorin 1964; Koh and Yeo 2002; Lewis 1928; Marx and Brocheriou 1961; Mucci and Dalgalarrondo 2000; Shore et al. 1978; Stannard et al. 1984; Yang et al. 1981).

A 24-year-old man was in jail for parole violation. After reading Matthew's biblical injunction to gouge out an eyeball and seeing a vision of Christ and a "gold ball" in front of his left eye, he pulled the eye out to "purify himself." He stated that he belonged to the "youthful cosmically enlightened movement." He decided to take out his eye because hate rays were emanating from it. He developed a Christlike affect and claimed that he was cleansed, at peace, and happy. He dated the onset of his problem to a period two and a half years earlier when he had freely used LSD and marijuana (Brown 1970).

A 19-year-old girl became psychotic when rejected by a man with whom she fell in love at a transcendental meditation camp. She thought that he was following her and that her parents were plotting against her. She wore glasses with reflecting lenses to hide her eyes. She slashed her throat and beat her face to destroy her eyes. During hospitalization, she jabbed at her eyes with a pen. She stated, "The radio said people would be better off if I were blinded." She intermittently attacked her eyes, saying such things as, "Everything I do is bad" and "Don't torture anybody but me." She said voices were controlling her. During the next seven months, her condition improved, and she made no further attempts to harm herself (unpublished case of Dr. Paul Horton 1971).

A 36-year-old man with chronic schizophrenia appeared before a nurse on the hospital ward holding his neatly dissected left eye in his hand. He stated that he had enucleated the eye because he wanted to "change" and to "save" the world, and because he could not find instruments for cutting off his genitals. At age 23, he had begun to deteriorate psychologically and felt that people could read his thoughts, especially about homosexuality. He feared he was turning into a woman. He joined a religious sect and said that he heard the voice of the Lord and that he would be able to talk with his dead father if he devoted his life to God. In discussing this case the authors equated the patient's eye enucleation with symbolic castration (MacLean and Robertson 1976).

An 18-year-old first-year college student who had no previous psychiatric history became increasingly withdrawn and preoccupied with religious ideas. He proclaimed himself an evangelist and ineptly acted out his homosexual fantasies within the dormitory, causing anxiety among the other students. When they rejected him, he felt guilty and became obsessed with a desire to expiate his sins.

In an isolated place, he sawed off his hand and then removed his eye with a screwdriver. He was taken to a hospital where he described his emotional state as free of pain, at peace with himself, and Christlike. He said that his actions were a mission for God. He was successfully treated and two months later was discharged from the hospital (Goldenberg and Sata 1978).

A 24-year-old arsonist and rapist was imprisoned, where he was sodomized by an inmate. He cut his wrists and blinded one eye to get transferred to a psychiatric hospital. He slashed his remaining eye with a razor blade in the belief that blindness would eliminate his anxiety about looking at people and would allow him to be a successful musical entertainer. On the ward he claimed that he was Jesus, and he was preoccupied with the size of his penis (Crowder et al. 1979).

A 25-year-old man blinded himself by attempting to scratch out his eyes while sitting quietly in a park. He calmly stated that "God told me to, to prevent people suffering." He claimed that God had talked with him, and he believed that he possessed some of the features of Jesus. During hospitalization he was restless, heard voices, tried to grasp "white birds flying around my head," and claimed that his eyes were healed. He improved with treatment but was unwilling to talk about his self-injury. Three months earlier, he had received treatment because he was eating his feces and acting belligerently (Tapper et al. 1979).

A 39-year-old single man took out his right eye with his fingernail in obedience to Matthew's biblical injunction to self-injure. He claimed that voices of devils, angels, and persons he had formerly known commented on his behavior in an accusatory tone and commanded him to injure his remaining eye. He believed that he had stolen the soul of a nurse seven years previously and that she exerted great control over him. He also believed that he possessed both male and female sexual organs and that he produced numerous babies daily (Ananth et al. 1984).

Major depression is an *affective disorder* characterized by symptoms such as depressed mood, appetite and sleep disturbances, feelings of worthlessness and excessive, inappropriate guilt, agitation or psychomotor retardation, and recurrent thoughts about death and suicide. Delusions and hallucinations may be present that often focus on themes of guilt, punishment, disease, and death. The following is a sample of cases of major depression involving eye mutilation. (For additional cases, see Adam 1883; Arons 1981; Bowen 1971; Brown 1970; Byrnes 1949; Dollfus and Michaux 1957; Gifford 1955; MacKinlay 1887; Pompili et al. 2006; Wackenheim et al. 1956; Wilson 1955).

A 48-year-old melancholy widow accused herself of being a great sinner. She was hospitalized after she went naked into the street and asked various men, including her minister, to marry her. She felt that her eyes were sinful because they had looked at worldly things. After reading Matthew's biblical injunction to gouge out an eye, she took out both of her eyes and asked the doctor to cut off her legs and feet. She felt that because Christ shed his blood, she must shed her blood to become saintly (Bergmann 1846).

Following discovery of her husband's conjugal deceptions, a 41-year-old woman became profoundly depressed and developed a desire to offer her sufferings to God. While delirious she ablated both of her eyes. One eye was found under her bed, the other eye on it. She was incoherent for two days, then she became calm and affable and regretted her actions (Terson 1911). In discussing the case, Terson referred to Blondel's thesis on self-mutilation (1906) in which seven cases of eye enucleation were listed. In five of the cases, the mutilation was performed by middle-aged women with a psychiatric diagnosis of Cotard syndrome, which is characterized by delusions of losing everything including one's possessions and body organs and thoughts of negation, nonexistence, and annihilation. Terson noted that his patient did not have Cotard syndrome; rather, he stressed the importance of paroxysmal delirium and of eye mutilators' need for expiation and martyrdom. He further noted that Blondel's use of the term *oedipism* to describe self-enucleators was not precise because Oedipus was not mentally ill when he took out his eyes.

A 50-year-old man became depressed with paranoid ideas following the death of his mother. He claimed that he saw the devil and that he had to atone for the sin of committing incest. He then took out an eye with his fingers (Harrer and Urban 1950; this article contains an interesting bibliography, especially of German works on self-mutilation).

A 44-year-old Egyptian immigrant from a strict Christian culture tried to scratch out his eyes because of guilt over going to topless nightclubs. Three years later, he said that a statue of Saint Mary commanded him to cleanse himself of sin by taking out his eyes. He was hospitalized after attempting to remove his eyes with a forceps. During psychological testing the next day, he shoved the test pencil into his left eye. He repeatedly attempted to take out his eyes for a week. He gradually improved with treatment, however, and was discharged six weeks later (Crowder et al. 1979).

A 28-year-old man was jailed for parole violations. He had become increasingly depressed and guilty over his antisocial behavior and over his mother's death (he felt responsible for her lung cancer). His girlfriend had threatened to leave him and had recently visited her ex-husband. He did not interact much with his cell mates, and his depression deepened. He felt that he was the world's worst sinner and was Satan incarnate. He thought about having killed birds as a young-ster, using his right eye to focus the gun, and about having sexually abused his sisters. He read the Bible constantly. After reading Matthew's words about goug-ing out an eyeball, he believed that God was telling him to remove his eyes to atone for his sins. While contemplating this, he noticed a bird outside the win-dow; for him this was confirmation of God's will that he remove his eye. He in-serted his fingers into his socket, pushed out his eye, threw it on the floor, and fainted (unpublished case of Drs. A. Favazza and M. Jayaratna 1982).

Bipolar disorder is another affective disorder characterized by symptoms such as elated mood, increased activity, distractibility, and inflated self-esteem. Delu-sions and hallucinations may be present that often focus on themes of power, privileged knowledge, and a special relationship with a deity or famous person. These manic symptoms may alternate with symptoms of major depression. The following cases demonstrate eye mutilation during mania. (For a well-documented additional case, see Green et al. 2000, which also involves mutilation of the hand, arm, leg, and genitals).

A 26-year-old woman bit a large piece out of her tongue and was hospitalized for acute mania. A year earlier, her 22-year-old manic brother had gouged out his eye. She claimed on various occasions that God ordered her to purify herself by tearing out her tongue, by fasting, and by burning herself. During a manic epi-sode, she deliberately wounded her arms, badly lacerated her vagina with her hand, and attempted to gouge out both her eyes, with resulting blindness in one eye (Howden 1882).

An 18-year-old girl rolled naked on the floor, screamed, sang nonsensical songs, and quoted the Bible. She was happy as she smeared herself with spit and urine. She imagined that she was in a castle and that a painter wanted to seduce her. In a calm moment she pulled her right eye out of its socket and twisted it, saying, "I have to die" (Axenfeld 1899).

During a manic episode, a 33-year-old woman tore up a picture of Christ, kissed it fervently, and proceeded to gouge out her left eye. She then cried, beat herself, spoke to imaginary persons, and insisted that she had to take out her remaining eye. She said that because she had always been bad, especially to her parents, and no longer believed in God, she needed to make a sacrifice. Her choice of an eye was made after reading the Bible. At age 56, she recounted her earlier enucleation. She admitted to sinning with her eyes and recounted that she used to sleep in the same bedroom as her parents, frequently saw her father's genitals, and often heard her parents' bed creak. On her wedding, day she dedicated can-dles to Saint Joseph and thought that a statue of Joseph had nodded to her just before she took out her eye. She admitted that "looking" at a man always excited her sexually. The author of this case believed the major psychological determinant to be the patient's premature hypersexuality and her tendency "to look" (which derived from her witnessing her parents in bed). She substituted Joseph for her father, and during her psychosis supposedly experienced the same affective states she had originally associated with her father (Hartmann 1926).

Obsessive compulsive disorder is characterized by persistent and unwelcome thoughts, images, or impulses and by repetitive ritualistic or stereotyped acts. The following two cases demonstrate eye mutilation associated with this disorder.

A 50-year-old Italian woman totally blinded herself and grotesquely disfigured her face by compulsively punching herself. Since the age of 16 she had been obsessed with irresistible impulses to touch, press, and hit parts of her head and neck. She battered herself so much that she felt no pain. She noticed certain "rhythms" of her eyes, teeth, and nose. Her destructive actions were linked to these "rhythms." She was never psychotic. Her compulsive self-destructive behavior was finally controlled following a surgical transorbital leukotomy. As a result of this operation, however, her thoughts and behavior became rigid and, in some ways, infantile; for example, she often held a doll in her arms and pretended that it was a baby (Balduzzi 1961).

A 30-year-old Jewish man was hospitalized because he had impaired the vision in both of his eyes by banging them repeatedly with his fists. He first exhibited ritualistic behavior at the age of 10. His parents had a stormy marriage, and he slept with his mother until he was an adolescent. At the age of 13, he masturbated after he saw his mother naked and then began to press his eyeballs to relieve his feelings of guilt. He developed a compulsive eye-touching ritual. At the age of 21, he was operated on for a congenital cataract in his left eye. Postoperatively he began to hit his face and eyes compulsively. He was helped somewhat by psychotherapy, and he married a psychiatric nurse. Following the death of his grandmother and the pregnancy of his wife, he again started hitting his eyes. He sustained a detached retina and eventual blindness in his left eye. He was hospitalized several times and gained some control over his actions, especially after developing a relationship with a rabbi. He was operated on for a traumatic cataract in his right eye. He recognized the absurdity of his behavior but felt powerless to change (Stinnett and Hollender 1970).

Hypochondriasis is a disorder characterized by an unrealistic fear or belief of having a disease despite medical reassurance. Desoff (1943) reported the case of a hypochondriacal patient who was convinced that his eye was cancerous. On several occasions, he popped the eye out of its orbit with his thumb but each time was able to have it pushed back in place. The eye became so damaged because of this trauma, however, that it had to be removed surgically.

The concept of *personality disorders* basically refers to engrained, inflexible, and maladaptive characterological flaws that impair social or economic functioning and cause subjective distress. Borderline personality disorder is the only mental illness in which, according to the official psychiatric nomenclature, the occurrence of physically self-damaging acts is a major diagnostic criterion. Additionally, this disorder is characterized by impulsivity, unstable relationships, inappropriately intense anger, brief mood swings, loneliness, chronic boredom, and uncertainty about one's self-image, values, loyalties, and gender identity. The following case demonstrates eye mutilation in this disorder.

An 18-year-old youth who had committed inexplicable acts of theft was hospitalized for occasional fainting fits and frequent subjective "attacks" characterized by a sensation of fear that originated in his abdomen and by the thought that his left eye was evil. Although the right side of his body was "good," he felt that someone evil was looking through his left eye and influencing his behavior. He begged the doctors to remove his eyes and began to savagely cut his wrists, forearms, and abdomen. Nineteen months later, he cut the conjunctiva and skin around his left eye. He made further cuts with a razor blade to his eyelid, cornea, and sclera. He said that he cut his eyes to gain relief from "attacks" and to demonstrate his suffering to the staff, who noted that his episodes of self-mutilation were often related in time to active planning for discharge from the hospital and to attempts to discuss his relationship difficulties (Griffin et al. 1982).

Antisocial personality disorder is characterized by continuous behavior in which the rights of others are violated. Persons who have this disorder typically demonstrate criminal behavior, disregard for the truth, irritability, aggressiveness, recklessness, and impulsivity. Especially when placed in a restrictive prison setting, persons who have this disorder are at high risk for self-mutilation. Segal et al. (1963), for example, reported on twenty-two young male prisoners in a Polish jail with "distinct pathologic personalities" who deliberately damaged their eyes repeatedly, leading to a total of 166 injuries to forty-three eyes. The most frequent method of injury was the placing of a toxic compound (ground-up pencil lead) into the eye, which often produced severe tissue damage and led to blindness, leukomas, and glaucoma. Other methods of injury included placing chlorinated lime, ground glass, or wood slivers into the conjunctival sac. Occasionally, a lighted cigarette was stuck into an open eye. As a rule, the prisoners injured their eyes on Saturday afternoons or on holiday evenings to delay detection and medical assistance. Some men inflicted their injuries within a few weeks of their scheduled discharge from prison. Many of the prisoners were terrified by the effects of their injuries, and they complied with medical treatment. Once they came under the influence of their fellow inmates again, however, they often repeated their injuries; nineteen prisoners mutilated themselves more than once, the maximum being seventeen times.

Factitious disorder is a fascinating mental illness. Persons who have this disorder deliberately display mental symptoms; when physical symptoms are present the disorder is called Munchausen's syndrome. Their motivation is linked to their need to assume a patient role, to have contacts with physicians, and to undergo medical procedures such as diagnostic tests and operations. A typical case is that of a 32-year-old nursing aide who reported that a fragment of glass had struck her right eye when she dropped a water glass into a sink. On ten different occasions over the next three months she had glass fragments removed from her eye, claiming that they all came from the initial accident. A nurse then saw her break a glass eyedropper and put tiny slivers of glass into her eye. The woman was popular with her co-workers, had a good work history, and appeared to be a reasonable person, working to help her husband get through medical school. She had a 12-year-old daughter and "all in all seemed to be a happy, adjusted person" (Wilson 1955). Rosenberg et al. (1986) reported cases of patients who burned their corneas with chemicals to gain medical attention. Also see Rogers and Pullen (1987).

A malingerer, similar to a person who has a factitious disorder, will deliberately produce and present symptoms. The major difference, however, is that the malingerer's goals for feigning illness are obviously recognizable, for example, to avoid an unpleasant assignment.

The literature on self-inflicted eye injuries by malingerers primarily deals with epidemics among soldiers. Cooper (1859, pp. 291–92) noted:

> It was scarcely possible to imagine a more humiliating picture of depravity than was presented by a ward filled with soldiers, labouring under ophthalmia, deliberately produced by their own hands. A regular correspondence had been detected, between these ophthalmics and their friends, requesting that corrosive sublimate, lime, and blue stone, might be forwarded to them through which and good luck, they hoped to get their eyes in such a state as would enable them to procure their discharge with a pension. . . . Ophthalmia, when counterfeit, is generally confined to privates of indifferent character, and does not extend to officers, women, or children, which is not the case with true ophthalmia.

Cooper also related a situation in 1809 when three hundred soldiers became affected with ophthalmia and were placed in a hospital. The commanding officer became suspicious, searched the ward and found small parcels of corrosive sub-limate concealed in the beds. "Means were taken to prevent a supply of this article, and in a very short time 250 of the men had recovered, and were then marched to their respective corps" (p. 293). Also see Somerset (1945).

In 1947, Somerville-Large reported on 375 cases of self-inflicted eye injuries among both British and Indian troops serving in India. The most commonly used irritants were jequirity and castor oil seeds; other substances included urine, to-bacco, sand, and leaves. "The ocular self-inflicted injury was considered to be a trivial thing among the Sepoys, and it was employed to escape for a few days from some unpleasant situation, perhaps following a rebuke or the refusal of permis-sion to do some desired thing" (p. 188). He also noted that French workers in Germany who wanted to escape penal servitude simulated the symptoms of tra-choma (an infectious disease causing blindness) by rubbing a certain compound in their eyes. "The Germans were so afraid of trachoma that many French work-ers were able to go back home owing to that trick" (p. 197).

As seen in these examples as well as in the previously mentioned report on Polish prisoners, epidemics of self-inflicted eye damage seem to be limited to persons in total-care institutions. Another example of such an epidemic is found in Anaclerio and Wicker's report in 1970 on twenty-seven chronic schizophrenic inpatients in a federal mental hospital who injured their eyes by frequently gaz-ing at the sun. Most stated that they sun gazed only when they were "sick" and that they did so to see or communicate with God or to make their eyes stronger. An ophthalmologist who has been examining eyes for twenty-five years at a large state mental hospital in Missouri told me that he has encountered only four cases of sun-gazing retinopathy; all were psychotic men who wanted to gain power from the sun. I am familiar with the case of a 42-year-old schizophrenic man with severe mutilative tendencies (self-amputation of his fingers and foot) who sus-tained bilateral macular burns as a result of staring at the sun. He thought him-self to be God and wanted to blind himself as an act of atonement to save the world. Deliberate sun gazing with an intent to cause blindness has also been re-ported in a "neurotic" 17-year-old girl (Eigner 1966).

Sun gazing left the German physicist Gustar Lechner (1801–1887) partially blind when he self-experimented on afterimage formation. Solar yoga has been popularized by Hira Ratan Manek, who claims that he has lived on only sun en-ergy and water for fifteen years. Spas and "wellness centers" often encourage sun gazing during the half-hour time when the sun rises or sets, although participants are encouraged to slowly work up to direct sun gazing for prolonged periods of time. Their belief is that, just as plants use photosynthesis to convert sunlight into food energy, human beings can transcend the need for food energy by absorbing sunlight through their eyes. The danger of doing this is damage to the retina and eventual blindness. In 2008, fifty Catholics in India were left with irreversible blurred vision after attempting to see the Virgin Mary by directly staring at the blazing sun. In 2009, the *Jerusalem Post* warned its Jewish readers not to stare at the sun during the once-in-twenty-eight-years Birkest Hahama or Solar Blessing ceremony. The blessing occurs at sunrise when the sun, earth, planets, and stars are supposedly positioned in exactly the same place as during both the creation of the world and the exodus from Egypt.

Self-inflicted eye damage does not constitute a specific syndrome but rather occurs among persons with a variety of diagnoses and a variety of motives. With the exception of one patient (a demented 85-year-old woman who enucleated an eye), the eye mutilators presented here range in age from 15 to 56 years. The average age of the male mutilators is 26 years, while the average age of the female mutilators is 28 years. Although most eye mutilators do not damage other parts of their body, case reports contain instances of additional mutilations to organs such as the tongue, head, ear, fingers, hand, abdomen, umbilicus, vagina, and penis. Also see Kennedy and Feldman (1994).

Eye mutilation may be associated with many different diagnostic categories, but in its most severe form it is most commonly encountered in psychotic depression, mania, schizophrenia, and drug intoxications. The reasons given by mutilators for their actions sometimes are idiosyncratic, for example, an attempt to dig out the brain through the eye or to decrease social anxiety and become a better musician. More often the stated reasons deal with the religious themes of atonement for sins, the casting out of evil spirits, the salvation of the world (frequently associated with an easily recognized identification with Christ), and obedience to God's will. The real or imaginary sins that must be atoned for become greatly magnified, especially in the minds of people who are depressed. Examples of such "sins" listed in the case reports include murder, incestuous desires, hostility toward parents, sexual abuse by others, physical abuse of others, and economic failure. Self-blinding is a suitable method of atonement because the eye is such a valuable organ.

Self-enucleation to rid the body of an evil spirit represents an extension of the ancient, widespread folk belief in the evil eye. The "spirit-infested" eye of a psychotic person becomes a terrifying, aggressive organ that can change the course of events, maim and kill others, and force one to look at tempting or forbidden persons and things. By isolating the evil spirit in an eye, the psychotic person gains some control over terror and aggression; should all other attempts fail to control the spirit, the desperate act of enucleation can remove it from the patient's body. In normal religious life, the struggle with devils may be won through prayer and healing rituals, but the demon of psychosis demands a more radical tactic.

Most people who have psychosis report a certain tranquility following self-enucleation, either because they have received the severe punishment they believe they deserve or because they have successfully rid their bodies of an evil spirit. In nine of the case reports, these patients assumed an identity with Christ-the-Sufferer and often stated that their enucleation served to save the world, thus identifying with Christ-the-Savior.

By far the most common motive expressed by self-enucleators is a literal interpretation of Matthew's biblical injunction that one can escape perdition by casting out an offending eye. The notion that one is achieving this sort of spiritual salvation may, in rare cases, spare a person from suicide. That many psychotic persons rationalize the mutilation of their eyes on the basis of a biblical admonition reflects the finding that deviant eye enucleation appears to occur particularly in Christian cultural areas.

The Link between the Eyes and the Genitals

Menninger (1935; 1938) articulated the classic psychoanalytic position that self-castration is the prototype of all self-mutilation and that any substituted organ is an unconscious representation of the genital. Freud noted in his essay *The Uncanny* that "a study of dreams, fantasies, and myths has taught us that anxiety about one's eyes, the fear of going blind, is often enough a substitute for the dread of being castrated." The notion that the eye represents the phallus originates in the belief that a vital fluid emanates from the eye just as sperm is emitted from the phallus; the glance of an eye then represents the male sexual function. Some amulets that counterbalance the force of the evil eye, such as the red chili horn, are thought to symbolize the erect penis.

In some cases, the damaged eye substitutes for the genitals; in other cases, the linkage between the two organs appears nonexistent. Greenacre (1926) found a "constant linkage of the eye-complex with disorders and conflicts of the sex life" (p. 557), but one might argue that the coexistence of sexual conflicts and eye disorders need not always imply a linkage. One of her astute observations was that "the eye may be held guilty for its own function, and the desire or fear of self-blinding appears as a wish on the part of the individual to punish himself for sexual looking, rather than as a direct self-castration wish. . . . The eye which is psychotically dimmed or blinded is generally the eye which has offended in its own right, rather than merely as a genital symbol" (p. 558). Also see Crowder et al. (1979).

Interpreters of the Oedipus myth have focused exclusively on the linkage between Oedipus's self-blinding and his discovery that he had bedded his mother; that is, the eye mutilation symbolizes self-castration. However, Oedipus's greater crime was that he caused the death of both parents. At the play's beginning, Oedipus curses the king's (his father's) murderer: "May he wear out his life in misery to miserable doom" (lines 245–49). Later on, Oedipus learns that Queen Jocasta had given up her child for fear of the evil oracle that "he should kill his parents" (line 1183). Oedipus rushes to find Jocasta, but by then she has committed suicide by hanging. He cuts the noose and proceeds to stick his eyes with the brooches from her robe, "shrieking out such things as: they will never see the crime I have committed or had done upon me!" (lines 1268–72). The Greeks regarded blindness as a terrible event. The blind seer who could perceive the future was a rare, paradoxical figure. Thus, Oedipus's self-blinding need not necessarily be interpreted symbolically. By causing the death of his parents, he became a victim of his own curse, and by his self-blinding he resigned himself to a life of miserable doom.

Although Freud was the first person to develop the eye-genital link and the concept of the Oedipus complex, the great French author Marcel Proust independently discovered the oedipal complex. In "The Filial Feelings of a Matricide," Proust tells the story of an acquaintance, Henri van Blarenbergh, whose father had recently died. Proust learned that his friend Henri had murdered his mother by sticking a dagger into her heart. "Soon afterwards," writes Proust, "four policemen, responding to an alarm, forced the bolted door and entered the murderer's room. He had inflicted wounds upon himself with the dagger, and the left side of his face was lacerated by a pistol shot. His left eyeball hung from its socket and rested on the pillow. . . . In this eyeball on the pillow I recognize the most frightful torment that the history of human suffering has relegated to us. It is the eye of the unfortunate Oedipus that I see" (see Zilboorg 1939, p. 293). Proust considered Henri to be a pious and tender son, an enlightened spirit driven by fate to crime and expiation. For Proust, the matricidal act demonstrated a certain purity and a religious atmosphere of spiritual beauty such as can be found in the Greek tragedies. Henri's mutilated eye was not linked with any sexual symbolism.

The Ears

Piercing of the earlobe to display jewelry is the most common form of body modification in the world. In one variation that is widely practiced in India and Southeast Asia, the earlobe is stretched in ribbonlike segments until it reaches shoulder length.

The ancient Egyptians pierced and stretched their earlobes, as can be seen in drawings of Queen Nefertiti and King Akhenaton. The biblical book of Exodus, chapter 21, refers to piercing the ears of faithful slaves. Even the Romans perforated and stretched their earlobes to accommodate jewelry. Celsus, the most famous Roman physician, devised surgical procedures for both men and women who wanted to repair the holes.

Sushutra, the Hippocrates of India, codified surgical procedures around 400 B.C. He described the procedure for piercing children's earlobes, which was done routinely for protection of children against evil spirits as well as for beautification. Majno (1975) concluded that plastic surgery was highly developed in ancient India for three major reasons: (1) unlike Greeks, Hindu warriors fought without helmets and were apt to have their noses and ears cut off; (2) the harsh laws of Manu prescribed amputation of body parts for offenders (a citizen who broke wind in the presence of the king was liable to be punished by having his anus mutilated); and (3) the use of heavy ornaments often resulted in torn earlobes. An elaborate system of classifying earlobes deformed by earrings was devised by Sushutra and gave rise to pedicle-flap reconstructive surgery.

The medical literature on ear mutilation is small. The most famous case is that of the artist Vincent van Gogh, who cut off his earlobe and presented it to a prostitute. The case is instructive because the forces that compelled his NSSI can be inferred from his paintings and his letters (Lubin 1961; Nagera 1967).

Vincent van Gogh was born on 30 March 30 1853, and died in infancy. Exactly one year later, another child was born to the van Gogh family. He too was named Vincent, and he would one day be known as one of the greatest artists of all time. It seems likely that the circumstances of his birth compromised his sense of identity. His mother idolized her dead child, and van Gogh became a substitute for his dead brother. Van Gogh became fascinated with the idea of resurrection, and he identified with Jesus. He often painted a halo around his own head in self-portraits, and in his painting *Pietà* he substituted his own image for that of Christ. His father was a minister, and, before devoting himself to art, van Gogh had spent several years as a fervent evangelist preacher.

The event that precipitated van Gogh's ear cutting was the threat of his housemate, the painter Paul Gauguin, to leave him. Van Gogh had invited Gauguin to share a house with him, but the two men had often argued bitterly. On 24 December, Gauguin left the house. Van Gogh, armed with a razor, followed him. Gauguin turned and looked at him, whereupon van Gogh went back inside, cut off his earlobe, wrapped it up, and gave it as a present to a prostitute he had frequented. The prostitute's name was Rachel, whose biblical namesake "mourns her children." Just as the biblical Rachel mourned her dead children, so too did van Gogh's mother mourn her dead infant. By presenting his earlobe to Rachel, van Gogh may have wanted her to grieve for and to love him. If one accepts the notion that a mutilated organ may be a genital substitute, then van Gogh's act was tantamount to a castration that left him helpless, wounded, nonthreatening, and in need of maternal comfort.

Another force that influenced van Gogh's self-mutilation was the news of his brother Theo's engagement to Johanna Bonger. Theo was much more than a brother to van Gogh; he was also the provider of money, of friendship, and of love. They spent every Christmas together, but when van Gogh cut off his earlobe on Christmas Eve of 1888, Theo was with his fiancée. The mutilation was not only an expression of his anger at Theo for abandoning him but also a successful, albeit desperate, method of effecting a family reunion. Theo came to see him as soon as he learned of the act.

Several months before cutting off his earlobe, van Gogh painted and then destroyed two paintings of Christ at Gethsemane in the Garden of Olives. He surely knew the biblical scene at Gethsemane in which Judas betrayed Christ: "At that moment they stepped forward to lay hands on Jesus, and arrested him. Suddenly one of those who accompanied Jesus put his hand to his sword, drew it, and slashed at the high priest's servant, cutting off his ear" (Matt. 26:51).

Clinical cases of ear mutilation are rare (Weinstock 1988). In one case, a 34-year-old man manually ripped off his right ear, saying that voices commanded him to do so to atone for his childhood sins. Before this event, he repeatedly removed small sections of skin from his arms, face, and ear, and had been hospitalized for many serious infections, including one so severe that maggots were removed from his right ear canal. He reported relief from tension and depression after removing the skin. He believed that his mother and relatives wanted him to suffer and that he deserved to be a famous world political leader because he had suffered through self-mutilation. He started cutting himself at age 12; shortly afterward he reported auditory hallucinations and persecuting and self-depreciating thoughts. His diagnosis was paranoid schizophrenia (Silva et al. 1989). Alroe and Gunda (1995) reported on three men who cut off large portions of their ears. One was diagnosed with schizophrenia and two with a personality disorder. They knew each other and the behavior seemed to be contagious.

The Nose

Self-mutilation of the nose is not common. A 31-year-old delusional Iranian woman believed that she was already dead and was only a soul that wandered in the desert and in lavatories. She felt that pools of cyanide and heroin had formed under her eyes, and that she had an ugly nodule on the tip of her nose. She happily and painlessly cut off the tip of her nose with a knife to become beautiful. She was hospitalized before she could remove her facial wrinkles with an iron (Ghaffari-Nejad et al. 2007). Plastic surgeons perform numerous rhinoplasties, thus affording a culturally approved procedure for individuals desirous of changing the shape of their noses. That so many persons are willing to undergo such operations, often at great expense, is understandable in light of the contribution of the nose to our perception of beauty. Indeed, the French essayist Pascal once observed that the history of the world might have changed totally if Cleopatra's nose had been a little longer! While surgical procedures performed in Western cultures serve to reduce the size of the nose, the Polynesians used to break and flatten their noses to achieve an enlarged effect. Some Australian aborigines still pierce the nasal septum and insert a piece of bone to flatten and widen the nose.

Nasal tissue has some properties of vaginal tissue in that it may become congested and even bleed as a form of "vicarious menstruation." Ritual nasal mutilation among males in Papua New Guinea is thought by the natives to serve the same purposes as female menstruation. In fact, Hogbin's book (1970) on this topic is titled *The Island of Menstruating Men* (also see Lidz and Lidz 1977; Newman 1965; and Read 1965).

The Gahuka-Gana and the Gururumba tribes of Papua New Guinea practice nasal mutilation on male adolescents in initiation rituals that mark the crossing over of young boys from the care of their mothers into the adult male division of society. Amid the shouts, chants, and flute music of warriors, the boys are confronted by a group of masturbating men who stick sharp leaves up their own noses until they hemorrhage profusely. The initiates also induce nasal hemorrhage. Each person then inserts a cane of reeds down his esophagus into his stomach to induce vomiting. The initiates spend six weeks secluded in the men's hut, where they learn the "secret" of the tribe's magic flutes. They then spend a full year in the men's hut, have little contact with women, and practice nose bleeding, vomiting, and flute playing. Several years later, they achieve full male status after a period of severe dietary restriction, intense flute playing, and instruction in the duties and rights of manhood.

The tribal men refer to the nasal bleeding as male menstruation. They are extremely frightened of a woman's menstrual blood, which they regard as a malignant force. They believe that each fetus is composed of womb blood and semen and that nasal bleeding rids the child of this womb blood and of menstrual contamination. Likewise, the induced vomiting is thought to get rid of any swallowed womb blood as well as any menstrual blood that may have been inadvertently eaten. Just as a young girl's hymen is broken ritually at the first menstruation, so too the cane used to induce vomiting is thought to break a membrane in a boy's body, permitting him to develop the sexual characteristics of a man. The men envy women's monthly, natural self-purification; therefore, they periodically induce nasal bleeding to maintain their health, strength, and attractiveness.

The nose-bleeding rites of the Sambia, a hunting and horticultural people of the New Guinea Highlands, have been detailed by Herdt (1982). The Sambia place great emphasis on the nose in regard to aesthetics and gender symbolism (the words for the penis contain the generic term for nose). They believe that menstrual-womb blood may be purged through initiatory nose bleeding. It is thought that a woman's air stream, emitted when speaking, defiles a boy's nasal orifice and interferes with the flow of blood and other bodily fluids. Even during coitus, men wear nose plugs to avoid absorbing foul vaginal odors. The most common method of inducing bleeding is to thrust stiff, sharp cane grass into the nostrils; alternatively, a strong salt solution may be injected into the nose. Both methods are painful and efficacious. Nose bleeding occurs during differing stages of developmental rites, for boys and men continue to practice it privately in later life when their wives go off to the menstrual hut.

The nose-bleeding practices serve important social functions. The boy separates from his mother, displaces female essences, and absorbs "maleness" by engaging in fellatio and filling up his body with semen. The aggression associated with the nose bleeding instills fear and avoidance of women, obedience to male authority, and bravado in battle. Nose bleeding results in constraints on male-female relationships, and the practice provides contexts for self-identity at different stages of the life cycle. As a result of pacification and a decreased need for men to be seen as fierce warriors, ritual nose bleeding is gradually being eliminated as a ritual practice.

The Ndumba, another Highlands group in New Guinea, have separate transition rites for young men and women (Hays and Hays 1982). In the *'ummansa* ceremony, young boys receive special knowledge and enter into male company for life. In the *kwassi* ceremony, young women who have reached menarche learn to control their natural power. Both ceremonies are stepping-stones in preparation for marriage and for male-female relations.

In the *'ummansa* ceremony the novice boys are restrained while sponsors shove stiff, sharp-edged leaves, stinging nettles, and salt into the boys' nostrils until they hemorrhage and the boys cry out for their mothers. The boys' bodies are rubbed raw with thorns. Later that day, they are made to lick rough leaves until their tongues bleed. After a nap, they are instructed in proper masculine behavior, especially sexual behavior. Groups of men visit the boys to provide further instruction and to rub their bodies with thorns, concentrating particularly on the boys' penises. The bloodletting in the ceremony makes boys "strong" and rids them of their "mother's blood." The nose bleeding is an act of purification and a prerequisite for entering into the men's house, learning the men's secrets, and participating in men's affairs.

Girls also must endure nose bleeding during the *kwassi* ceremony following a girl's first menstruation. There is much dancing and singing, a repeated refrain being, "Men are the enemy." At the end of the ceremony, the girl is led to a stream where her mother's brother shoves sharp leaves into her nostrils to induce hemorrhage. Why is this done? One interpretation is that it is a way for men to assert social dominance. Even the nose bleeding of boys may be "a symbolic statement of control over society instead of merely a physical purification" (Hays and Hays 1982, p. 235); that is, ridding the boy of his mother's blood may represent freedom from women's power.

Young boys of the Awa tribe in New Guinea develop into men by engaging for ten to fifteen years in a series of rituals. The purging ritual includes being beaten with a cudgel, inducing nasal hemorrhage and vomiting, cutting the penis, and being stuck with nettles. The Awa regard physical growth as a process in which a basically amorphous, watery body is transformed into a well-formed, firm body by the removal of liquid. "Bleeding, then, directly stimulates the drying, strengthening processes of tissue growth" (Newman and Boyd 1982, p. 257). Vomiting is another way of removing liquid.

The ritual of severe penis cutting is associated with betrothal. The young men first go through intense nose bleeding in which the sharp leaves are pounded into the nostrils with a hammer to cause copious bleeding. The penis is then gashed open with a knife. Wedges of flesh are removed, and sometimes the urethra is penetrated. The wounded organ is repeatedly struck with a knife and vigorously rubbed with salt or nettles. The profuse bleeding and intense pain endured during this ritual are thought to enhance the life force in the initiates' bodies, to strengthen them against the dangerous and powerful female substances that are contacted during intercourse, and to induce the production of semen. The married men attending the ritual are invigorated by having their own penises punctured by a stone-tipped arrow shot from a tiny bow. This procedure (penis shooting) is undertaken several times yearly by adult men to prevent and to treat illness and "to combat simple lethargy." The men then gather to instruct the initiates in the details of proper sexual conduct.

Young Awa women must also go through a special ritual at the time of their betrothal. Their noses are bled by their mothers' brothers to stimulate their life force, and they are instructed about their sexual obligations and responsibilities. After the betrothed young man has completed his ritual, he joins his bride in public. The completion of the ceremony takes place at night. The bride is taken to a special ritual site where she engages in intercourse with a group of her husband's relatives while their wives look on. The men copulate with her as often as they wish. The copulations are to force harmful fluids out of the bride's vagina and to increase her reproductive potential.

The most famous psychiatric case of nasal self-mutilation is that of Freud's obsessive patient, the Wolfman (a name given to him because of a dream he had). He had a fixed idea that he was the victim of a nasal injury caused by electrolytic treatment of obstructed sebaceous glands, that he had a scar, hole, or groove in the tissue, and that the contour of his nose was ruined. Dr. Ruth Brunswick, another psychoanalyst who treated him, stated that "nothing whatsoever was visible on the small, snub, typically Russian nose of the patient" (Gardiner 1971, p. 264). In 1923 he observed a black wart on his mother's nose. The following year, he had two teeth extracted and began to have queer thoughts about his nose. When his mother returned to Europe, he noticed a small pimple on his nose. He scratched it out, looked in a mirror, and saw a "deep hole" where the pimple had been. He became obsessed with the hole and felt obliged to stare at it with a mirror every few minutes to observe the progress of healing. His life was embittered because, according to his perception, the hole never healed. He consulted numerous dermatologists, when told that nothing could be done, he was seized by despair and was on the verge of suicide: "thus mutilated he could not go on living." When another physician used an instrument to press the spot on the Wolfman's nose, he experienced "an acute ecstasy" at the sight of his own blood. But he was not satisfied with the outcome and sought more medical opinions. His nose was treated with electrolysis, and when he complained of a scar he was told that scars never disappear. He looked constantly in his pocket mirror, attempting to establish the degree of his mutilation. Brunswick felt that his nasal symptoms represented a mother identification and an expression of his repressed, bisexual femininity. She noted that he purchased a woman's compact case and used it to observe and powder his nose. She recognized sadomasochistic trends in his character and linked his demands for treatment of his nose with a castration complex (Gardiner 1971).

The Mouth

Self-mutilation of the mouth, particularly lip and tongue biting, is often seen in children with relatively rare organic disorders such as Lesch-Nyhan syndrome, de Lange syndrome, autism, neuroacanthosis, and Tourette's syndrome (these disorders are discussed in chapter 9 in the section on stereotypic self-mutilation; animal models have been presented in chapter 4). Spencer et al. (1999) present a case of gingivitis artefacta; their report has an extensive bibliography.

Congenital indifference to pain with anhidrosis (markedly decreased sweating), congenital sensory neuropathy with anhidrosis, and familial dysautonomia (Riley-Day syndrome) are genetic autosomal recessive disorders in which self-mutilation results from an inability to perceive pain normally. Such children with deficient pain perception accidentally may chew off parts of their tongues, lips, or fingers; they may pick off part of their noses, extract teeth, break bones, and sustain numerous bruises and ulcerations (Gadoth and Mass 2004). Shelley (1962) described a girl with insensitivity to pain "who painlessly enucleated herself one night and then in the morning told the nurse nonchalantly that her eyeballs had 'dropped out' during the night" (p. 339). The management of such patients is highly problematic.

The dental literature contains a few brief case reports of various types of oral self-mutilation in which psychological factors were paramount (Golden and Chosack 1964; Goldstein and Dragan 1967). Hoffman and Baer's psychiatric study (1968) of three children who indulged in gingival self-mutilation revealed that the children developed organic lesions when they experienced a strong sense of deprivation e.g., the birth of a sibling or abandonment by parents. The oral lesions affected family dynamics in that the children became the center of attention. On discovering that the lesions brought both attention and gratification of dependency needs, they continued to aggravate the lesions by scratching and denuding their gingiva.

Culturally sanctioned mutilation of the teeth is done for a variety of reasons, the most common being beautification. In some African, South American, and Pacific Island cultures, teeth are blackened with burnt oil and filed. The incisors may be filed or broken to create a desired shape or inlaid with metal. In Western culture, models and actresses have their teeth straightened, whitened, and treated to fulfill an ideal of beauty.

The knocking out of teeth has also been associated with mourning and with the propitiation of the ghost of a dead ruler, as among the Sandwich Islanders. An African Bantu myth holds that death enters the human body through the teeth; to allow death a chance to exit, a triangular gap or notch is created by filing the teeth. Many Australian aborigines include tooth evulsion among the physical ordeals of male initiation rites.

Based on interpretations of dental folklore as well as on clinical cases, psychoanalysts have noted that the teeth may be associated with sexual symbolism. In *General Introduction to Psychoanalysis*, Freud wrote: "A particularly remarkable dream symbol is that of having one's teeth fall out, or having them pulled. Certainly its most immediate representation is castration as a punishment for onanism" (164). The concept of the *vagina dentata* refers to a rarely held male fantasy that the penis may be mutilated during intercourse by teeth hidden within a woman's vagina (Elwin 1943).

Although it is difficult to consider the tongue as "the primal organizer of the self" (Bonnard 1960), the possible phallic symbolism of the tongue is more readily comprehensible (Flugel 1925). The tongue, like the phallus, is a vascular organ that can be protruded and used intrusively during sexual acts. The following cases of self-mutilation of the tongue demonstrate sexual symbolism.

A 23-year-old woman said that a physician told her she needed throat surgery to cure her stutter. At the age of 26 she had episodes of nervousness and uncontrollable slurping and had trouble holding food in her mouth. After four minor auto accidents she lost her job and started to bite her lips, which became infected. She was hospitalized for three months for severe depression. At the age of 29, single, unemployed, and very unhappy, she appeared at a psychiatric emergency room saying, "I keep biting my tongue!" She stuffed a bloody, saliva-soaked rag in her mouth and gnashed her teeth in it. She had bitten off the tip of her quivering, macerated, beefy-red tongue. She explained that her teeth were trying to destroy her tongue and that she used the rag to keep her teeth away from her tongue. She was malnourished and dehydrated. Her fingers, used as wedges to pry apart her teeth, were sore and denuded of skin. Each time she bit her tongue she cried out in pain, protruded it, and exposed chunks of freshly lacerated, bleeding tissue. She begged for help and fell to the floor in agony. Many types of therapy were tried including electroshock, medication, hypnosis, and psychotherapy. None proved successful.

The psychiatrists who reported the case (Slawson and Davidson 1964) considered the patient to be immature because she rejected marriage. Because marriage "involves acceptance of the genital role and the reality of a penis," her tongue mutilation symbolized rejection of the penis and implied "an unconscious wish to destroy that threatening organ" (p. 587). Additionally, they noted that the mouth may symbolize the female genitalia; there are some anatomical similarities in that they are both cavities lined with moist, mucosal tissue surrounded by muscle, and both have lips (or labia) at the mucocutaneous junction. Both may possess teeth—the one in fact, the other in fantasy (*vagina dentata*). The bloody rag in the patient's mouth may represent a sanitary napkin that controls the blood of a fantasized castration. Thus tongue, penis, mouth, and vagina may be equated symbolically, and the mutilation may demonstrate "an oral sadistic attack on the incorporation of an organ both feared and desired" (p. 588).

Michael and Beck (1973) described a 33-year-old man who had schizophrenia and who cut out his tongue during a psychotic episode. As a child, he did not speak clearly until the age of 9, when his teacher "showed me how to use my tongue." He married a schoolteacher and one year later he began exposing his genitals in public. He spent many of the following years in a state mental hospital (he once tried to electrocute himself as punishment for exposing himself). His wife divorced him, and he took up with a female patient but was confused over wishes to be with his ex-wife. He decided to "correct" his bad decision of choosing the female patient over his wife by purchasing a knife with the intention of cutting off his hands, then his feet, then his tongue, and finally gouging out his eyes. Instead, he cut off two-thirds of his tongue and flushed it down the toilet. He felt relieved and asked his brother to call his wife to see what he had done.

The psychiatrists believed that the patient's exhibitionism resulted from profound feelings of rejection and that the tongue mutilation resulted from fear of emerging homosexual impulses. They equated the mutilation with symbolic self-castration in that it was an attempt to correct a defect (exhibitionism) that caused his wife to leave him and to accomplish a merging with his mother, who apparently cared for him more when he had a speech impediment. In fact, his mother said that after the mutilation he sounded much the way he did as a child.

Book 6 of Ovid's *Metamorphoses* contains a frightening story of tongue mutilation linked with sexual violence. The Greek hero Tereus married the beautiful Procne, and they had a child named Itys. At Procne's flirtatious insistence, Tereus traveled to Athens to bring her sister, Philomela, for a visit. With one look Tereus fell madly in love with Philomela. On the journey home he raped her. She pleaded to be killed, but Tereus instead cut out her tongue: "He thrust sharp tongs between her teeth, her tongue still crying out her father's name. Then as the forceps caught the tongue, his steel sliced through it, its roots still beating while the rest turned, moaning on black earth. As the bruised tail of a dying serpent lashes, so her tongue crept, throbbed, and whimpered at his feet. This done, the tyrant renewed his pleasure on her wounded body."

Tereus kept Philomela locked up and told Procne that she had died. Philomela, however, wove a coarse tapestry depicting her fate and had it delivered to her sister. Procne freed her and said, "Now is no time for tears; we need good steel. . . . This is my day for crime, to take a torch to all rooms of the palace and to push Tereus into its flames, or chip away his tongue, tear out his eyes, cut off the genitals that injured you." Just then her son, Itys, appeared, and she noticed how much he looked like his father. With tears in her eyes and despite Itys's pleading, she slaughtered him, cooked his body parts, and served them to Tereus for dinner. After he had eaten, she tossed the boy's bloody head into his face. The women escaped the anger of Tereus by changing into birds with red spots among their feathers. Shakespeare's gruesome play *Titus Andronicus* is based on Ovid's story and additionally contains instances of self-mutilation; for example, one character chops off his hand.

Not all tongue self-mutilation occurs within a sexual setting. Prince (1960) described several strange and fatal cases of self-mutilation of the tongue among the Yoruba of Nigeria. The first case was that of an 18-year-old student who acted strangely in school. When brought to the hospital he held his head in an odd posture and kept protruding his tongue. He began biting his tongue so severely that he was given electroshock treatments and a major tranquilizer. He subverted all attempts to keep him from destroying his tongue, which turned into a necrotic mass from the constant, savage biting. The dead tissue was removed surgically. He was given antibiotics and was fed through a tube. He did not hemorrhage much, and his blood pressure stayed within normal limits. He lost a great deal of weight, however, and his temperature rose; within ten days he was dead.

The second case involved an 18-year-old female student who was psychotic as manifested by shouting, auditory hallucinations, and the delusion that she had eaten her parents and her girlfriend. She was given a major tranquilizer. After two days she postured her head oddly and then bit off her tongue. She died within three more days in a manner similar to the previous case. A third case, about which little was known, was that of a psychotic young man who intentionally bit his tongue and almost totally severed it. He was brought to a hospital, and his tongue was sewn back in place. He pulled out the stitches, continued to bite his tongue, and died shortly afterward.

According to Prince (1960), in these cases a curse or invocation was the most likely factor precipitating the patients' psychoses and influencing their symptomatology. Among the Yoruba, words may be omnipotent: "To utter the name of something may draw that something into actual existence . . . not only within the mind and body of he who utters and he who hears the word, but also in the physical world as well" (p. 66). Among the Yoruba, for example, if someone is verbally abused by another or laughed at, he or she may retaliate by saying, "You will bite off your tongue and never speak again," or "You will laugh yourself to death." Because curses can be effective only when words are spoken, the destruction of a person's tongue is a particularly effective method; the victim no longer possesses the physical capacity to utter a retaliatory curse.

The Tlingit Indians of the Northwest Coast (North America) had a custom described by a French traveler in 1799 as "the most disgusting perhaps that exists on the face of the earth. . . . [Women] have the lower lip slit close to the gum the whole width of the mouth, and wear in it a kind of wooden bowl without handles which rests against the gum, and which the slit lip serves as a collar to confine, so that the lower part of the mouth projects two or three inches. . . . This whimsical ornament not only disfigures the look, but causes an involuntary flow of saliva, as inconvenient as it is disgusting." The initial ritual slitting occurred at menarche and was a rite of passage signifying that a girl was available for marriage. The piercer was the girl's future mother-in-law. When the girl married, a larger labret (the ornament that was inserted into the slit lip) was provided; each change in a woman's status was accompanied by a different labret. The symbolism of this custom is rich and refers to social relations, eating, the potlatch ritual, and sexuality. The sliced lip represents a vagina, which is filled by a labret representing a tongue-phallus. In Tlingit art, figures "often unite with each other by sharing a tongue in what might be interpreted as a symbolic representation of sexual union . . . maleness and femaleness are united by the appearance of the labret when worn" (Jonaitis 1988). By the mid-1800s, large labrets were no longer used by the Tlingit, largely because of negative reactions by European visitors. They were replaced by small silver or bone pins that were inserted into the lower lip.

Finally, mention should be made to removal of the uvula (tissue that hangs from the soft palate) by tribal medicine men in Ethiopia and Eritrea. The surgery is done supposedly to prevent throat infections (Fleischer 1980; Hartley and Rowe-Jones 1994).

CHAPTER SIX

The Limbs

The arms, legs, hands, feet, toes, and especially the fingers are body parts well suited anatomically for self-mutilation. The amputation of a finger joint, for example, can be accomplished rapidly and accurately with minimal loss of blood, with little loss of function for many tasks, and with good healing of the wound. Further, the deformed finger stump is readily available for public display. In fact, the most ancient form of ritual mutilation is finger amputation. It was practiced twenty thousand years ago and has been practiced ever since (Janssens 1957; Moodie 1920). The first graphic evidence of finger mutilation is found in late Paleolithic imprints in the cave at Gargas in southern France. Although hand imprints have been found in many local caves, only in the Gargas cave do the imprints show finger mutilation. Of ninety-two recognizable imprints, the most common mutilation is absence of the tip of the four fingers, with the thumb being spared. The most plausible explanation is that the amputations were part of religious rituals associated with mourning or healing.

The antiquity of finger mutilation is also demonstrated in aboriginal populations. In 1886 an African Bushman family was "exhibited" in Berlin. Four of the six family members had digit tips amputated. Virchow made drawings of their hands and noted that "in every sickness of what kind soever it is usual with them to take off extreme joints of the fingers, beginning with the little finger of the left hand." Gardner and Heider (1968) presented striking photographs of current finger mutilation among the Dugum Dani tribe of New Guinea. Young girls have their fingers cut off as a sacrifice at funerals; after a hard blow to the elbow to deaden the pain, the fingers are chopped off with a stone adze. Many Dani women fondle their children "with hands that are mostly thumbs."

Two Swedish anthropologists, Lagercrantz (1935) and Soderstrom (1938), wrote lengthy articles on finger mutilation. Many studies, often with startling photographs by respected nineteenth- and early-twentieth-century anthropologists, are included in their references.

In West Africa, finger amputation was sometimes performed on corpses. If the deceased had been impotent, his little finger was cut off and inserted in his anus to horrify the dead man so much that his spirit would seek reincarnation as a woman so as to have children in a new life. The Bushmen amputated a corpse's finger in order to facilitate passage into a blessed afterlife. Among the Ashanti parental love turned to anger if an infant died in the first week of life. The dead body was beaten, and a finger was cut off. The body was then buried in the village garbage dump. When a firstborn child died among the BaBoyes, all subsequent children underwent amputation of the first joint of the little finger. The severed fingers were then buried in the grave of the dead child to placate the evil spirit who killed it.

Among the Xhosa, a sickly child might be treated by amputation of a finger joint. Sometimes the operation was performed to help the child "grow up strong and brave." Schambaa mothers cut off the fingertip of a child with eye problems and dropped blood from the severed fingertip into the affected eye. An interesting Mashona legend tells of ogres who killed a boy and a girl, then cut off parts of the genitals, the lips, and the first joints of the little fingers. These parts were taken by the chief, who secretly prepared medicine from them that was eaten at a feast to ensure a fruitful harvest.

The Hottentots amputated fingers as a sign of engagement and marriage. A widow, for example, would cut off a finger upon remarriage, thus releasing herself from all bonds with her dead husband. A number of tribes cut off specific fingers as a sort of surname or badge of the clan. Among the Zande, a person accused of magically willing another's death was forced to eat a dish that contained a small-finger joint from the deceased.

In Oceania and the Pacific Islands, finger mutilation was endemic and likely persists today in remote places. One reporter in New Guinea noted in 1900 that "the custom of amputating in some cases the first, in others the second, joints of the index and middle fingers is very common after the death of a near relative. . . . A mother will cut off the first joint for her children and the second for her husband, father, or mother" (Soderstrom 1938, p. 26). Finger amputation was performed, sometimes on a large scale, at times of mourning; one hundred fingers might be amputated for a king's burial. If the deceased belonged to a rich family, tribesmen sent their fingers to the survivors, who were expected to reward such signs of mourning. In Hawaii, the mutilations were especially fierce; survivors of the deceased might, in addition to finger amputation, pull out their teeth, burn themselves, tattoo their tongues, and cut off their ears.

In Polynesia, Captain James Cook found many natives with amputated fingers and wrote that "this operation is performed when they labour under some grievous disease and think themselves in danger of dying." Among some aboriginal groups in Australia, the tip of a woman's left little finger was bitten off at the time of her engagement to warn off suitors. In order to bring luck in fishing and to

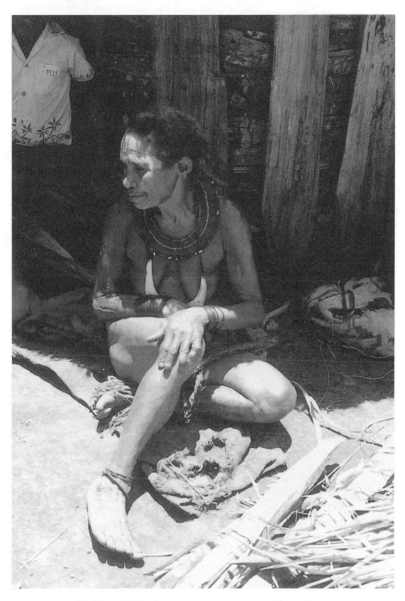

A woman from Chimbu Province, New Guinea highlands, who chopped off her fingertips in mourning for deceased male relatives. (Photo courtesy of Dr. Wolfgang Jilek)

make winding of the fishing lines easier, girls had their fingers removed. A band around a finger was tightened daily until the joint dropped off. Another procedure was to bind the fingers with coarse spiderwebs until the joint started to die. The girl then placed her hand in an anthill until the ants ate off the joint.

Finger mutilation was also prevalent among North American Indians. The relatives of a young Crow Indian warrior, for example, mourned at his death by prolonged severing of finger joints, cutting off their hair, and gashing their bodies. The Mandan Indians cut off the first and fourth fingers of the left hand during religious rites. In their quest for a guardian-spirit protector, many Plains Indians underwent a period of fasting, exposure to the elements, and amputation of a finger as an offering to the sun.

The Hands and Arms

In both history and folklore, the human hand has been associated with special powers. In Athens, the hand of a person who committed suicide was cut off and buried separate from the rest of the body to prevent the ghost of the deceased from haunting the living. Biblical accounts of Jesus's ability to heal by touching led to the European belief that the touch of a king could cure diseases, especially a form of tuberculosis called scrofula. The "hand of glory" refers to the folk belief that the severed hand of a hanged man possessed healing qualities. In eighteenth-century France, thieves often carried such a hand with them because it supposedly put people to sleep, thus making burglary easier. The Bloody Hand of Ulster, an old heraldic symbol, is an erect, red palm of a severed left hand on a silver background. It represents the hand of the brave O'Neill, forefather of the Irish princes of Ulster. The legendary story is that several Celtic warlords were on an expedition when they sighted land. They raced because the first to touch the land could claim it for his clan. When O'Neill's ship fell behind, he chopped off his left hand and flung it to the shore a moment before his competitors landed.

A legend reminiscent of Saint Lucy, who cut out her eyes to cool the passions of a suitor, is that of the tenth-century British saint Wilfreda. King Edgar was in love with her. He pursued her to a church, where, on bended knee, he proposed marriage. She refused, however, leaving behind her hand in the king's grasp. Unnerved, he pursued her no longer.

In European jurisprudence during the eighth to twelfth centuries, the use of a sworn oath to determine guilt and innocence was superseded by the ordeal in which the accused underwent a test whose outcome depended on divine intervention. It was believed that God protected the innocent from injury during an ordeal. In the ordeal of boiling water, the accused put his or her hand into a cauldron of boiling water and tried to retrieve a small stone or ring at the bottom. The more serious the crime, the deeper the water. The hand (or arm) was then carefully wrapped in a bandage and sealed with the signet of the judge. After three days, the bandage was removed, and guilt or innocence was determined by the physical condition of the limb. The water was thought by Christians to represent the biblical deluge in which the wicked were punished, while the fire under the caldron represented Judgment Day.

The most widespread European ordeal was one in which an accused person carried a red-hot iron bar and walked nine feet; the more serious the crime, the heavier the iron. The hands were then wrapped and examined for evidence of healing after three days. Persons of high rank often requested this ordeal voluntarily to prove their innocence. A famous story involves Bishop Poppo, who went as a missionary to Denmark in A.D. 962. The pagan Danish king Harold Blaatland dared him to prove his faith in God. Poppo underwent an ordeal of red-hot iron before the royal court. His hands were not injured, and as a result of this miracle the Danes converted to Christianity.

During the trials of the Inquisition, an accused person was presumed guilty, was usually not told the charges, and was tortured as a means of forcing a confession. Perhaps the most popular torture was the strappado. The accused person's hands were tied behind his or her back. A cord was fastened to the wrists, and a 125-pound weight was attached to the feet (the weight was increased to 250 pounds during "extraordinary" torture). With a pulley the accused was lifted into the air and dropped rapidly. The rope was secured before the feet touched the ground, thus dislocating the joints of the person's arms. The procedure was usually repeated three times. Insane persons, children, and pregnant women were exempt from the strappado, and Inquisitors also were supposed to stop the torture if the accused's life or limb was endangered. It was practically impossible, however, not to dislocate the arm joints. The accused were warned that if they died or were crippled by the strappado, they had only themselves to blame for not confessing the truth (Lea 1973a and b).

The Feet

In 1882, Dr. R. A. Jamieson, of Shanghai, presented a pair of feet to the British Royal College of Surgeons. The feet belonged to a Chinese beggar who extracted much pity and made a profitable business in Shanghai's foreign settlement by displaying the mutilated stumps of his legs while carrying his feet on a string around his neck. To make himself as attractive as possible to the charitably disposed, he had fastened cords around his ankles, tightening them every two days. After two weeks, he felt no pain; after six weeks, he was able to remove the feet by partly cutting and partly snapping the bones. The stumps healed, and the feet became black and mummified.

In ancient China a severe method of ensuring feminine virtue was developed: women's feet were deliberately modified (Levy 1968). Literally and figuratively, Chinese men made sure that wives and mistresses would not "run around."

Chinese foot binding started out fairly innocuously during the eleventh century A.D. when court dancers bound their feet with tight shoes. Their tiny feet became objects of admiration, and a more effective binding procedure for creating tiny feet was soon developed. Following an old palace tradition, a beautiful and elaborate pedestal in the shape of a lotus served as a dance floor; the term *golden lotus* became synonymous with bound feet.

At that time, Chinese attitudes toward women were relatively liberal. Widows and divorced women could remarry, and courtesans wrote frank poems about their feelings. A conservative backlash developed during the Sung dynasty. The "total" woman of this period was the one who stayed at home, was docile, worshipped her husband, and had tiny feet. Foot binding became a visible sign of the upper classes, signifying that a woman was so refined that she was incapable of doing anything useful except satisfying her husband. Officials sometimes ordered excessive foot binding to enforce morality among the lower classes. In the Fukien area, for example, one governor ordered that all women's feet be crippled to change their unchaste behavior. These women could hardly move, and when they attended celebrations or funerals, the gatherings were referred to as "A Forest of Canes."

The process of foot binding began in early childhood. A bandage two inches wide and ten feet long was tightly wrapped around each foot, sparing only the large toe. The object was to break many of the bones in the foot, to bend the toes into the sole of the foot, and to bring the sole and heel as close together as possible. The flesh often became putrescent and sometimes one or more toes sloughed off. The pain continued for about a year, until the feet became numb.

Children who attempted to loosen the wrappings were beaten, and every few weeks the bound feet were compressed into new and smaller shoes. The following was written by a woman who endured the bindings: "In the summer, my feet smelled offensively because of pus and blood; in winter, my feet felt cold because of lack of circulation and hurt if they got too near heat. Four of the toes were curled in like so many dead caterpillars; no outsider would ever have believed that they belonged to a human being. It took two years to achieve the three inch model. My toenails pressed against the flesh like thin paper. The heavily creased plantar couldn't be scratched when it itched or soothed when it ached. My shanks were thin, my feet became humped, ugly, and odiferous; how I envied the natural-footed!" (Levy 1968, pp. 27–28).

Deformed, tiny feet became a standard of beauty. Poets praised them; men demanded them in their wives; courtesans without them were shunned. The tiny foot contained the beauty of the entire body: it glistened like the skin; it arched like the eyebrow; it pointed like jade fingers; the deformed heel was soft and rounded like the breasts; it was small like the mouth, mysterious like the vagina, and its odor was more seductive than that of the armpits. Lotus lovers reveled in smelling, rubbing, chewing, licking, and washing tiny feet. "Eating Steamed Dumplings in Pure Water" was the Chinese term once used to describe foot licking. One connoisseur noted that the flavor of the lotus foot was "the greatest flavor of mankind, beyond sweet and sour, unnameable." Another wrote: "Every night I smell her feet, placing the tip of my nose in the deepest recesses of her plantar. I am extremely excited by the smell. I only regret that I cannot swallow down the white chestnut with one mouthful. But I can still place it in my mouth and chew the plantar" (Levy 1968, p. 142).

The ecstasy experienced by Chinese men on seeing or fondling a lotus foot was the equivalent of that experienced by Western men on seeing or fondling a female breast (Suh-ho 1915). The Chinese also believed that foot binding had a special bonus; it caused layers of folds to develop in the vagina, resulting in a "supernatural exaltation" during intercourse. The inability to walk supposedly also caused women's thighs to become sensuously heavier and caused the vagina to tighten.

Foot binding persisted for a thousand years. The Manchu conquerors in the seventeenth century passed laws against it but with little effect. Not until the end of the nineteenth century did attacks against foot binding become widespread. Western travelers criticized it as barbarous. Chinese intellectuals demanded that foot binding be ended because of the loss of face and prestige it engendered internationally. In 1894, an Unbound Foot Association was started in Canton, and branches emerged in many cities.

Christian missionaries zealously denounced the custom. Some refused to let women who had bound feet enter a church; others would accept only girls who had natural feet into boarding schools. A missionary named Gladys Alward worked as a provincial foot inspector, attacking the custom everywhere she went. A group of prominent Western women living in the Far East influenced the Empress Dowager Tz'u-ksi to issue an anti–foot binding edict in 1902.

Resistance to change was stubborn; for a millennium the Chinese people equated tiny lotus feet with perfect beauty. Laws against foot binding were not enough. Millions of leaflets and placards were distributed, and writers produced poems and popular songs that attacked the custom and proclaimed the beauty and virtue of natural feet. In 1911, the Chinese revolutionary leader and physician Sun Yat-sen prohibited foot binding. Officials forcibly removed women with bound feet from their homes and publicly ridiculed them. Bounties were paid to women who turned in their bindings. The Japanese vigorously prohibited foot binding on Taiwan. Because women who had bound feet often hid at home, the Japanese did house-to-house searches and destroyed all chamber pots, thus forcing women to be seen when they went to a public toilet.

Foot binding was finally eliminated in the 1930s. Chinese attitudes toward women had changed drastically in the face of liberal reforms. Women who had bound feet were divorced and deserted by their husbands. Many who tried to "let out" their feet found that they were unalterably crippled and hobbled along with canes, the permanent victims of a terribly cruel custom.

Clinical Cases

Deviant self-mutilation of only the upper limbs is associated mainly with many disorders such as tertiary syphilis, encephalitis, major depression, and schizophrenia (wrist slashing is discussed in chapter 7). Religious delusions often are prominent. In the newly proposed body integrity identity disorder, persons deliberately amputate their fingers, hands, toes, feet, arms, and legs or seek surgeons who will do it for them.

Medical and Hereditary Disorders

Urechia (1931) described the case of a 39-year-old alcoholic man who was admitted to the hospital with symptoms of syphilitic dementia. He was treated by inoculation with malaria (the high fever caused by malaria is effective in destroying the spirochete of syphilis). He proceeded to develop convulsions, however, and in his confusion he bit off and ate several of his fingers without feeling the slightest pain. When asked why he did it, his response was that they itched. He died within several days. An organized meningeal hemorrhage was found on autopsy.

Conn (1932) reported the case of a 21-year-old woman who complained of sharp, penetrating, shooting pains in various parts of her body and of hallucinations that accused her of autoerotic practices. Her pains were relieved by a placebo. While at home one week later, she placed her right hand under the bed spring and deliberately fractured the phalangeal articulations. At the same time, she fractured the bones in her left hand and the left little toe, and then dislocated both thumbs. She displayed her malformed, bleeding hands to her mother, who fainted. The patient explained that she mutilated her limbs to relieve the terrible pains. Over the next six months, she pulled out her fingernails, lacerated her ear, and kept banging her hands. In the hospital, she proudly displayed her hands to anyone who was interested. She had several neurological signs, such as unequal, irregular pupils and a passive tremor of her left arm. Conn concluded that her symptomatology, observed over an eight-year period, strongly resembled an acute, descending, radicular type of encephalitis. He felt that her autoerotic conflicts resulted in mutilative acting out, conflicts that came "to the surface" because her organic pathology weakened her protective psychological inhibitions.

Self-mutilation of the hands and feet is associated with neurological lesions and diseases (Gadoth and Mass 2004). For example, people who have congenital indifference to pain often accidentally injure themselves severely and may present with marked skeletal and soft tissue damage in their hands and feet. Their inability to perceive pain may stem from a cortical lesion. Landwirth (1964) described a 22-year-old man who had a congenital sensory neuropathy manifested by an inability to appreciate pain, temperature, proprioceptive stimuli, and other surface sensations. Several of his fingers and toes were surgically amputated because he was often unaware that he had injured them, resulting in chronic infections. Because he ignored his wounds, picked at them, and refused to change dressings, an irate surgical staff sent him to a psychiatrist. The patient explained that he felt overwhelming disappointment and anger when attempts to heal his wounds failed; by deliberately making his wounds worse, he at least could predict the outcome with certainty. By the age of 21, his right leg had been amputated and he had developed a chronic osteomyelitis in his left leg, which was sure to lead to another amputation. He began to cut his wrists and forearms in different locations. His arm cutting was a sort of experiment to determine the ability of his body to heal itself. He developed chronic osteomyelitis of his left index finger and asked that it be amputated. When the surgeon refused, the patient stuck his infected finger through a hole in a shoe box, calmly cut it off with a hacksaw, and put it in a plastic bag in a freezer for later "study." Feeling helpless and victimized by his untreatable medical condition, he mutilated himself in an attempt to establish control over part of his body. Instead of waiting passively to lose his finger, he actively destroyed it. "He could then feel that he was losing body parts because this was his wish" (Dubovsky 1978; Dubovsky and Groban 1975).

Other inherited conditions, in addition to congenital insensitivity to pain, are associated with peripheral neuropathy and self-mutilation. Acanthosis is caused by defects in the membranes of red blood cells as well as brain cells and is associated with a wide variety of symptoms, including tics, abnormal muscle tone, muscle wasting, strange facial and mouth movements, Parkinsonism, and dementia. Perhaps its most recognizable sign is tongue and lip biting. Onset occurs mostly in adult life. In type 1 tyrosinemia the blood level of the amino acid tyrosine, a building block for most proteins, is elevated due to a deficiency in an enzyme needed to metabolize tyrosine. Among its many symptoms are liver and kidney failure as well as peripheral neuropathy. It is particularly common in Quebec, Canada. Hereditary sensory and autonomic neuropathy type IV is a disorder with both congenital insensitivity to pain and lack of sweating. It is associated with mental retardation, bouts of unexplained fever, temper tantrums, self-extraction of fingernails, and self-amputation of fingers and toes that often are deformed or infected (Axelrod and Gold-von-Simson 2007).

Lesch-Nyhan syndrome is an inherited disorder found only in boys. Due to reduced or lack of the enzyme hypoxanthine-guanine phosphoribosyl transferase, uric acid accumulates in the blood and leads to gout, kidney stones, involuntary writhing, facial grimacing, repetitive limb movements, mental retardation, and compulsive biting of the fingers, hands, and lips. The biting is remarkable for its awesome rapidity; upon release from restraints, a child's hand may go instantly into his mouth (Christie et al. 1982). Symptoms usually appear in the first few years of life but may be delayed until adolescence. Those affected with this syndrome "usually plead with their parents or other caretakers to keep them in restraints and they are extremely upset when the restraints are removed" (Jankovic 1988).

Classical autism is one of the pervasive developmental disorders and has a strong but not fully understood genetic basis (Abrahams and Geschwind 2008). Often associated with mild/moderate mental retardation, it is characterized by marked and sustained impairment of social interaction and communication as well as restricted, repetitive, stereotyped behavior, interests, and activities. Head banging occurs as well as biting of the wrists, hands, and fingers.

The brachial plexus consists of nerve fibers that run from the spine from below the fifth cervical and first thoracic vertebrae through the neck to the armpit and the upper arm. Damage to this plexus due to complications of childbirth may result in severe biting of fingertips of the damaged limb at about two years of age. A retrospective U.S. study found a self-biting incidence of 3 percent (McCann et al. 2002), while a prospective study in Saudi Arabia found an incidence of 4.7 percent (Al-Qattan 1999). Traumatic cervical spinal cord injury at any age may result in severe biting of the fingers and hand; the causes of this behavior are both biological and psychological (Couts and Gleason 2006).

Psychosis

Religious delusions are prominent in all of the reported cases of hand mutilation by people who are psychotically depressed or schizophrenic. Lewis (1928) described a highly educated and cultured widow who had a happy marriage, a fine career, and no history of mental illness. At the age of 57, she said that the Second Coming of Christ would take place at Christmas. Later, the world was going to be lost. She took a knife and almost severed her left hand at the wrist. The surgeons who treated her found it necessary to amputate her hand. She declared that she "must have been misled by Satan" and regarded hospital staff as devils. She had lucid moments interspersed with confused ones. She groaned and prayed continually, spat on the floor, refused food, and drank water from a bucket to wash away her sins. She died suddenly. An autopsy showed only "an appearance of exhaustion in the adrenals"; it was surmised that her death was due to a profound psychic or endocrine disturbance. Lewis concluded that "since this self-amputation was evidently done as a punishment for sin . . . the incident may be classified with those symbolizing self-castration at the somatic level" (p. 194).

A 37-year-old man had several psychiatric hospitalizations after a bad conduct discharge from the military. While on a ship, he developed delusions that his shipmates were going to torture and kill him. After a number of abortive suicide attempts, he decided to overcome his torturers by emulating Christ, who overcame adversity by enduring the torments of his captors. The patient burned his index finger to a crisp to prove he could withstand pain. Then he ate the distal and middle phalanx. When he discovered the difficulties involved in burning his wrist (he intended to eat his hand) and armpit, he abandoned the attempt, now confident that he could vanquish his tormentors. He attempted to control his aggression by identifying with the powerful figure of Christ and by destroying a part of his body rather than committing suicide. Eating his finger may have reflected the gratification of frightening homosexual impulses—the finger symbolizing a phallus—which were, in part, the source of his psychological decompensation (Mintz 1964).

In the section on eye mutilation in chapter 5, I described the case of an 18-year-old schizophrenic college student who felt guilty about his homosexual interests; he sawed off his right hand with a hacksaw and removed an eye with a screwdriver. He was a self-proclaimed evangelist and regarded his mutilation as a special mission for God. In the same article in which this case was noted (Goldenberg and Sata 1978), the authors also reported the case of a young man who was increasingly preoccupied with religious thoughts after he participated in a Bible study group that discussed Matthew's famous injunction to remove an eyeball. After several attempts to saw off his hand and to chop it off with an ax, he finally shot it with a rifle and requested surgical amputation, "saying that he was acting on God's commandments." Schlozman (1998) also reported two cases of self-amputation of the arms in patients with psychotic feelings of guilt and concrete religious preoccupations.

Arons (1981) told of a 30-year-old man with schizophrenia who sawed off his right hand. Preoccupied with the passage from Matthew, he considered the amputation "a necessary act." He considered removing his eye but decided on the hand amputation instead. He had attempted suicide previously and often felt hopelessness. He had derogatory auditory hallucinations about his homosexuality and delusions of persecution. He spent twelve years in the hospital with little improvement and continued his homosexual activities with other patients. While on a pass, he stood in front of a moving train and was killed instantly.

I am indebted to Dr. M. K. Au, of Hong Kong, for the following case of a 32-year-old schizophrenic Chinese man whose self-amputation of a hand was related to his participation in a martial arts cult known as god-sent kung-fu, or magic boxing. This cult believes that fighters who master the mystic power of being possessed by a god (usually the Monkey God) become immune to injury.

The patient and a woman friend were cult members. After swallowing charm papers, they believed evil spirits were after them. Confused, they ran naked through the countryside, where the police arrested them. They posted bail and were released. The next day, while at a restaurant, the patient chopped off his left hand. He was rushed to a hospital but, against medical advice, he fled, leaving his hand behind. That afternoon the couple, certain that they were being chased by evil spirits, jumped out of the window of their third-story apartment. Because they were god-sent kung-fu fighters, they did not believe they would be injured by the fall; evidently neither suffered real physical damage, but both were brought to a mental hospital, where they admitted to ideas of reference, auditory hallucinations, and paranoid delusions. When asked why he had chopped off his hand the man stated, "I wanted to show my determination to abstain from gambling. . . .

I could not be harmed because of protection by the god-sent kung-fu." The woman responded well to treatment and was discharged within two months. The male patient made a much slower recovery. His hand was surgically reimplanted and worked fairly well. The woman's mental condition remained stable, but the male patient deteriorated. He gave up magic boxing and frequented various Christian churches. He hoarded rubbish at home, often walked backward, neglected his personal hygiene, and continued to have persecutory delusions and auditory hallucinations. The situation was one of a folie à deux in which the patient, who was clearly schizophrenic, "induced" psychotic symptoms in his mate.

Body Integrity Identity Disorder and Love of Amputation

Perhaps the most shocking behavior reported widely on the Internet, on television, and in the print media is the desire of persons, most of whom appear to be rational and nondelusional, to have a limb amputated. The 9 June 2008 edition of *Newsweek* magazine, for example, published a piece titled "They'd give their right leg," which contained a photograph of a one-legged man on crutches with the caption "Victims of body-integrity identity disorder have a relentless desire to amputate healthy limbs."

To better understand this behavior, we need to clarify some terminology that is often confusing to both health professionals and the public. The word *apotemnophilia* was coined by Money et al. (1977) to refer to a paraphilia that involves sexual arousal dependent on a person's becoming an amputee. The more recent word *acrotomophilia* refers to sexual arousal by persons dependent on a partner who is an amputee. Body integrity identity disorder (BIID) refers to a rare but provocative condition in which persons desire amputation of a limb that is perceived to be extraneous to their bodies ("It really isn't part of me"). BIID in some cases involves the sexual behavior of apotemnophilia and acrotomophilia. In addition to requesting a limb amputation, persons who have BIID may seek to acquire a disability such as blindness or total paralysis below the waist for psychological rather than financial reasons. Veale (2006) described a woman with a poor sense of self who had a persistent desire to become deaf; she stuffed plugs in her ears and learned sign language as a way to establish an identity as a member of the deaf community.

Money et al. (1977) reported two cases of men who demanded a leg amputation. Neither man was psychotic, and their conditions were thought at that time to be conceptually related, but not identical, to transsexualism, bisexuality, Munchausen syndrome, and masochism.

The man in the first case stated that he was a "cryptic transsexual" but that his problem centered on his leg rather than his genitals. He requested referral to a surgeon who might be willing to amputate his leg. He wrote: "Since my 13th year, my conscious life has been absorbed, with varying intensity, in a bizarre and prepotent obsessive wish, need, desire to have my leg amputated above the knee; the image of myself as an amputee has as an erotic fantasy (each one different) that accompanied *every* sexual experience of my life: auto-, homo-, and hetero-sexual, since, and beginning with, puberty" (emphasis per original). He had had sexual experiences with two amputees; the first, with an older man, was satisfactory while the second, with a woman, was not pleasurable. He used pictures of amputees as a visual aid during masturbation. Between his two marriages he admitted to "promiscuous sexual activity," especially with adolescent males. He loathed himself on those occasions when he felt "like a woman" and noted that he wanted "to make real the fantasy that I am an amputated homosexual adolescent, for in possessing my stump I can, concurrently, possess my penis."

Because he could not find a surgeon willing to amputate his leg, he deliberately injured himself in the hope of forcing an amputation. He hammered a steel pin into his left tibia and infected the wound by placing facial acne pus and nasal and anal mucus in it. He did this repeatedly, and he also tried to get rid of his leg by placing a tourniquet on his thigh. Unfortunately, from his point of view, his leg healed with medical treatment. He eventually sought counseling for his problems and took courses that would enable him to have a career fitting amputees with prostheses. Although he thought psychotherapy was helpful, he was frequently depressed over his inability to rid himself of his leg. He thought his condition resulted from pathological family relationships (he described his mother as extremely overprotective, his father as repressive and hypercritical of his relationship with his mother, his adult older brother as having been a chronic bed wetter, and his younger sister as a lesbian) and from early childhood incidents. When he was 2 years old, his left foot and leg were so severely burned in a kitchen accident that he was unable to walk for almost a year. When he was 5 years old, his mother was severely burned in another domestic accident. He wrote that he had a savagely forbidden wish to be like a girl and that an amputation might both secure his father's love and sympathy and establish his male identity: "One of the anticipated 'pleasures' [for me] of being an amputee is the possibility of a genuine experience of identification."

The second case involved a man who requested amputation of his right leg. He thought it would be sexually pleasurable to fondle a man's stump. During sexual activity, he fantasized both himself and his partner as amputees. He also had fantasies about amputees who overcame their handicaps, for example, by waterskiing. Frustrated that no surgeon would cut off his leg, he wrote, "It is interesting that transsexuals can obtain sex change [operations], people obtain cosmetic surgery to meet the norms of society, and I cannot obtain my fulfillment legitimately." Through "underground" ads in newspapers he contacted persons who had the same desires but who were successful in obtaining amputations. Their method was to contrive a leg injury that required surgical amputation. He rejected this approach as too brutal and painful. He gained some gratification by doing volunteer work with amputees. He considered three reasons for his apotemnophilia. The first was that the amputation might represent a sacrifice of atonement (presumably for his sexual activities) based on his early childhood experience as a devout church member. The second was that the amputation might represent a way to avoid homosexuality because "most amputees, one way or the other, do get married." The third, and most significant, stemmed from childhood experiences. He was born with a mildly clubbed right foot and was severely criticized by his father for his faulty gait. The condition was corrected surgically, but he received no praise for walking correctly. At the age of 15, he fractured his right leg: "I didn't mind the pain at all. I didn't mind the cast. In fact, I rather enjoyed this experience of cast, crutches, and means of mobility."

Wakefield et al. (1977) reported on a 28-year-old married man who was sexually excited by the sight (or photographs) of female amputees, was fascinated by men who had lost a digit or a limb, and wished to undergo an amputation. Two years earlier, he had experimented with amputation to see if it would be enjoyable. He deadened a finger by submerging it in dry ice. After it became necrotic, he told a physician that it had been damaged at work. He experienced pleasure during "the ultimate act" of amputation by the surgeon. A few months before seeking treatment, he put a rubber band around a toe and amputated it with a razor blade. As a child, he used to tie strings around his fingers, toes, and hands; he felt pleasure when they became discolored and fantasized about their amputation. At the age of 13, intrigued by a photograph of a boy who had lost a leg, he constructed and wore a peg leg. While wearing this apparatus, he experienced his first orgasm. He felt sexual excitement in cutting the hand or leg off photographs of women as a prelude to masturbation. He established contact with members of an underground group who indulged in self-amputation and referred to themselves as "hobbyists." On one occasion, both the patient and a fellow hobbyist put on sandals to expose their amputated toes and walked through a shopping center for signs of public reaction.

The patient said he was happily married and had a "normal" sexual relationship with his wife, who accepted his "hobby" even if she did not understand it. His mental status examination was normal. He recognized the bizarre nature of his symptoms even though he described them in a matter-of-fact, almost blasé manner. He had weekly therapy for nine months and he thought of his desire for amputation as "doing to myself what I might have wanted to do to her [mother]." The examining psychiatrists concluded that his self-mutilative acts were counterphobic responses to castration anxiety and that his reaction to the stump of female amputees belied an unconscious belief that women possessed a penis. Further, they felt that his "crippled woman fetish" was linked to hostility toward women and that his symptoms served as a safety valve for his unconscious rage and destructiveness. They also reported that between May 1973 and January 1975 the widely distributed erotic magazine *Penthouse* published twenty letters on "monopede mania," in which readers described their sexual experiences with amputees. They also cited a popular comic book called *Amputee Love* that contained ambiguous drawings that made it difficult to distinguish a woman's stump from a penis.

Beresford (1980) reported the case of a 29-year-old man who was hospitalized for an elective amputation of his right lower leg. Two years earlier, he had shot himself in his right foot and calf. He described the shooting as an accident but his stepfather and the emergency room physicians believed it was done purposefully. When he was 5 years old, his mother had remarried, and he had began to regard his right leg as bad and alien. Periodically, he had tried to injure his leg, and during adolescence he put his leg in a plaster cast he had constructed. His favorite playmate as a youth was a young girl whose right leg was crippled from polio. His current complaint was that his leg was extremely painful. He sought a complete amputation but the surgeon recommended only a below-the-knee amputation.

During a psychiatric consultation, he described himself as a loner who lived in a cabin in the woods with a dog. His hair was shoulder length, and he wore a shirt with an antidraft slogan. He described an episode in which he angrily threw a man out of a third-story window as the most frightening time in his life. He was diagnosed as being a schizoid person who used counterphobic mechanisms, isolation, fantasy, hypochondria, and projection to defend against his feelings of aggression and who projected his aggressive impulses onto his right leg and desired to have the aggression removed surgically. After much discussion, he had a below-the-knee amputation. Although he refused psychotherapy, the patient reported no pain at a six-month follow-up and ambulated well with a permanent prosthesis.

The complete history of the fascination with disabled persons has yet to be written. The first worldwide conference on this fascination was held in 1985, and since that time gatherings have focused on disability and issues such as education, music, cinema, art, religion, and sexuality. The Internet has emerged as a major portal for information, chat rooms, and forums about both on-demand amputations and sexuality. A virtual community has developed. One of its major Web sites is called Overground: A Site for the Disabled and Their Admirers, the Devotees and the Wannabees (its motto, "Disability is a feature, not a defect").

In 1998, a widely circulated news story reported on a man who had failed to amputate his healthy leg but found a notorious surgeon (an article in *Forum* magazine labeled him "the worst doctor in America") who performed the amputation in a Tijuana, Mexico, motel room. The man died and the surgeon was convicted of second-degree murder.

The year 2000 saw a major increase in attention to on-demand amputation. In Scotland a surgeon amputated the healthy legs of two patients who had requested it, stating, "It was the most satisfying operation I have ever performed. I have no doubt that (it) was the correct thing for these patients." In a BBC documentary on the topic, two psychiatrists noted that psychotherapy "doesn't make a scrape of difference in these people," and that "this is a potentially fatal condition because people may unintentionally harm or kill themselves by performing self-amputations." Carl Elliott's *Atlantic Monthly* article, "A New Way to be Mad" (2000), created an intellectual stir. Also in 2000, Wise and Kalyanam published the first case of a man with acrotemnophilia who cut off his penis twice (the methodology was obtained on the Internet; limb lopping kits with "the Amazing Van Gogh Ear Remover" were advertised both on the Internet and on television) because of a fascination with the image of his penile stump. Surgeons had reattached it the first time. The patient had no desire to change his gender and admitted to spending many hours masturbating to his amputee pornography collection. Furth and Smith published their book on apotemnophilia in 2000.

The term *body integrity identity disorder* was coined by a social worker; she described the case of a man who used a shotgun to damage his healthy right knee to force a surgical amputation (Horn 2003). In 2005 Michael First, a psychiatrist at Columbia University, published the first serious, non–single case report study titled "Desire for Amputation of a Limb." He interviewed fifty-two subjects self-identified as having a desire to have an amputation. None were delusional. They reported that during childhood or early adolescence they developed a desire for an amputation because it would correct a mismatch between their anatomy and their sense of "true" self (identity). Neither psychotherapy nor medication diminished their desire. Six subjects self-amputated a limb, while three had healthy limbs amputated by a surgeon. Those whose amputations were at the precise, desired site reported feeling better than they ever had and had no interest in further amputations. First concluded the condition is "an unusual dysfunction in the development of one's fundamental sense of anatomical (body) identity."

Despite its relative rareness, BIID has stimulated thoughtful articles in publications such as *Quarterly Journal of Speech* (Jordan 2004); *Journal of Applied Philosophy* (Bayne and Levy 2005); *Journal of Law, Medicine, and Ethics* (Bridy 2004); *Neuroethics* (Ryan 2008); *Continuum: Journal of Media and Cultural Studies* (Sullivan 2005); *Sexuality and Disability* (Solvang 2007); and *Psychology Today* (Adams 2007). In general, these articles are sympathetic to the plight of persons who have BIID. (Also see the informative Web site at www.biid.org.) They note that healthy tissue is removed or modified on a large scale by surgeons (e.g., circumcision, breast reduction or augmentation, rhinoplasty, and sex reassignment). Those who have BIID do not want to change their gender, do not seek attention by physicians or cosmetic repair for a defect in body appearance or participation in the body modification subculture or financial gain. They are not delusional and do not respond to psychotherapy or medication. Legal surgery seems to be the only effective treatment, and persons who have BIID embrace their resulting disability as preferable to living with a limb that they do not recognize as part of their true body.

Several psychological theories have been proposed to explain the disorder, but the latest research points to a neurological cause, namely a failure to represent one or more limbs in the right superior parietal lobe in the brain. This amazing discovery is discussed in detail in chapter 10, as is the latest nonsurgical treatment in chapter 11.

CHAPTER SEVEN

The Skin

The skin is a thin layer of tissue that encloses the body. Physiologically, it is a fairly simple organ; socially and psychologically, however, it is highly complex. Persons may be judged and much of their fate determined, for example, by the color of their skin. Although we sometimes merge our sense of self-identity with that of another person or entity when we fall in love, participate in an intense group experience, or achieve some sort of mystical state, we normally live within our skins. All that is enclosed by my skin is me; everything else is not me. The skin is a border between the outer world and the inner world, the environment and the personal self.

The skin is also a message center or billboard. Through scarification and tattooing, for example, permanent messages about one's beliefs and social status are communicated. Temporary emotional states are also often communicated via the skin. Rage may be displayed by flushing, embarrassment or shame by blushing, and fear by blanching. Deliberate self-injury of the skin, a morbid self-help behavior, indicates that a person is attempting to cope with some form of emotional distress such as intense anxiety, depersonalization, suppressed rage, or fear of abandonment.

This chapter examines both culturally sanctioned body modification practices involving the skin, such as tattooing, branding and piercing, and deviant behaviors such as skin picking, cutting, carving, and burning.

Tattoos

Although tattooing is a universal practice of great antiquity, it reached its apotheosis in the Pacific Islands. Charles Darwin noted, "Not one great country can be named, from the Polar region in the north to New Zealand in the south, in which the aborigines do not tattoo themselves." The word *tattoo*, first recorded by Captain Cook, derives from a Polynesian word for knocking or striking (a sharp needle was dipped into pigment and knocked into the skin).

Polynesian tattooing, or *moko*, was done by a professional artist and symbolized social rank. Although the entire body was tattooed, special attention was given to the face, which was covered with circles, curved lines, and scroll-type indulged in tattoos to enhance their sense of self-pity; a woman who put the name or likeness of her pimp on her arm might be trying unconsciously to evoke the jealousy and wrath of her customers, so as to encourage mistreatment and further justification for self-pity. Parry believed that male homosexuals got tattooed as a method of admitting or even extolling their "perversion;" one man had the words *Open All Night* and *Pay as You Enter* inscribed on his buttocks. He also noted that some men tattooed their penises to facilitate seduction, and Asian prostitutes tattooed their sexual organs to ward off venereal disease. The pain of flogging was thought to be lessened if a sailor had a Christian cross tattooed on his back, and the tattoo of a pig on the left foot supposedly protected against drowning.

Ferguson-Rayport et al. (1955) considered tattoos to be akin to a projective psychological test. Personality disordered patients were more apt to have multiple tattoos that dealt with pornographic, sentimental, bombastic, and pseudo-heroic themes, for example, tattoos of cartoon characters or the words *Fuck the Army* on the hand used to salute superiors. Schizophrenic patients were more apt to have solitary tattoos, sometimes placed on unusual sites, that dealt with idealistic or magical themes (also see Goldstein 1979; Goldstein and Sewell 1979).

In modern times, tattoos have become mainstream in Western cultures and tattoo parlors can be found in small towns just about everywhere. Even among a small but growing subculture within evangelical Christianity the term " Marked for Jesus" refers to religious tattoos as a legitimate expression of individuality, identity, and faith (Flory and Jensen 2000). In 2003, the American Museum of Natural History, in New York City, had an exhibition surveying four thousand years of skin decoration titled "Body Art: Marks of Identity." The overwhelming majority of tattoos are innocuous—a butterfly on the ankle, decorations across the lower back of females (sarcastically called a "tramp stamp")—with little or no significance except possibly to demonstrate that a person is faddishly modern or is tweaking his or her parents gently. Undoubtedly athletes, especially professional basketball players, have served as models for young men with dreams of glory. In an interesting interview (Hochman 2009) the currently most tattooed team, the Denver Nuggets, described their unique markings—"I'd never get the same tattoos as the next guy unless we win the NBA trophy championship, and we all get that trophy tattooed on us." One player has "Mama's Boy" on his chest because his mother is his best friend and offers good advice. Other players have slogans such as "Hustle" on one leg and "Harder" on the other, or "No pain" on one arm and "No game" on the other. One player, known as "The Birdman," has wings tattooed on both arms as well as a host of other possibly meaningful tattoos such as "Honkey-Tonk" in large letters on his lower chest. Mike Tyson, the boxer, self-tattooed a Maori *moko* warrior design around his left arm and eye.

Tattoo enthusiasts hold conventions to admire and outdo competitors. There are many tattoo Web sites, and the print and television media have given undue coverage to persons who have unusual markings all over their body. My impression is that most persons with tattoos that are excessive beyond the typical mores of Western tradition have little insight, usually say, "I just like the way my tattoos look," and become angry at the suggestion that their tattoos might reflect psychological "issues." In the not so distant past, psychiatrists used the word *neurosis* to describe persons who have unresolved mental and emotional conflicts, often going back to childhood, that exist in the unconscious but affect current behavior. Some excessively tattooed persons are in it for show business, and many for subtle or not so subtle fashion adornment, but many others use their tattoos to gain the attention that perhaps was denied them in the past, to live out a fantasy, and to resolve, albeit indirectly, unresolved conflicts. This formulation seems evident in the cases of a meek young man with tattoos of ferocious animals on his chest and arms, and of the daughter of a conservative rabbi who is heavily tattooed despite strict prohibitions against her behavior.

Scarification

Scarification, the process of cutting the skin to produce scars, is done for aesthetic and social reasons. While the traditions of Christianity, Islam, and Hinduism accept mortification of the flesh as a worthwhile and holy practice, they do not encourage permanent lesions. Darkly pigmented skin is not particularly suitable for tattooing, but its tendency to form keloids, or hypertrophied scars, accentuates scarification.

Scarification is less common in Africa now than in the past and many governments have passed laws prohibiting it. It is done for aesthetic reasons, to produce distinctive tribal marks, to fulfill ritual requirements, and even for medical purposes—e.g., a star cut on the skin over the liver is thought to prevent hepatic disease (Brain 1979).

The Tiv of Nigeria scarify themselves primarily for aesthetic reasons (Bohannon 1956). Some designs on Tiv females are characteristic and immutable over generations, while others change just as Western clothing fashions do. Lincoln (1981) uncovered another extremely significant purpose. The key to Tiv social organization is genealogy; it determines territorial rights, suitability of marriage partners, land usage, and much personal behavior. The Tiv who live in a territorial segment (called a *tar*) consider themselves to be descended from a common patrilineal ancestor. When a *tar* is threatened by conflicts, rituals involving a decorated sacred object are performed by a secret group of elders. The fertility of the land and the well-being of the *tar* depend on this sacred object. When it must be replaced or repaired, the elders use sacrificial blood of an aborted fetus from a woman who is pregnant for the first time, as her fertility is concentrated in the fetus. The blood is poured through the central hole of the sacred object and then is scattered onto the fields and into wells, thus ensuring a good harvest.

The sacred objects of the Tiv are carved statues of women. The decorations on the objects roughly duplicate the scarification patterns inscribed on females at puberty. These scars represent Tiv family, heritage, land, traditions, genealogy, and myths. Thus, according to Lincoln, the scarification "may represent the structure of time, placing the pubescent girl at the intersection of past and future. Beyond that, it may be taken as a picture of genealogical descent, whereby she is shown to be heir of the ancestors, bearer of descendents, and guarantor of the lineage's continuity" (p. 48). The scarification transforms the girl both into a woman and into a sacred object on whom the *tar*'s fertility depends. The scars anchor time and space and to ensure the continuity of life.

Scarification is associated with rebirth and with the development of masculinity during initiation ceremonies among the Kagoro of Papua New Guinea. On the day of the ritual, teenage boys are beaten with sticks as a reminder of their submission to the tribal elders (among the Elema tribe, initiates let the chief urinate in their mouths). The painful skin-cutting ritual is held in the men's ceremonial house. Razor blades are used to "cut double circles around the boy's nipples and to make a wide band of incisions in a curved serpentlike pattern symmetrically on the right and left side of the body, first on the upper arms, chest, and abdomen, then from the shoulders down the back to the lateral aspect of the thigh" (Jilek and Jilek-Aall 1978, p. 255). A crocodilelike skin pattern is formed over much of their bodies, which are then covered with oil and mud to produce raised scars; such a pattern is associated with the belief in huge, reptilian monsters that embody the masculine-aggressive principle. Amid the noise of drums and bull-roarers, the boys' pet dogs are clubbed to death and "carried off dangling from a pole like slaughtered pigs." When the wounds are healed, the boys emerge from the ceremonial house and go on public display while the women of the village rejoice and dance. The boys are reborn as men and are strengthened by bloody ordeals to compensate for the perceived lesser biological endurance of the male sex. They also are rid of the polluting female blood that accumulated in their bodies during gestation and suckling.

In many cultures, branding is a form of scarification in which the skin is heated to produce a scar. The traditional method is to apply a hot piece of metal, but new methods employ electrocautery and lasers. Like tattoos, branding has been used as a mark of identity (slaves, military deserters, criminals, etc.) but in modern times is chosen electively as a form of permanent body modification. The process of branding is far more complex than tattooing and depends on the temperature of the heat, the amount of time that the heat is applied, the pressure used, the placement of the brand, and a person's skin type. Some African American college fraternities crudely brand new pledges as an initiation rite and some people get branded to mark a meaningful life event, but the majority consider branding for aesthetic reasons. Branding is not a procedure to be taken lightly, and the number of professionally trained branders is few. Although many tattoos can be removed (a costly and time-consuming procedure), branding is almost always forever.

Body Piercing

The centrality of ritual piercing reached its apotheosis among the Olmecs, Aztecs, and Maya of Central America. In addition to elaborate tattoos, head molding, and teeth filing, these groups were prodigious piercers of the penis and of the tongue with stingray spines, needles, flint blades, and bones (Christensen 1989; Schele and Miller 1986). The purpose of their piercings was to draw blood to atone for their sins and to appease the gods. By piercing his penis, from which flowed royal blood, the Maya believed that their king nourished the land and its people. Men anointed roadside idols with their penis blood. In a temple ceremony, priests had their penises pierced with a needle whose thread attached them to each other to produce a cascade of blood. Intricate carvings show kings piercing their penis while their wives simultaneously pierce their tongues. The great Aztec god, Quetzacoatl, did penance by piercing his legs and established his right to rule by piercing his penis.

Tamil Hindus' body piercing is central to their worship of Lord Murugan, whose conveyance is a peacock and whose symbol is a *vel* (a sacred lance). At his Thaipusam festival devotees, after a period of training, go into trance and pierce their cheeks and tongues with replicas of the *vel*. Some honor him by carrying a kavati, a heavy mini-alter festooned with flowers to mimic a peacock, which is attached to their bodies by multiple fish hooks. Festivals similar to Thaipusam have become popular with tourists who enjoy the joviality of the environment and are shocked that the piercings are, despite the vascularity of the tongue, bloodless.

Piercings for sexual reasons using hypoallergenic metal rings and bars include the nipple, penis, scrotum, and external female genitalia. In nipple piercing, a ring is usually centered horizontally and inserted through the base of the nipple. Healing in men takes a month or two, while in women it may take a year. The rings can be painful if the breasts become engorged during menses. Difficulties such as blocked milk ducts and problems with sucking the nipple may result from breast feeding with the piercings in place (Deacon et al. 2009). The baby's gums, tongue, and palate also may be injured.

Piercings of the penis and scrotum use rings or barbells. There are at least forty types (see the BME Web site, www.bmezine.) so I shall mention only a few. The apadrayva involves a painful process in which a barbell is inserted through the glans (tip) of the penis from front to back and may take up to a year to heal. It is mentioned in the Kama Sutra (A.D. 700) and supposedly is the piercing that provides the most pleasure for women. The ampallang also involves piercing the glans, but from side to side and also may pass through the urethra; the passage of urine helps to clean the piercing and facilitates healing. Some women find this piercing irritating and may damage their back teeth and soft palate during fellatio. In the so-called Prince Albert piercing a carved or circular ring is inserted near the frenulum and exits through the urethra. It is perhaps the most common penis piercing, although it usually does not enhance a woman's pleasure and it causes urine to spray haphazardly. A guiche piercing is placed through the skin between the anus and the scrotum. Weighted beads or attachments may be added to this piercing to enhance pleasurable sensations. Scrotum piercing can be done with a wide variety of jewelry. Some men may have ten or more scrotal piercings. They are just for show, however, because they provide no sexual stimulation to either the man or his partner.

Among the many types of female genital piercing, the most common is the horizontal hood (often mistakenly called a "clit ring"), in which a ring is inserted with its bead resting on the clitoris, thus providing continual stimulation. It is both easy to do and fast healing. Both the inner and outer labia can be pierced; the Princess Albertina piercing passes through the urethra. There is even a Princess Diana piercing, in which two small rings or bars are placed under the hood next to the clitoris.

I have described only a few of the many different types of piercings that are available nowadays, mostly at the same shops that offer tattoos. Piercings, also, may result in minor (20%) and major (3%) medical complications (Ross 2000; Stewart 2001). Allergic reactions—especially to jewelry containing nickel—can cause skin to itch, weep, and form crusts. Any piercing can become infected and bacterial seeding may affect heart valves. Unsterilized piercing instruments can transmit viruses such as HIV, hepatitis, and genital warts. Hypertrophic scars (keloids) can be ugly and difficult to repair. Jewelry can migrate from its original site and be rejected by the body; this is often caused by direct trauma to the jewelry and by pressure or friction from tight clothing. Thick gauge rings should be used in the navel to prevent migration or rejection. Some penis piercings can become problematic unless the jewelry is sized when the penis is erect. Piercings in areas with poor blood supply, such as ear cartilage, can result in serious infections with abscess formation, decayed tissue, and ear deformation. Tongue jewelry can result in gingival injury and chipped teeth. (For studies about medical complications see Boardman and Smith 1997; Koenig and Carnes 1999; Samantha et al. 1998; Smith 1997; Widick and Coleman 1992). The BME Web site lists 154 risks associated with piercing and modification. Among those that I had not anticipated are anal buttplug capture, reduced ejaculatory distance, divorce, and psychiatric commitment! The last actually may be significant. In an unpublished talk at the 2005 annual meeting of the American Association of Suicidology a well-known research psychologist, David Lester, reported on a survey of 4,700 persons who had frequented the BMEzine site. The median age of the respondents was 21 years; 88 percent were white; 45 percent were students; 56 percent were heterosexual, 38 percent were bisexual, and 5 percent homosexual. Only 34 percent had never contemplated suicide, while 39 percent had contemplated it, and 27 percent had made one or more attempts. Among those who had attempted suicide were 27 percent of men and 46 percent of women with pierced eyebrows, 24 percent of men with a tongue piercing, and 39 percent of men and 48 percent of women with shoulder or upper arm scarifications.

I will discuss the issues of body modification and of "body play" in chapter 9.

Human Pincushions

Gould and Pyle (1896) compiled medical reports on a nineteenth-century European phenomenon, namely, the practice by "hysterical" women of sticking pins into their bodies. In one case, 217 needles were removed from the abdomen of a young woman during an eighteen-month period. Her physician first thought that she swallowed the needles during an epileptic seizure, but after removing one hundred additional needles from a tumor on her shoulder he discovered that she was sticking them into herself. Another case described a 26-year-old woman who, while in prison awaiting trial, pressed thirty pins and needles into her chest. She used her prayer book as a hammer. On autopsy, needles were found in her lungs, mediastinum, and liver. Her descending vena cava was perforated, and her left ventricle had a needle sticking in it.

There were probably two cultural influences on the behavior of "needle girls." The first was a fascination with media reports from the Near East about holy men who placed their bodies on beds of nails. More significant was the popularity of entertainers who called themselves human pincushions. The best known was Edward H. Gibson, a vaudeville performer who invited audience members to thrust pins into any part of his body except his abdomen and groin. He offered $5,000 to any physician able to detect signs of pain. On one occasion, he erected a wooden cross on the stage and prepared to have himself crucified. An assistant hammered a spike through the palm of Gibson's hand, but the act was stopped when some people in the audience collapsed. Gibson had a congenital indifference to pain (Dearborn 1932).

The practice of sticking needles into the skin is still encountered although not written about very much. A colleague in England told me of a 32-year-old man whom he saw in a hospital emergency room. The patient went there because "one of his needles" had become embedded in his chest wall. At the age of 10, he used to sew his fingers together with needle and thread. He progressed to sticking sewing needles into his body, especially his chest, in a compulsive manner. The needle sticking was described as painful and bloody. It caused his nipples to become erect and was followed by masturbation. Alfred Kinsey, the great sex researcher, allegedly stuck pins into his scrotum while masturbating. All of the needle-sticking patients I have encountered personally also cut and burned their skin. Their usual practice is to stick sewing needles under the skin of their arms, legs, chest, and abdomen. They then massage the area so that the needles migrate from the point of entry, thus hampering any attempts to remove the needles surgically. The needles may get into the blood stream and become inserted into the heart (Jagmeet et al. 1992; Mihmanli et al. 2002).

Inert charm needles, or *susuks*, are inserted under the skin of the face, neck, and skull of some women in Southeast Asia to enhance or preserve beauty, youth, charisma, health, or success in business. They show up on radiographs usually as an incidental finding (Lim and Seet 2005; Nor et al. 2006). In a type of acupuncture called *hari*, hundreds of small needles are permanently inserted under the skin in various parts of the body. These needles may cause serious injury when they migrate into patient's brains, hearts, bladders, chests, abdomens, and spinal columns. (Baek et al. 1992; Gerard et al. 1993; Hama and Kaji 2004; Kim et al. 2006; Roy J 1974; Shiraeshi et al. 1979; Ullroth and Haines 2007).

"Needle freaks" are well known within the drug subculture. They seem to de-

rive so much gratification from injecting themselves that the act of sticking themselves with a needle is as important as the drug itself. Some heroin addicts, for
example, are able to obtain pleasure and to reduce withdrawal symptoms merely
by sticking a needle into their arms. Some therapists note that many addicts request acupuncture as part of their treatment. Regardless of what physiological
process (if any) took place, the needle sticking itself gratifies some basic need in
these addicts.

A brief media frenzy ensued in 2008 when William Shiels, a radiologist in
Ohio, reported on nine teenage girls and one teenage boy who collectively had
inserted more than fifty objects—needles, staples, paperclips, glass, wood, plastic, pencil lead, crayons, and small stones—under the skin of their arms, ankles,
feet, hands, and neck (Fauber 2008). Nine of the subjects had a history of nonsuicidal self-injury (NSSI), four had been sexually abused, and all had psychiatric
diagnoses such as bipolar disorder, depression, post-traumatic stress disorder,
or a borderline personality. Both the physicians involved and the media tried to
make the case for "self-embedding disorder," but the insertion of objects into the
body is widespread and hardly new. It is a behavior, not a disorder, associated with
many mental illnesses. Skin cutting, for example, is a far more common behavior
but is not recognized as a mental disorder in its own right.

Skin Lesions

Obsessive-compulsive disorder is a well-defined mental illness, but many psychiatrists believe that there are other conditions with recurrent or intrusive thoughts,
impulses, images, and behaviors that fall within the category of obsessive-
compulsive spectrum disorders. Two of these are psychogenic skin excoriation
(Stein et al. 1993) and trichotillomania.

In psychogenic skin excoriations (aka neurotic excoriations, dermatillomania),
persons repetitively and excessively scratch, rub, dig at, squeeze, and gouge mostly
normal skin tissue but also skin tissue that was once problematic, such as old
acne lesions, scars, scabs, or insect bites (Cyr and Dreher 2001). Every part of the
body except for areas that cannot be reached is victimized. Girls with acne start
early, but the majority of cases involve women over the age of thirty years. Exco-
riators simply cannot resist the urge to damage their skin. Many are anxious and/
or depressed. The worst case I ever saw was a 25-year-old man whose entire body,
except for his back and genitalia, was scratched raw. After prolonged excoriations
the affected areas may become hard and coarse (chronic lichen simplex). Some
patients bite off and eat the skin of their finger joints and nails. This condition is

associated with both infections and social morbidity (e.g., shame or embarrassment at being seen in public). The act of excoriation may provide momentary relief from itching (the differential diagnosis of itching is long and ranges from dry skin to renal and liver failure to diabetes); in some persons it has a pleasurable component. Skin picking is also seen in body dysmorphic disorder but it is focused on an anatomical spot, often on the face, that is normal but is perceived to be ugly or deformed (Phillips et al. 2008). This disorder may have a higher rate of suicide than any other mental illness.

Trichotillomania (hair pulling) is another obsessive-compulsive spectrum disorder (although it is officially classified as an impulse control disorder). The scalp, eyelashes, and eyebrows are the most common targets, but hair may be pulled from the pubis and other body areas as well. The behavior may occur automatically outside of a person's awareness or it may be done intentionally in response to a distressing urge, thought, or sensation such as itching or burning in a hairy area. Some people eat the hair; a large enough hair ball (trichobezoar) can result in failure to absorb food properly, anemia, weight loss, intestinal obstruction, and even death. Comorbid disorders include anxiety and depression. In severe cases lifestyle restrictions and intimacy problems are prevalent, sometimes resulting in suicidal thoughts.

Factitious dermatitis (dermatitis artifacta) is another NSSI involving the skin. In this disorder persons create all sorts of lesions on their skin for the purpose of assuming the sick role and receiving medical attention, usually from dermatologists. The lesions often are created in areas that can be reached by the dominant hand and are produced by scratching, pinching, eroding, blistering, gouging, burning, applying caustic chemicals, glass shards—just about any means imaginable. The disorder has been reported in both pediatric and geriatric patients but mainly in young adult females. Some lesions mimic known skin disorders but typically are odd and have an unusual distribution. Misdiagnosis may have disastrous consequences. As noted by Hollender and Abram (1973, p. 1284), "The extreme occurs when the diagnosis is missed and a consulting surgeon, intending to be helpful, adds his mutilating procedures to the patient's own." Perhaps the most dramatic of these cases is that of a 31-year-old woman who suddenly developed gangrene of her left little finger, resulting in its amputation. Tricking her physicians, she was able to produce more gangrenous lesions and underwent thirty-three surgical amputations until her entire left arm had been removed (Thomas 1937). Patients who have this type of NSSI both enjoy being a "difficult" case while displaying a certain indifference to their illness. They almost always deny producing their lesions and go doctor shopping. Many may be diagnosed with a borderline personality disorder. The course of the disorder ranges from brief to chronic. (See Gregurek-Novak et al. 2005; Koblenzer 2000; Nielsen et al. 2005; Saez-de-Ocariz et al. 2004; Shah and Fried 2006; Urgulu et al. 1999; Verraes-Derancourt et al. 2006.)

A more serious type of NSSI occurs in persons who have delusions of parasitosis (Trabert 1995). These individuals are convinced that their skin is infested with parasites, insects, or tiny organisms. To rid themselves of these imaginary bugs, they gouge their skin with fingernails, knives, and needles, and even caustic solutions. Examination of the skin may reveal discrete lesions or linear tracks where "parasites" have been pursued. The typical patient is a middle-aged or older woman who, when she seeks help, brings a bag with pieces of her skin, dried blood, and dirt for the physician to inspect (Frances and Munro 1989). Unlike neurotics, these patients do not experience relief from excoriation. Psychological assessment reveals delusions of persecution as well as concern over sexual contamination (Zaidens 1951). Guilt and resentment, often stemming from a fantasized relationship with a parent, are projected onto the skin. This focusing on the skin—a circumscribed delusion—may be, in fact, a defense against more global psychological deterioration.

Delusions of parasitosis may be singular. or as with other tactile hallucinations, may be associated with schizophrenia, depression, drug use (especially cocaine and methamphetamine), and a host of medical conditions (diabetes, multiple sclerosis, cancer, vitamin B12 deficiency, hypothyroidism, etc.) in which patients seem to experience bugs crawling on, burrowing into, or residing in their skin. Persons who have this disorder may convince other family members that they too are infested by parasites. The European literature refers to patients who have chronic feelings of insects falling or crawling on their skin as well as biting and prickling sensations in the absence of other psychiatric findings or the usual delusions of parasitosis (Conrad and Bers 1954).

A related condition was proposed by a woman in 2001 who reported that she found red, white, blue, and black fibers emanating from sores on her 2-year-old son. She called it Morgellons disease after a one-line description in a 1690 letter written by the English physician-writer, Sir Thomas Brown, of an endemic distemper in French children "called the morgellons; wherein they critically break out with harsh hairs on their back." The literature on this condition is recent and highly controversial. The "fibers" that people pull out of these lesions have never really been identified and many experts believe they come from clothing. Passions about this putative disorder run high, and there is a large virtual community of persons linked by the Internet who believe they have this disorder. Due to congressional pressure, the federal Centers for Disease Control and Prevention formed a task force in 2006 to do research on Morgellons and has been joined by medical organizations. Theories about its cause range from infection with an organism (agrobacterium) that induces cellulose fiber production in plants, a mass hysteria propelled by the media and the Internet, a reaction to pesticides, and even a form of alien bioterror. (See Murase et al. 2006; Savely et al. 2006.)

Case Studies of Skin Cutters

The case of Helen Miller is among the best-documented cases of self-cutting (Channing 1877–78). At the age of 29, after two years of incarceration, Miller was discharged from the New York Asylum for Insane Criminals. A few months later she was sent to jail for stealing a stuffed canary and a microscope lens from a physician. At least a dozen physicians treated her for opiate addiction and for dysmenorrhea. To gain admittance to the asylum, she began to "cut up." She

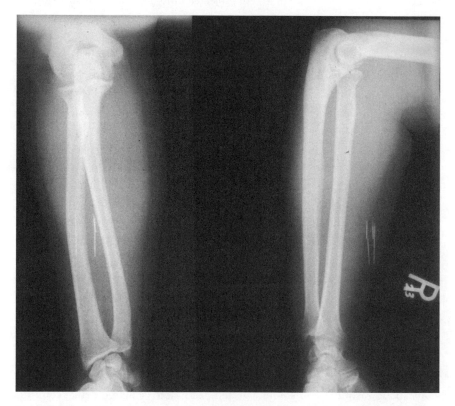

X-ray of the arm of a woman who inserted sewing needles under her skin.

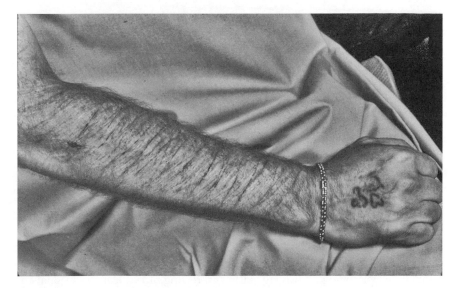

The arm of a 39-year-old man, much of whose life has been spent in institutions, including orphanages, prison, and mental hospitals. He said, "I reach out for help by cutting myself. It may be stupid, but I get results. People help me when I cut."

periodically slashed herself; at final count ninety-four pieces of glass, thirty-four splinters, four shoe nails, one pin, and one needle had been removed from her arms. On one occasion, "the skin and superficial fascia were cut in a straight line and as cleanly as if done by a surgeon, but the muscular tissue below was hacked in every direction and nearly to the bone" (pp. 370–71). She felt no pain when inflicting her wounds and seemed to experience erotic pleasure when the doctors probed her flesh to remove objects. She had episodes during which she cursed and abused other patients, neither ate nor slept, and begged to be left alone. These outbursts terminated after several days either in continued NSSI or utter exhaustion. At the age of 30, her delusions of persecution intensified and indications of dementia emerged. While it is likely that she had neurosyphilis, her self-injury was diagnosed as hysterical in origin. Her psychiatrist mistakenly considered her self-injurious acts to be attempted suicides. This important theme is discussed in chapter 10.

The early psychoanalytic literature viewed self-cutting as symbolic castration in order to avoid real castration, as Rado (1933) put it, "the choice of the lesser evil." Novotny (1972) regarded cutting as a masochistic phenomenon. Because both rage and sexual gratification result from the cutting, he surmised that guilt may follow, which, in part, is atoned for by the injury, much in the same way

Sioux warriors cut their chest muscles to atone for the unconscious wish to bite the breast of the frustrating mother, according to Erickson (1950). Novotny found that many cutters, when stress is intense, project "oral rage" onto the environment. Rather than suffer passively from some fantasized attack, they take control and cut themselves, reconstituting their ego functions to a certain degree; for example, cutting helps patients distinguish between reality and fantasy, between what is "inside" and what is "outside."

Winnicott (1958) discussed a woman who, fascinated by autocannibalism, had fantasies about lost Arctic explorers who ate parts of their bodies to survive. The woman mutilated herself by eating pieces of her fingers. Winnicott considered her act to be one of "experiencing." He noted that each person who reaches "the stage of being a unit with a limiting membrane and an outside and an inside . . . [has] an inner reality . . . an inner world which can be rich and poor or can be at peace or in a state of war" (p. 230). An intermediate part of the life of a human being is "experiencing . . . [which] exists as a resting place for the individual engaged in the perpetual human task of keeping inner and outer reality separate yet interrelated" (p. 230). Kafka (1969) developed the theme of experiencing in a psychoanalytic study of a young woman who had the "exquisite border experience of sharply becoming alive" at the moment of cutting herself. She described the flow of blood as being like a voluptuous bath whose pleasant warmth spread over her body, molding its contour and sculpting its form. She was at a loss to understand why everyone did not indulge in blood baths, especially because they were readily accessible simply by "unzipping" one's skin. The patient described her blood to Kafka as a transitional object, "a potential security blanket capable of giving warmth and comforting envelopment," which was linked to her internalized mother. Because the patient did not always consider her skin to be her own, cutting it was a "transitional choice between the sadistic and masochistic object." Kafka felt that the elimination of skin cutting might result when the patient re-formed a more bodily-ego-syntonic skin membrane. The process he recommended was the working through of the transference and, especially, of the countertransference; for example, the patient decreased her NSSI when Kafka "experienced fully my inability to save her life."

Kwawer (1980) reported on his intensive psychotherapy with a 23-year-old cutter who had borderline personality disorder. In childhood her family was exceptionally attentive to her physical appearance. Her parents fought, sometimes to the point of physical violence and separation. She worked with several therapists who treated her with medications but were unable to help her stop cutting herself, pulling out her sutures, and setting fire to her bandages. When she entered the hospital, treatment was exclusively psychotherapy. She cut herself badly when her therapist went on vacation. She experienced shame over her bodily functions and described her menses as disgusting. She collected her blood and saved it; in stressful times the jar of blood had a calming effect on her. Therapy focused on her feelings and fears of being alone and abandoned and on her sexual identity: "Becoming more openly erotic in her attachment to me, she stared at my groin in treatment hours, trying to visualize my genitals, and had fantasies about my sexual relationships" (p. 212). The nursing staff dealt with her cutting matter-of-factly, treated her injuries as medical problems, and did not capitulate to her demands for "caring." Kwawer felt that her angry demands for demonstrations of his concern were an insistence that he "take responsibility for behavior we both knew only she could control." She developed a vampiristic ritual— sipping or drinking her blood every night, mixing dried blood with water if no fresh blood were available. Her requests for medication were denied, and she became more open in psychotherapy, where her fantasies about homosexuality, prostitution, masturbation, and abnormal sexual urges were explored. She was elected chairman of the patient community group, learned to drive, bought a car, secured a part-time job, actively pursued her interest in pottery, and planned for her discharge. She went to live in a halfway house, continued outpatient therapy, and stopped cutting. Kwawer concluded that "only after a direct confrontation in the treatment with her self-mutilation, vampiristic rituals, and psychotic mother, was it possible to carry on a therapeutic inquiry into the developmental issue of womanhood around which [her] adult life had faltered" (p. 215)

The importance of depersonalization in some instances of skin cutting is clear in the case of a 20-year-old man who was hospitalized for the first time after cutting his wrists (Miller and Baskhin 1974). His symptoms of mutism, negativism, confusion, disorientation, and psychomotor retardation resulted in a diagnosis of catatonic schizophrenia. Three weeks after discharge, he went on a drinking binge and awoke in a jail to learn that he had assaulted, robbed, and nearly killed a man. He spent the next four years in prison, where he cut himself a dozen times. Upon release from prison, he planned to marry, but at the last moment his fiancée changed her mind. The patient decompensated and was hospitalized for two years (which is when the article was written). He incessantly cut himself on the arms, legs, chest, and abdomen. His chest cuts exposed his ribs, while the limb cuts went deep into muscle; once he even cut into his peritoneum. His psychiatrists determined that he "mutilated himself to terminate states of acute depersonalization characterized by feelings of unreality, deadness, and depression, of being outside himself and not in full control of his actions" (p. 641). He was unable to recount the events of his life in a meaningful chronology; because of innumerable episodes of depersonalization, he experienced life as a series of discontinuous episodes. His "claim that he could tell when each wound was inflicted and what the circumstances were surrounding the mutilation leads to the conclusion that he preserved in the flesh, in a dramatic and conspicuous manner, the history of events he could not integrate into the fabric of his personality" (p. 647).

Bliss (1980) reported on self-cutting among women with the rare diagnosis of multiple personality. The cuttings—sometimes brutal ones—were done by alter egos. One patient reported while hypnotized: "When I was 19, Sarah [a personality] cut my foot [a deep gash with a broken piece of glass]. She couldn't hurt my stepfather so she hurt me. She just gets angry, and I get hurt. . . . She cut my wrist with a big long knife to punish me because I'm weak" (p. 1392). Bliss had only female cutters in his sample. He felt that while women usually direct their rage against themselves, men direct their anger against others who presumably symbolize brutal relatives in early life. Another study of one hundred patients with this disorder found that seventy-one had a history of suicidal gestures. "Internal homicide" behavior in which one personality attempted to kill an alternate personality was found in fifty-three patients, while NSSI, which was usually inflicted on one personality as punishment by another, was observed in thirty-four patients (Putnam et al. 1986).

Siomopoulos (1974) regarded skin cutting as an impulse neurosis strongly linked with sexual symbolism; for example, skin cutting supposedly represents the creation of multiple little female genitalia on the skin, "which become available for uninhibited touching, handling, and all sorts of manipulations" (p. 90). In one case report a young woman had a history of intense masturbations in childhood. At menarche she was preoccupied with religious ideas. She was sent to a convent school where she cut her breasts and abdomen. The impulse to cut followed periods of extreme tension and was irresistible. She cut herself frequently, "with mixed feelings of pleasure and guilt." She dreaded sexual contacts and avoided dating. She was hospitalized but continued cutting. The behavior became less frequent as she participated in therapy that dealt with her fears about sexual relationships and her early masturbatory activity.

In recent decades, stories about individual, mainly female, cutters have appeared only in the lay press. One of the best, about an attractive, blonde, upper-middle-class cheerleader at a Catholic school, was featured on the cover of the *New York Times Magazine* (Egan 1997). Many brief, dramatic stories are told in *The Bright Red Scream* (Strong 1998). Caroline Kettlewell's *Skin Game* (1999) is both a minor literary masterpiece and an insightful memoir of her life as a cutter and of her recovery.

Group Studies of Skin Cutters

Self-cutting, especially wrist cutting, became a focus of psychiatric interest in the 1960s, and pioneering studies helped to shed light on the characteristics of cutters and the reasons for their behavior. They set the foundation for an understanding of the skin-cutting phenomenon. A number (Asch 1971; Burnham 1969; Grunebaum and Klerman 1967; Pao 1969) portray the typical wrist slasher as "an attractive, intelligent, unmarried young woman, who is either promiscuous or overtly afraid of sex, easily addicted and unable to relate to others. . . . She slashes her wrists indiscriminately and repeatedly at the slightest provocation, but she does not commit suicide. She feels relief with the commission of her act" (Graff and Mallin 1967, p. 41). These investigators considered most self-cutters to be schizophrenic or borderline.

Nelson and Grunebaum (1971) reported on twenty-three wrist slashers, mainly white females, who were seen for follow-up five to six years after the initial contact. Six were diagnosed as psychotic, eight borderline, and two neurotic. Three intermittently psychotic patients had committed suicide. Only two psychotic, four borderline, and both neurotic patients had improved. Patients attributed their decline or cessation in cutting mainly to increased ability to cope with sexual and angry feelings, to marriage with its responsibilities, and to therapy. Improvement was associated with increased verbal expression of feelings, with new constructive behavior, and with control of psychotic symptoms; insight into the genesis of slashing behavior was not helpful.

Twenty-four hospitalized women who repeatedly cut their wrists had the following characteristics: (1) a history of NSSI, such as rubbing glass fragments into their faces, carving initials in their skin, repeatedly traumatizing fresh fractures, and cutting themselves on the legs, abdomen, and face; (2) a history of surgery, hospitalization for serious illness, or lacerations requiring multiple sutures before the age of 5; (3) irregular menstrual periods, frequent amenorrhea, and a negative reaction to menarche; (4) confused sexual identity; and (5) complaints of depression, chronic feelings of emptiness, and eating disorders such as anorexia and/or bulimia. Most of the wrist cutting done in the hospital was a reaction to separation or rejection; for example, it occurred during active planning for discharge or just before the therapist's vacation. The patients described themselves as numb, unreal, or empty immediately before cutting. During and after the cutting episodes, they felt satisfied, relieved, and even happy and fascinated at the sight and warmth of their blood. Rosenthal et al. (1972) interpreted these findings to mean that the patients experienced mounting anxiety that led to frightening depersonalization; cutting terminated the depersonalization—"a primitive way of combating the feelings of unreality and emptiness." Further, because 60 percent of the episodes occurred during menses, wrist cutting was possibly a means of dealing with genital trauma and conflicts about menstruation. The cutting thus represented a form of vicarious menstruation that was regulated and predictable rather than passive and frightening.

In England, Gardner and Gardner (1975) did a controlled study of female habitual self-cutters. The most common experience leading to self-cutting was an unpleasant feeling of tension that intensified until the patients experienced relief by cutting their skins. Only seven of twenty-two patients had depersonalization before cutting.

Simpson (1975) compared twenty-four Canadian wrist cutters with a control group of persons who had attempted suicide by self-poisoning. Each group had twenty females and four males. The cutters differed significantly from the controls in having major mood instability; complaints of "emptiness"; a strong interest and/or job in a paramedical field; excessive use of alcohol and drugs; a history of compulsive overeating and/or anorexia; negative reactions to menarche and menstruation; a history of surgery or hospitalization in early childhood and of a home broken by divorce, death, and parental deprivation; difficulties in verbalizing emotions and needs; and a pattern of painless cutting and bleeding after a period of depersonalization, followed by relaxation and repersonalization.

Another English study (Roy 1978) compared twenty nonpsychotic inpatients, who had cut themselves at least twice, with a control group. The cutters (thirteen women and seven men) were significantly more introverted, neurotic, and hostile, had more sadomasochistic fantasies, made more suicide attempts, and reported excessive physical punishment in childhood. Personality disorder was diagnosed in eighteen cutters. The main reasons given for cutting were self-anger (seven patients) and a need to relieve tension (six patients).

Simpson and Porter (1981) studied twenty children and adolescents (sixteen girls and four boys) hospitalized for NSSI. Their average age was 15 years. Although all of the subjects were periodically suicidal, none intended to commit suicide through self-injury. Most of the girls cut their arm or wrist; several cut their breasts, burned themselves with cigarettes, or punched themselves until bloody or bruised. The boys typically cut their arm and/or penis. General characteristics of the group included eating disorders, abuse of alcohol and drugs, a history of physical abuse by family members (often including sexual abuse), and a sense of abandonment, isolation, and unlovability. The authors felt that the acts of NSSI were (1) a form of stimulation that enabled the person to "feel something" other than terrifying isolation; (2) a method of satisfying physical and sexual needs that historically were met through violent and bizarre activity; (3) an outlet for anger and rage; (4) a means of self-punishment for real or imagined transgressions or for loving fantasies toward parental figures; (5) a dramatic request for help; and (6) a relatively safe, controlled method of reducing painful emotional trauma. NSSI neither killed the patient, as would suicide, nor physically harmed others who contributed to the patient's survival.

New types of group studies emerged in the late 1990s and are discussed in chapters 9 and 10. These studies are more focused, focusing, for example, on the roles in cutting of impulsivity, childhood trauma, interpersonal communication, and the like, and offering behavioral, developmental, biological, and other models for understanding self-injury.

Self-cutting in Total Institutions

Mental hospitals and correctional facilities are high-risk areas for NSSI, most commonly cutting. A good predictor of such behavior among prisoners is the presence of scars on the wrists and arms upon entering prison (Jones 1986). Major self-mutilation is rare. A seventeen-year case review of inmates at a Canadian regional penitentiary uncovered only seven cases of attempted or successful self-castration. Four were transsexuals who had been refused sex reassignment surgery (Conacher and Westwood 1987).

The increased incidence of NSSI is due to both the presence of individual psychopathology and the nature of life in total institutions. Living where behavior is closely scrutinized by staff and where basic functions such as eating and sleeping are regulated twenty-four hours a day encourages regression and may worsen mental symptoms. Forced institutionalization, such as commitment to a mental hospital or imprisonment, often creates feelings of desperation, demoralization, despair, and boredom among inmates, who may resort to NSSI to deal with these feelings. Also, the crowding together of persons over extended periods of time facilitates the outbreak of epidemics of NSSI.

An epidemic of self-cutting occurred on a psychiatric inpatient unit for emotionally disturbed adolescents. It began when a girl cut herself, tried to make her thumb fall off by wrapping a rubber band around it, and began to push pins into her body. After eight months, she was discharged from the unit when she inserted pins near her eyes. Another girl began to cut herself at the same time; after swallowing pins, nails, and glass she too was discharged. A month later, a boy cut crisscross designs on his hands. Eleven adolescents were caught up in the cutting. It was discovered that several boys had cut secretly a month before the girls. The adolescents took their cutting patterns from the first boy and girl who initiated the behavior. The epidemic was prolonged by two girls who vied to produce the more severe symptoms; it ended with the transfer to another unit of four cutters with antiadult feelings. The transferred patients did well. "It would appear that each needed a period of acting out to be followed by a more controlling environment, and it proved impossible to provide both situations in the same unit" (Matthews 1968, p. 132).

In a Canadian correctional institution for adolescent girls, 86 percent of inmates carved their skin. The average number of carvings was 8.9 per girl. Most of the episodes (71%) involved carving initials in the skin of a parent or a "lovelight" (a close and intimate girlfriend; the term did not necessarily have any sexual connotation). Most carvers cut themselves when angry or depressed. Forty-eight percent reported that the carving was related to the lovelight system, where the act was regarded as a demonstration of affection, a sealing of a pact, a demonstration of anger over rejection by a lovelight, a jealous response to a lovelight's behavior, or a method of getting more attention from a lovelight. Girls who carved were thought by their peers to be "sharper" and more popular than noncarvers. "Carving was the girl's way of expressing independence, autonomy, and personal freedom. It was more than just a symbol of adolescent striving for independence or their way of opposing adult infringement on their personal freedom" (Ross and McKay 1979, p. 134). Carving provided the girls with a sense of power, satisfaction, and control over their lives.

Podvoll (1969) argued that self-injurers in a hospital quickly assume an identity equated with their acts. The label *cutter* or *slasher* confirms a distinctive, functional role. Although self-cutting may lead to a personal sense of calmness, it evokes "feelings of unbearable intensity" in caretakers and challenges staff roles and hospital structure. The hospital unit that contains a cutter must engage in a struggle of caring versus punishment. Relationships exist among self-injurious behavior, the rituals and ceremonies of a hospital unit, the meaning and coherency of its social organization, and its therapeutic effectiveness. Kroll (1978) demonstrated that a marked reduction in the incidence of NSSI on a psychiatric ward occurred only after "problems were dealt with from a consistent framework, and the staff pulled together as a unit" (p. 433).

Prisons are hotbeds of NSSI and contain many psychopaths (persons who have an antisocial personality disorder). Hare (1970) found that psychopaths have a lowered state of cortical arousal and when thrust into prison may seek extra stimulation through NSSI because of their inability to tolerate the routine and boredom of prison life. In his classic book, *The Mask of Sanity* (1964), Cleckley noted that bored sociopaths may engage in self-damaging behavior in order to experience novel, stimulating experiences.

Johnson and Britt (1967) examined self-injuring prisoners and found that few were motivated by factors external to prison life, such as relationships with family or loved ones. "Normal" motivations resulted in 42 percent of NSSI; that is, they were consistent with an inmate value system intended to outwit officials or to disrupt usual administrative procedures. Most normal motives involved a desire to manipulate a transfer to a particular prison or to a certain cell block (sometimes to establish a homosexual relationship), and to gain access to narcotics.

Fifty-eight percent of self-injurious acts resulted from "abnormal" motivations not consistent with prison culture in that they reflected efforts to evade pressures from other inmates and an inability to withstand the stresses of prison life. Inmates with these motivations were more likely to injure themselves while in the hospital or in nonpunitive settings, thus highlighting their maladjustment to the prison environment. Abnormal motives included a desire for medical or psychiatric attention, fear of homosexual attack, anxiety over admission to prison or subsequent reassignment, a wish for reclassification, and fear of being killed if one was suspected of informing on other prisoners.

Self-injury done in anger typically involved two to four deep, painless lacerations over the fleshy parts of the arms or legs. The inmate was somewhat relieved by the sight of his blood and called for help. The manipulative inmate typically made a small, single, painful, horizontal cut requiring a few sutures. If the manipulation did not work the behavior might escalate, even to the point of sawing off toes with razor blades. The fearful inmate typically made one or two small, painful cuts on his arms. If this "cry for help" did not produce results, he might injure himself more severely. Inmates who were in mental turmoil displayed a variety of NSSI acts, ranging from superficial cuts to facial lacerations. The cutting was not painful and often gave a pleasant sensation of relief.

One of the most sympathetic studies of self-injurious behavior among prisoners is Toch's *Men in Crisis* (1975). His book catalogs the feelings, thoughts, and behaviors of prisoners caught up in a spectrum of despair. It considers self-mutilation a unique index of "breakdowns" among prisoners. In an institution for youthful offenders Toch found a self-mutilation rate of 7.7 percent; in adult male prisons the rate was 6.5 percent; in a women's prison the rate was 10.8 percent. Most acts of NSSI are recorded only when severe medical problems arise, and when bizarre, psychotic patterns emerge. In most instances the "inmates are disinfected, bandaged, and discreetly sent back to their cells."

Toch considered self-injury by prisoners to be a form of coping. Many inmates regarded both the world and the prison as overpowering, unfair, and malevolently arbitrary. Problems were seen as predestined by some greater power, and self-injury was an expression of disengagement or self-exoneration. Prisoners placed in solitary confinement sometimes panicked; for them NSSI became a demand for release. Some inmates felt a desperate need for support, understanding, or help that could not be provided by untrusted, unsympathetic, or incapable peers or staff. NSSI served to bring such inmates to the attention of medical staff, who were often perceived to possess magical powers.

Self-injury was a simple statement of bankruptcy among some prisoners who perceived themselves as "inescapably relegated to the junk heap of life." NSSI was a form of moral or psychological surgery that removed the basis for feelings of shame and guilt: "It might sound strange to you, but after I done it, the next day I felt different. For some reason . . . it made me feel better. It made me feel that I had cut something out of myself, I started making a new thing" (p. 61). Inmates who thought that an important relationship was dissolving sometimes cut themselves as a demonstration of the depth, sincerity, and intensity of their affection.

The psychosocial backgrounds of eight inmates at a special facility for habitually violent prisoners were the focus of a study by Bach-Y-Rita (1974). These men averaged ninety-three scars each. They frequently cut themselves without feeling pain while in isolation. The cutting was preceded by a feeling of depression and mounting tension and was followed by a sense of relief. Bach-Y-Rita felt that "the constellation of withdrawal, depressive reaction, hyperexcitability, hyperreactivity, stimulus-seeking behavior, impaired pain perception, and violent aggressive behavior directed at self or others may be the consequence of having been reared under conditions of maternal social deprivation" (p. 1020).

Hillbrand et al. (1994) compared fifty-three male self-injurers in a maximum security hospital with a control group. During the two-year study, 17 percent of patients engaged in NSSI. They were younger, more verbally and physically aggressive, received higher doses of neuroleptics, and had more diagnoses of personality disorder or mental retardation. Almost half the cases were confined to one incident. More than two incidents were an indication that the behavior would be repeated, and the more the incidents, the greater the likelihood of severe self-injury. "Thus, there appears to be a window of opportunity for treatment after the first incident. . . . After that time, self-mutilation appears to be refractory to treatment." Some patients self-injured more than fifty times.

To test Turner and Toffler's hypothesis (1986) that self-mutilation in prisoners indicates severe psychiatric morbidity rather than the a natural response to the privations of the institutional environment alone, Wilkins and Coid (1991) examined women when they were admitted to a London prison: 7.5 percent had a history of NSSI, especially cutting; 27 percent had self-injured two to five times, 32 percent six to ten times, 19 percent more than ten times, and 15 percent more than fifty times. A quarter said that their self-harm was entirely precipitated by the stress of life events (arrests, arguments, loss of property, etc.), while another quarter had no explicable reason; half offered both reasons. Many said their self-injury was a sudden impulse; 69 percent said that the self-harm relieved their symptoms of tension, dysphoria, and irritability; and 26 percent felt relief from depersonalization. In comparison with a control group, the women with a pre-prison history of NSSI had "a depressing picture of early deprivation, family disruption, and physical and sexual abuse . . . poor adjustments in their sexual development, uncertainty in later sexual orientation and identity, failure to develop stable relationships, and evidence of polymorphous perversity."

In a second paper on the same inmates, Coid et al. (1992) identified two groups. One was characterized by five or more episodes of self-harm; teenage onset and no identified external precipitant for the behavior; multiple body areas affected; symptom relief achieved; history of overdoses, alcohol abuse, fire setting, and other impulsive behaviors; personality disorder diagnosis (especially antisocial and borderline); multiple previous convictions with first court appearance as a teenager. The other group had fewer than five episodes of self-harm; onset at age 20 or later; frequently identified precipitants for their behavior; little symptom relief; uncommon history of overdoses, alcohol abuse, fire setting, impulsive behaviors, or personality disorder diagnosis; and few previous convictions with first court appearance as an adult. The authors concluded that the poor prognosis of the first group was due to a deficit in impulse control combined with a severe underlying affective disorder. This conclusion was based primarily on an association between borderline personality disorder (the most common diagnosis given to women in the first group) and depression.

In 1939, Dollard et al. hypothesized that persons who are frustrated are more likely to demonstrate aggression when certain internal characteristics and external factors are present. A study of male inmates at medium/maximum security prisons who had been referred for mental health services upheld this frustration-aggression hypothesis. Shea (1993) found that self-injurers had higher levels of internal characteristics that increased the likelihood of self-harm than did non-self-injurers; for example, they had higher levels of hypersensitivity to stress, intense response to frustration, social alienation and impulsivity, as well as poorer insight and coping skills. Among the external factors present were a highly restrictive environment, the prevalence of sharp objects and matches that could be used for self-harm, substance abuse, changes in relationships or living quarters, real or perceived losses, extremes in temperature, and a reaction of staff that facilitated secondary gain from self-harm.

Although exposés of prison conditions and prisoner behaviors appear frequently in the media, the high prevalence of self-injury is rarely reported. A remarkable example of such a report is the forty-eight-page article "Rock-a-Bye-Baby: The Life and Death of Marlene Moore," written by Anne Kerhsaw and Mary Lasovitch for the Kingston, Ontario, *Whig-Standard Magazine* (25 November 1989). A victim of childhood physical and sexual abuse, Marlene became a bully and was placed at the age of 13 in a juvenile corrections facility, where 86 percent of the girls were skin carvers. The majority of her adult years were spent in correctional and mental health institutions. Her life was marked by aggression, assaults, thefts, rape, alcohol and drug abuse, lesbian encounters, and at least a thousand episodes of self-cutting. Her body became a mass of scars. Many well-intentioned persons, including social workers, psychiatrists, lawyers, and parole supervisors, tried to help but without success. At the age of 32, during her final stay in jail, Marlene joined other prisoners in cutting themselves. While in a punitive segregation cell, she collected her blood, threw it at the guards, and hanged herself. Her story shocked the sensibility of an entire nation.

An interesting report on self-mutilation in a "labor correcting camp" in the Soviet Union was provided by Yaroshevsky (1975), himself an inmate who worked as a prison surgeon. He treated inmates "who cut their veins, sewed up their mouths, sewed buttons on their bodies, disemboweled themselves, slashed off their fingers, toes, genitals and ears, swallowed foreign objects, and so on" (p. 443). One prisoner urinated on his feet and put them through a broken window until they froze. Yaroshevsky regarded these self-mutilative acts as a way of both expressing grievances and gaining transfer to the medical unit. Political prisoners did not mutilate themselves, despite the fact that their conditions were much worse than those of the other prisoners. Rather, they went on hunger strikes, a passive mode of protest by which they asserted control over their own fates and bodies.

Self-cutting in Schools

Hundreds of studies have looked at cutting in adolescents (e.g., Jacobson and Gould 2007; Nock and Prinstein 2005; Petersen et al. 2008). A community sample of 633 adolescents completed anonymous surveys; 18 percent endorsed minor forms of NSSI (hair pulling, skin picking, self-biting) and 28 percent endorsed skin cutting, carving, and burning. The average number of NSSI incidents was about 13 in the past year. The cutters, carvers, and burners were more likely to have a history of psychiatric treatment, hospitalization, suicide attempts, and current suicidal thoughts (Lloyd-Richardson et al. 2007).

Few studies have specifically targeted students in middle and high schools, although I suspect that the vast majority of teachers have personally encountered at least one cutter in their classrooms. Hundreds of brief articles are accessible online for teachers wishing to identify and deal with students who self-injure. The S.A.F.E. (Self Abuse Finally Ends) *Manual for School Professionials* (2008) and *Student Workbook* (2008) are excellent resources. The most cited study has a sample of 440 Canadian high school students, but some results do not seem quite right. Sixty-one percent admitted to NSSI with a girl-to-boy ratio of about two to one. Skin cutting (41 percent) was the most common behavior, followed by self-hitting (33 percent), skin pinching (6.5 percent), biting (5 percent), and burning (3.3 percent). Amazingly, 13 percent said they engaged in NSSI daily, while 28 percent said several times a week, and 19.6 percent several times a month. Eighteen percent self-injured only once. Other amazing findings were that the age of onset of NSSI was age 12 or earlier for 24.6 percent, and 61 percent said they had stopped their NSSI (Ross and Heath 2002).

Barry Walsh (2006) has problems with some of these findings, as do I, although he notes, and I agree, that the current generation of young student self-injurers has changed greatly. He finds that they have lower rates of childhood sexual or physical abuse; show strengths in the areas of family, peers, and school; are psychologically healthier; and stop their NSSI more rapidly (6 months to 2 years). Shaw (2002), in a study of six female college students who extensively engaged in NSSI for one to five years with a range of episodes from ten to fifty, reported that, while they still experienced much distress in their lives, all six were doing well in college and had stopped their NSSI; several were in serious relationships. Two had no treatment at all while the others responded well to therapy. True, the study is selective and small, but I never would have imagined such success when I started my studies of self-injury in the late 1980s.

I have encountered self-injury by contagion in many high and some middle schools. One school even had a "cut of the month" club where students would compare their cuts and scars. Adolescent wrist cutting also has been reported as a dare game (Lena and Bijour 1990). Walsh (2006) has proposed thoughtful reasons for the contagious spread of self-injury in schools. While acknowledging the importance of individual psychopathology, his focus is on interpersonal issues. Because of their limited communication skills, for example, students may demonstrate their emotional distress concretely and forcibly through cutting rather than words. Cutting may also be done to make others feel guilty and to coerce them (especially parents) to "give me what I want or else!" Students may be influenced by lead cutters who may be admired for their ability to upset teachers and who serve as role models. They may also pick up on the extra attention/ therapy, medication, etc., that cutters get and decide to follow suit, especially if they feel neglected. Students enjoy being members of an exclusive clique or club; some may base their exclusivity on joining an athletic team or cheerleading while others band together on the basis of being a cutter. Such exclusive groups share an intimate, unique experience that may encourage disinhibition—"Try it, you might like it"—as well as the competition I saw in the "cut of the month" club. For most students, the thrill of shared cutting experiences wears off after a while, but some, particularly those who have problematic personality, anxiety, and depression issues, may be unable to give up and may go on to develop a deliberate self-harm syndrome (see chapter 9) that will make their lives miserable for a decade or more.

CHAPTER EIGHT

The Genitals

This chapter considers the many forms of male and female genital self-injury and body modification found in culturally sanctioned practices and among people who are mentally ill. Psychoanalytic theory in the older literature holds that the self-injury of other body parts is symbolic of or a substitute for castration.

Castration

In the beginning, there was Chaos. Then Gaea, deep-breasted Earth, appeared, as did Eros, who influenced the creation of beings and things. Gaea gave birth to Uranus, the sky, whom she made her equal. The Sky covered the Earth, and Gaea and Uranus produced the twelve Titans, the first race. Uranus kept the children captive in the depths of the earth. Gaea, an angered mother, fashioned a sickle and planned vengeance against Uranus. The children refused to take part in the plot, except for Cronus, the last-born Titan. With Gaea's help, Cronus took the sickle and castrated his father, Uranus, casting his genitals into the sea. They splashed into the water; from the resulting sea foam, Aphrodite was born, and from the wound blood that dropped to the earth, the Furies were born. Cronus released his siblings and ruled the new dynasty. He married his sister, Rhea, and they produced six children. Fearful of being deposed, Cronus ate the first five children as soon as they were born. When she was pregnant with her sixth child, Rhea went to her parents (Uranus and Gaea) for help. She gave birth in a secret cave and fooled Cronus by wrapping a stone in swaddling clothes. He ate the stone, thinking it was his child. Rhea reared the child, who grew up and vanquished his father, Cronus. The child's name was Zeus.

This famous story from Greek mythology demonstrates several themes associated with castration that have been incorporated into Western psychological perceptions. A son deposes his father by castrating him, thus establishing a prototype of adolescent rebellion against tyrannical authority. When the father's mutilated genitals were cast into the sea, the sea foam formed into Aphrodite, the goddess of fertility and the personification of the power of love, thus demonstrating the linkage between the sexual and aggressive drives. The blood from the father's genital wound fell to earth and gave rise to the Furies, the terrible forces that can drive a person to madness.

Castration originated at least five thousand years ago when humans learned that it made some animals more docile, larger, and tastier to eat. The Caribs, fierce Indians for whom the Caribbean area was named, are the only known group suspected of applying this reasoning to other humans. They reportedly castrated prisoners and kept them in stockades for fattening and tenderizing before being eaten. Culturally accepted castration of men throughout the world tends to fall into several major categories, namely, punishment and prevention of adultery and sexual crimes, enhanced religious spirituality, and institutionalized eunuchism.

In Western nations, castration has sometimes been employed as therapy for sex offenders and as a means of preventing the propagation of criminal rapists and mentally retarded persons. One of the most virulent proponents of preventive castration (Barr 1920) noted that "the very life blood of the nation is being poisoned by the rapid production of mental and moral defectives, and the only thing that will dam the flood of degeneracy and ensure the survival of the fittest, is abrogation of all power to procreate" (p. 234). Barr called for mandatory castration of "the scum and dregs of mankind . . . the hereditary irresponsible . . . degenerates, imbeciles, defective delinquents, and epileptics—the very nightmare of the human race, ever with sexual impulses exaggerated" (p. 234).

Bowman and Engle reported in 1957 that in Denmark 600 male sex offenders were castrated between 1929 and 1952 with the consent of the prisoner, his wife, and close relatives. In Norway 243 men were castrated between 1934 and 1950: "If the patient fully realized the purpose of the operation and accepted it voluntarily, the results were good" (p. 81).

To understand the linkage between religion and castration, we must turn to Phrygia in Asia Minor, where the cult of Cybele was formed in the fifth century B.C. and extended into the early Christian era (Engle 1936; Frazer 1958; Hays 1964; Vermasseren 1977). Cybele was the Great Mother goddess, the mysterious power that awakens everything to life. She had many names, including Aphrodite, Artemis, Persephone, and Demeter. She was compared with Isis and was known as the "life-giving, frenzy-loving, joyful one, gratified with acts of piety." Her cult spread throughout Asia Minor and into Greece, where she was described in the Homeric hymns as being surrounded by howling wolves and roaring lions.

Cybele consorted with only one man, Attis, and he pledged eternal fidelity to her. But then he had an affair with a nymph. Enraged, Cybele killed the nymph. Attis became insane and, thinking himself pursued by the Furies, emasculated himself, whereupon he was changed into a pine tree.

Attis's emasculation was immortalized by the great Roman poet Catullus (first century B.C.). He described how Attis, moved by madness,

> Lopped off the load of his loins with a sharp flint.
> Woman now, and aware of her wasted manhood,
> Still bleeding, the blood bedaubing the ground still,
> With feminine fingers she fetched the light drum
> That makes the music, Great Mother, at your mysteries.
>
> *(Poems of Catullus* 1969)

Festivals in honor of Attis were held in the month of March. On the Day of Blood (24 March), the cult priests, in mourning for Attis, flagellated and castrated themselves, and ran through the streets proudly holding their bloody genitals, which they eventually threw into a house. The honored household was then duty bound to supply the emasculated priests with women's clothing and ornaments, which they would wear for the rest of their lives. Many spectators, caught up in the intense emotionality of the occasion, the frenetic music of cymbals and drums, and the sight of flowing blood, followed the priests' example and castrated themselves. This day of sorrow and irrevocable sacrifice was followed by the Day of Joy, the Hilaria, which celebrated Attis's resurrection. Secret ceremonies were also held, the most famous being a baptismal rite in which a devotee climbed into a pit. A bull was placed on a grating over the pit (the taurobolium) and was slaughtered. The bull's blood fell through the grating and covered the person in the pit, washing away his sins and granting him a new life. The main sanctuary of Cybele, where this bloody baptismal was performed, was located in Rome on the grounds of the Vatican Hill, near what is now Saint Peter's Cathedral (Vermasseren 1977).

About 204 B.C. the statue of Cybele was carried to Rome, where she was worshiped as Mother of the Trojans, the founders of Rome, and where she protected the Roman state. As the Roman empire expanded, so did her cult, and temples dedicated to her were erected in Spain, France, Germany, Britain, and all the Roman provinces. When the Romans accepted the statue of Cybele into their city they knew little of these wild rites. In fact, they were shocked by the strange appearance of the priests of Cybele who flocked to Rome. They had long, bleached hair, wore ornaments, and walked like women. They told fortunes for money, engaged in trance dancing, and flagellated themselves. Although the emperor Julian called emasculation "that holy harvest," most Romans thought the priests were insane and mocked their effeminacy. But some Romans were fascinated by their burning faith, ascetic life, and austere discipline. According to the French historian Graillot (1912), "Many troubled souls were drawn toward these inter-preters of the divine word who appeared superior to other men, who listened to companions and examined consciences and gave consolation and divine hope."

The growth of the early Christian church coincided with the period of cult worship of Cybele and Attis, and Christian priests assumed some of the higher characteristics of the eunuch-priests. Many temples devoted to Cybele were taken over by Christians, who converted them into shrines of the Virgin Mary. And, as Hays (1964) pointed out, "the carefully desexualized figure of Christ is more than a little reminiscent of Attis."

Although the Christian church did not encourage castration, some followers interpreted literally the words of Matthew 19:12: "For there are some eunuchs which were so born from their mother's womb: and there are some eunuchs which were made eunuchs of men: and there be eunuchs which have made themselves eunuchs for the kingdom of heaven's sake."

The most famous castrate was the theologian Origen (A.D. 185–254), who later lamented his action. Another was the presbyter Leontius, who castrated himself so that he could continue his relationship with the virgin Eustolium. His act angered the church hierarchy, who deposed him from his high office and protested when the Arian Christian sect ordained him bishop of Antioch. There is some evidence, too, that a sect known as the Valesians, active in the third cen-tury, supposedly castrated themselves and forcibly castrated others. In A.D. 325, the Church Council of Nicea prohibited priests from becoming eunuchs, and this became the official position of the Roman church forever after. A singular exception was castrating young boys to preserve their voices for performing in the church choirs where their sweet singing rendered great public good. A num-ber of theologians and popes objected to the practice, which finally was stopped in 1880 by Pope Leo XIII.

Castration for religious reasons among Western Christians has occurred in-frequently over the centuries. One of the most famous religious castrates of the nineteenth century was George Rapp, founder of the utopian, Christian, Har-mony Society (1785–1847) in Pennsylvania. Rapp was troubled by sexuality and strongly encouraged the members of his community to live in celibacy. He cas-trated himself and was accused of castrating his son and several men who were unable to control their sexual urges.

Within the Eastern Orthodox tradition, the secret sect known as the Skoptsi, or eunuchs, included castration as a central religious practice (Goldberg 1930). The sect, which flourished in Russia throughout the nineteenth and even into the twentieth century, was founded in 1757 by a runaway peasant named Selivanov.

He cut off his testicles because he could not follow his ideal of complete sexual abstinence. He was exiled but was recognized as Christ by a small band of disciples and achieved "perfection" by cutting off his penis with a red-hot knife. He interpreted Matthew 5:27–29 (the text referring to cutting off one's hand and gouging out one's eyes) to mean that the genitals should be cut off so that a person would not be tempted to commit adultery. Selivanov believed that Adam and Eve were created sexless and that after the Fall, the halves of the forbidden fruit were grafted onto them, forming testicles and breasts. In his view, removal of these organs restored persons to a more pure state and relieved them of the burden of following Adam and Eve's sinful indulgence in sexual intercourse.

The cult spread among all social classes and at one time may have numbered a hundred thousand. The Skoptsi practiced chastity and fasting and abstained from games, feasts, and strong alcoholic beverages. They uttered prophecies and violently danced after the fashion of dervishes. They were ardent proselytizers; members who brought in twelve converts willing to undergo genital mutilation were given the rank of "apostle." They supposedly visited condemned prisoners under false pretenses and castrated them in their cells. They lent money at high rates and forgave debts if borrowers agreed to enter the sect and accept mutilation.

Male Skoptsi were readily identifiable because castration rendered them beardless and corpulent. The Russian government actively tried to suppress the cult, but the task proved difficult. The publicity attached to persecution attracted people to mutilate themselves to become martyrs. Some Skoptsi were shut up in monasteries, but with their ardent faith and powers of persuasion they succeeded in converting Orthodox monks to their ranks. Trials against cult members were reported as late as the 1890s.

Eunuchism, the large-scale practice of castration for social reasons, became important in the Eastern Roman empire. The Byzantine emperors chose eunuchs for high political offices, and not infrequently, noblemen volunteered to become eunuchs. The law recognized three types of eunuch: those whose testicles had been cut off (*spadones*), those whose testicles had been crushed (*thlassiae*), and those whose penis and testicles had been cut off (*castrati*). Although the majority of eunuchs were *castrati* (over six thousand a year were sold as slaves and lust objects in the markets of the Eastern Roman empire from the seventh to the ninth centuries), many of those who achieved high positions underwent less-mutilative procedures.

With the rise of Islam, the institution of eunuchism did not overly prosper, initially. Muhammad told a follower who asked for permission to castrate himself to avoid the temptation to fornicate, "He who castrates himself or another does not belong to my followers, for castration in Islam may consist only in fasting." The early Arabs, however, purchased castrated slaves who were employed as harem keepers. Beginning with the mid-thirteenth-century Mameluke period in Egypt and with the fourteenth-century Ottoman empire in Turkey, eunuchs not only served in harems but also married and held the highest political positions. Muslims did not perform the castration themselves but rather purchased eunuchs. Some Christian monasteries in Egypt supported themselves by becoming "eunuch factories." Another center was Khartoum, where slave raiders brought their captives to barbers, monks, and physicians to undergo castration. The trade in eunuchs was brisk and profitable, castrati being the most desirable harem employees.

In the Far East, Buddhist countries have little history of castration. The countries that follow Islamic precepts used eunuchs as in the Middle East, and those that follow Hindu precepts institutionalized eunuchism among some entertainers and dancers. Curran (1886) described castration of adults and children among Indian Hindus, apparently for religious reasons and financial gain. He noted that a ligature was tied tightly around the base of the scrotum, and the penis, testes, and scrotum were cleanly cut off with a sharp barber's knife.

During the sixth century B.C. in China, eunuchs were employed as servants for imperial concubines and carried out household functions. Only the royal family had the right to employ eunuchs, a practice that continued through the nineteenth century. Chinese men voluntarily accepted castration to improve their social status, including men who were married and had children. The operation was performed by royal surgeons who were themselves eunuchs. Once accepted into the royal household, eunuchs were forbidden to leave; some achieved political prominence. Jamieson (1882) described castration operations performed outside the palace gates. A man who volunteered for castration was solemnly asked if he would ever repent of his decision. If he appeared doubtful, he was released; if not, his genitals were swiftly cut off by one stroke of a small, sickle-shaped knife. A pewter plug was inserted into the urethra. For three days the volunteer received nothing to eat or drink. Healing took one hundred days.

In India, Pakistan, and other South Asian countries there are "third gender" persons known as hijras who are intersex or males but act and dress as females. They live in households of their peers and worship Bahuchara Mata, a manifestation of the Mother Goddess. Some are born with ambiguous genitalia while others have a "rebirth" operation involving castration of their penis and testicles.

They have a low social status and earn money by telling fortunes, begging, prostitution, and by showing up, uninvited, at weddings, where they sing, dance, and demand fees for not causing a commotion. Because of sometimes brutal discrimination against and high rates of HIV among hijras, organizations such as the All-India Eunuchs Welfare Association and the Benazir Income Support Program (Paskistan) have been formed to provide financial, health, and welfare benefits (See Nanda 1999; Reddy 2003). In 2003, the case of an American male who cut off his penis in order to become a hijra was reported (Master and Santucci, 2003).

Elective self-castration in current Western culture is discussed in chapter 9.

Monorchy

Monorchy, the ritual destruction of one testicle, ranks among the strangest forms of genital mutilation. The earliest descriptions came from European explorers among the Bushmen and Hottentots of South Africa in the 1600s. While it is tempting to dismiss these as misinterpretations or flights of fancy, one cannot dismiss references to the custom by highly regarded twentieth-century anthropologists such as Evans-Pritchard and Seligman.

Lagercrantz's review (1938) revealed differing methods and motives for monorchy. In one tribe the right testicle of each young boy was crushed between two flat stones. In another, the mother of each boy removed the right testicle with her teeth and ate it. In yet another, a tribal "surgeon" cut open the scrotum and pressed out and cut off one testicle. A ball of healing herbs was wrapped in sheep's fat and inserted into the scrotum. Then the wound was sewn closed. The primary reason given by natives for monorchy was that it made the boys swifter, more agile hunters. Other reasons stated that it prevented both sickness and the birth of twins (an evil omen) and that it was sexually attractive to women. Interpretations offered by Europeans were that it curbed the sexual appetite of young men, served as a method of birth control, and established a measure of social control; for example, a rapist would be punished by having his remaining testicle removed. As late as 1938, an anthropologist reported that "it is practised at the present day by people who are certainly not of Hottentot blood, but who must have derived their language as well as many of their customs from Hottentot conquerors in by-gone times. It stands to them in the same relation that circumcision does to many Bantu clans, that is, among them a youth cannot enter the society of men or take to himself a wife until he has become a monorch" (pp. 200–201).

Cutting the Penis

Penis cutting is an extremely ancient practice that takes different forms, ranging from the simple slicing of the foreskin to the splitting of the penis from tip to base of the urethra. The reasons given for this practice are diverse and include such notions as sanitation, substitution for human sacrifice, symbolic castration, desire to be like women, elevation to the status of manhood, sexual differentiation, enhanced fertility, contraception, resolution of identity conflict, permanent incorporation into a social group, control of sexual urges, a mark of caste, a test of endurance, a covenant with God, and so on.

Subincision, the slitting open of the urethra, exists mainly among aborigines in the northwest and central areas of Australia. It frequently is the last ordeal a young man must endure as he is initiated into manhood. Gould (1969) described these initiatory ordeals among the Yiwara. The youth first has an incisor tooth knocked out and his nasal septum pierced. Amid dancing and singing that re-enact episodes of the totemic kangaroo, the boy lies on his back across a living table of men, who are on their hands and knees, and undergoes subincision, during which his urethra is cut open, with a sharp stone fluke, from the urethral meatus to a point about halfway to the scrotum. During these ceremonies some subincised men enlarge their old cuts.

Rivers (1926) reported that in Fiji subincision was performed to evacuate pathogenic bad humors. In New Guinea, Wogeo men periodically incise themselves in emulation of the purification women experience during menstruation. Margetts (1960) reported a strange situation among the Kenyan Samburu, where prepubertal boys perform subincisions on themselves in private without any ritual, during the lonely job of herding cattle.

Many investigators have tried to explain why Australian aborigines practice subincision. Basedow (1927) thought that the operation was done for contraception or for sanitation, e.g., to relieve or prevent urethral inflammation caused by dirt or insects. Another theory is that subincision is done to simulate the female genitals (Roheim 1949). Indeed, some groups use the slang word for vagina when referring to the subincised penis. This argument is enhanced by the fact that men often gash the subincised penis to draw blood during rituals: "Seeing that in the female the blood originated from the vulva, what is more natural than to make it come from the analogous organ in the male" (Montagu 1946–47, p. 432). Bettelheim (1955) used Australian examples to support his notion of vagina envy in men. He asserted that an unconscious purpose of male initiation rites may be to assert that men, too, can bear children and they try to acquire sexual apparatus and functions equal to women. Another theory is that the subincision results in a broader erection, thus enhancing the sexual act for women. Comments obtained from some aborigines—"Girls tell you straight away: you got big *burra* [subincised penis], I won't go to any other man" (Cawte 1974, p. 126)—would seem to support this theory.

Many anthropologists favor a more general theory: circumcision, subincision, and initiation rites validate membership in a cult lodge, are a badge of increased ritual status and physical courage, bind the tribe together, and counteract disruptive tendencies inherent in aboriginal social and spiritual life (Elkin 1945; Gould 1969). Walbiri aborigines have explained that the practice of subincision derives from their kinship kangaroos and other marsupials who have a bifid penis, and from sacred myths. Thus, subincision may have evolved out of a reverence for totemic marsupials as godlike ancestors whose characteristics men should imitate (Cawte 1974; Cawte et al. 1966).

Male Circumcision

Circumcision is a very old form of body modification, as evidenced by its practice among aborigines, by Paleolithic cave drawings of circumcised men, and by the emphasis on the use of a stone or flint knife for circumcision rites among Semitic and other groups. Joshua 5:2, for example, reads: "The Lord said to Joshua, 'make flint knives and circumcise the Israelite nation.' " Egyptians practiced the procedure as evidenced by circumcision scenes painted on the walls of tombs and by circumcised mummies. The practice has been widespread but not universal. The Mongols have never circumcised, nor is there any mention of it in the Sanskrit literature. Except for Athabascan tribes, circumcision was not widely practiced by North American Indians, and among South American Indians it is found in only a few tribes.

The most basic form of circumcision is a simple gash of the foreskin, as commonly reported among Pacific Islanders. The most brutal form, known as *salkh*, has been reported among Arab tribes in Yemen (Chabukswar 1921). To marry, a young man had to first undergo *salkh* without anesthesia under the careful scrutiny of friends. The ordeal consisted of flaying and removing all of the skin of the penis and the abdomen from the umbilicus to the scrotum. If the young man complained or flinched the procedure was stopped. The victim was deemed unfit for marriage and full membership in the tribe and was sold into slavery or killed.

If he survived without flinching, the crowd rejoiced, and he received treatment for his wounds, which generally required several months to heal. Some youths died as a result of the *salkh*, while others developed urethral fistulae.

The saga of circumcision among Christians and Jews has produced a vast literature. The first biblical reference is Genesis 17, in which the Lord appears before Abraham, establishes a covenant with him and with his descendants, and promises that he will multiply exceedingly: "Circumcise the flesh of your foreskin, and that shall be the mark of the covenant between you and me." Every male child was to be circumcised at the age of eight days, as were all male slaves. Why circumcision was chosen is puzzling because all other forms of bodily modification are prohibited to Jews.[1] Further, circumcision was a widely practiced pagan custom; Jeremiah 9:25–26 lists "Egypt and Judah, Edom and the Ammonites, Moab and the desert dwellers" (Arabs) as nations that are circumcised in the flesh although not in the heart. If anything, circumcision would have made the Jews more like the Egyptians, from whom they probably learned the practice during their subjugation by the Pharaohs.

A grisly biblical story involving penis cutting is that of David, the slayer of Goliath. King Saul, displeased with David's popularity, set a strange bride-price for the hand of his daughter, Michal. He told David to bring him the foreskin of two hundred Philistines, reckoning that David would be killed in the attempt. But, as recounted in 1 Samuel 18, "David arose and went, he and his men, and slew of the Philistines 200 men; and David brought their foreskins . . . that he might be the king's son-in-law. And Saul gave him Michal his daughter to wife." Another circumcision story is told in Genesis 34, which entails Dinah's rape by Shechem, who then wanted to marry her. Her family agreed to the marriage on the condition that Shechem and all of the men of his village first be circumcised.

---

1. Of all of the commentators who have tried to explain this enigma, Isaac (1967) seems to make the most sense. He notes that the Lord actually made two covenants with Abraham. In Genesis 15, Abraham is told that he will inherit Canaan. He asks for a sign and is told to split several animals in half. He then has a dream vision identifying that his descendants will indeed inherit the promised land. In the second covenant, Abraham is promised offspring (even though he is 93 years old and his wife is 90) who will multiply and establish a great nation if he agrees to cut his foreskin. In each case, cutting occurs, and Isaac believes that biblical circumcision may be "a special case of the ancient custom of using cutting or dismemberment rites in connection with treaty and covenant obligations" (p. 54). Although we usually associate treaties and covenants with binding, this was not always the case; for example, Alexander the Great bound Asia and Europe together when he cut the Gordian knot. Even today, silk ribbons are cut to inaugurate bridges and highways, and cutting symbolizes the joining together of plans that once were separate. The ancient ritual of cutting worked *backward*, indicating that the covenant partners had been bound together in the mythical past; it also worked *forward*, indicating that the now separate partners belonged together as part of an original whole. Thus, the circumcision cut recreated a mythical past "to give substance and status to an alliance directed to the future." In this context, Isaac's argument may have substance.

While they were recovering from the circumcision and were still in pain, Dinah's brethren "took each man their swords, advanced against the city without any trouble, and massacred all the males."

Milah, the Jewish circumcision rite practiced for about two millennia, involved a simple cut and removal of the tip of the prepuce. During the Hellenic period many Jews converted to paganism and undid their circumcision through a surgical procedure known as *recutitio* or by using a funnel-shaped copper instrument, the *pondus Judaeum*, which covered and stretched the foreskin. Jewish rabbis of that time were angered and a new procedure was developed, the *periah*, in which the entire foreskin was removed, making a cover-up impossible.[2]

Early theories about the origin of circumcision focused on hygiene. However, most Jewish writers have presented purely religious arguments that suggest it is an act of faith. In addition, Moses Maimonides (A.D. 1135–1204) wrote in part 3, chapter 49, of his *The Guide of the Perplexed* that circumcision is done to weaken the penis in order to decrease sexual intercourse. "The bodily pain caused to that member is the real purpose of circumcision. . . . It is hard for a woman with whom an uncircumcised man has had sexual intercourse to separate from him; in my opinion, this is the strongest of the reasons for circumcision."

The procedure was controversial in the early Christian church, with some factions advocating and others denying its necessity. Saint Paul had Timothy circumcised "because of the Jews of that region" (Acts 16) but eventually decided that the ritual was immaterial. "It is the same God who justifies the circumcised and the uncircumcised on the basis of faith" (Rom. 3); "Circumcision counts for nothing and its lack makes no difference either" (1 Cor. 7); and, "Be on guard against those who mutilate. It is we who are the circumcision, who worship in the spirit of God and glory in Christ Jesus rather than putting our trust in the flesh" (Phil. 3). At one point Paul was so angry at the agitators who were turning Christians against each other over this issue that he is said to have wished they would castrate themselves (Gal. 5:12)!

As the church matured, circumcision rarely was problematic; indeed, January 1 is a holy day, the Feast of Jesus's Circumcision. A strange chapter in the history of Christianity deals with the status of Jesus's foreskin. At one time, twelve

2. In the sixth century A.D., a change was made in the ritual; the circumciser moistened his lips with wine and then sucked the child's penis. This procedure, called the *metsitsah*, although widely practiced, did not become universal. In fact, in the last half of the nineteenth century many physicians and others objected to the health hazards of the *metsitsah*. The use of a glass tube was advocated instead of direct mouth-penis contact. In spite of this recommendation, illnesses such as tuberculosis undoubtedly were spread by traditionalists who transmitted the organisms through their mouths. Weiss (1962) published an investigation of Jewish circumcision throughout the world, his "attention having been called to the death of two newborn male infants shortly after their circumcision" (p. 31).

churches in Europe claimed possession of this sacred relic, which was venerated for its ability to cure impotence and infertility and to ease labor pains. Among the mystical nuns who contemplated the foreskin was Saint Birgitta, who had a vision of Mary holding it in her hand, and Saint Agnes, who had visions of swallowing it. Various legends developed; one was that the foreskin was left to Saint John, Mary Magdalen, or the Apostles and was eventually possessed by Charlemagne. Another legend was that Mary was circumcised (various cults held that all the events in Jesus's life were duplicated in Mary's).

Psychoanalysts have written widely on circumcision. In *Moses and Monotheism*, Freud theorized that circumcision evolved as a defense against the bisexual, orgiastic tendencies of pagan religions. The cult of Cybele, for example, required actual castration of priests and devotees. The Judaic God demanded an end to these orgies but accepted circumcision as a token of castration. In the words of the psychoanalyst Schlossman (1966), "Circumcision appears to be the last phase of a particular evolutionary process of sacrifice to the gods. The Toltecs and the Maya of Mexico sacrificed adults, the Phoenicians sacrificed children. In another phase the genitals were offered to the Mother Goddess, and finally the foreskin was offered to Jehovah as a sacrificial token" (p. 351). Glenn (1960) proposed a relationship between circumcision and anti-Semitism; the circumcised Jew is supposedly perceived as a mutilated person who seeks revenge and wants to circumcise others, giving rise to anti-Semitic prejudice.

Male Infibulation

Male infibulation is the practice of putting a clasp (fibula) or string through the foreskin. The major treatise on this topic is Dingwall's book (1925). Once the fibula is in place, the foreskin is unable to retract over the glans, making erection either painful or impossible.

Roman singers and actors were infibulated because it was believed that forced abstinence benefited their vocal ability. This notion was first written about by Aristotle: "For in those who are wont to indulge their lust the voice changes to that of a man, which is not so in those that restrain themselves." Actors were voluntarily infibulated also because it made them sexually attractive to women who reckoned that a man denied sexual activity for prolonged periods of time would be an ardent lover when the fibula was removed. Some athletes and gladiators were infibulated because sexual acts were thought to weaken them for competition. Only recently have professional athletes been allowed to travel with their wives. Paintings on Greek vases depict athletes with strings through their fore-skins, ostensibly to preserve their vitality.

In medical practice infibulation was prescribed to prevent illnesses thought to result from masturbation and nocturnal emissions. Karl August Weinhold, a German professor of surgery, proposed in 1827 that the human race might be bettered and the world population problems solved if the majority of men were infibulated; anyone who attempted to remove his clasp without the proper ap-proval would be subjected to severe punishment.

Bauer, a physician in St. Louis, described the successful use of infibulation as a remedy for epilepsy and seminal losses (1879–80). His patient was a debilitated young man whose mind was greatly agitated and who lived in constant fear of insanity because of frequent nocturnal seminal emissions, petit mal epileptic attacks, and headaches. His condition was believed to have been caused by ex-cessive childhood masturbation. Treatment consisted of a bland vegetarian diet, little heat in his bedroom, cold baths, a hard mattress, avoidance of lascivious reading, prompt evacuation of his bowels with cold water enemas, and, finally, infibulation with silk strings. The strings were tied at night to prevent erections and were loosened during the day. A one-year follow-up revealed that the patient was free from all symptoms.

Female Genital Modification

A most severe form of modification, introcism, was formerly practiced among Australian aborigines and was last reported in 1938. The vagina of a pubertal girl was slit with a knife or torn open by the fingers of the operator to enlarge the vaginal opening. This painful operation was immediately followed by forced in-tercourse with a group of young men. The spilled semen and the vaginal blood were collected and drunk as a tonic by the feeble, sick, and aged members of the tribes. Groups that practiced introcism also practiced male subincision.

Female genital modification remains a major public health problem in Africa affecting several million girls yearly, according to the World Health Organization. Most commonly midwives perform the surgery and may operate on thirty young girls in a day. Simple circumcision, known as Sunna circumcision in Muslim countries, consists of cutting off the clitoral prepuce and is analogous to male circumcision. Excision consists of cutting off the prepuce and the tip of the clito-ris, and may include scraping away part or all of the labia minora. Infibulation, known as Pharaonic circumcision, involves removal of the clitoris, the labia minora and majora, and the mons veneris. The vagina is then sewn shut except for a small opening to permit the exit of menstrual blood.

Boddy (1982) witnessed infibulation as it was performed before 1969, when local anesthetics became available and more sterile procedures were followed. A young girl was made to sit at the edge of a hole in the ground while her adult female relatives held her arms and legs. A midwife scraped the external genitalia with a razor. The raw tissue was pressed together, and the wound was closed by inserting thorns into the skin. The thorns were held in place by thread or bits of cloth. A piece of straw or a reed was inserted so that the vaginal scar tissue would not obliterate the opening. The girl's legs were then tied together, and she was left immobilized for a month. Boddy also witnessed the procedure in 1976 and noted the changes: a local anesthetic was injected into the genital area, and the clitoris and labia minora were cut away with scissors. The midwife then sewed the labia minora together with a surgical needle and sutures, leaving a small opening. Antiseptic lotion was liberally applied.

Although the procedure seems gruesome from a Western perspective, it is a cause for celebration in African societies where it is performed. The young girls may be dressed as brides and receive money, gold, and clothing as presents. In urban areas, printed invitation cards may be sent to guests. Singers and dancers often provide entertainment during the celebration.

Verzin (1975) listed the medical complications of these operations. Immediate or early complications include shock or death secondary to hemorrhage, infection, urinary retention, and injury to the urethra and anus. Later complications include malformation of the external genitalia that hinders or prevents medical examination, implantation dermoid cysts (some as large as a football) with subsequent abscesses, urinary tract infections, chronic pelvic sepsis, and dyspareunia. Additionally, the rigid circumcision scar often creates obstetrical problems, because during birth the baby's head can be forced backward and causes severe perineal lacerations. In addition to a posterolateral episiotomy, an anterior cut has to be made. If not done properly this may result in fistulae to the bladder and urethra.

Special problems occur for infibulated women at the time of marriage because the sewn vagina must be opened in order for consummation to take place. El Dareer (1982) noted that the customs and traditions about this matter vary widely. In one village, on the wedding night a friend of the bridegroom ties the woman to a bed. Her husband opens her vagina with a razor blade, knife, or scissors and attempts to have intercourse. Sometimes the nervous husband accidentally cuts into the rectum. The most common method is for the husband simply to keep pushing into the small vaginal opening with his penis. After a few weeks complete penetration can be achieved; the vaginal tears and bleeding associated with this method are considered normal. If this method fails, the couple may go to a midwife or a physician to open up the vagina surgically.

Although the age at which female genital operations are performed ranges from 7 days to 11 years, most are done between the ages of 6 and 10 years. Excision is practiced in a large number of African countries, ranging from the west coast through central Africa to the east coast (Hosken 1978). Surveys taken at girls' schools in the Sudan, exclusive of Khartoum, showed that practically all girls are infibulated by age 12. Surveys in Kenya showed that 40–80 percent of girls are circumcised. Almost the entire female population of Somalia is said to be infibulated, while in Upper Volta 70 percent of women appearing at one hospital were found to have undergone excision. Out of a sample of 3,210 rural and urban Sudanese women, 98 percent admitted to having been operated on. Of these, 83 percent had been infibulated, 12 percent had been excised, and 2.5 percent had been simply circumcised. The remainder were uncertain of the type of operation they had had.[3]

Huxley (1931) recounted that native misunderstanding of the arguments of Christian missionaries has contributed to the problem. For example, in Kenya the word *virgin*, as in the Virgin Mary, was translated *muiritu*, a Kikuyu word signifying a girl who had been circumcised and initiated but yet unmarried. As Huxley noted, "So the native Christian is confronted with a puzzle. He finds the mother of Jesus extolled and blessed in the faith he has embraced; but she is described in the Bible as a young woman who has been initiated and circumcised. And now the missionaries tell him that female circumcision is wrong" (p. 197). Efforts by Church of Scotland missionaries to forbid excision were credited by Jomo Kenyatta as being a major factor in the rise of anticolonial political activity. Kenyan men resented British interference with ancient tribal customs, especially those that threatened their domination over women. Thus, the rite of excision became an emblem of patriotism.

Gruenbaum (1982) and many others have tried to understand why these practices persist despite governmental laws prohibiting them and public health campaigns against them. The mutilative rituals serve a major purpose; they are an

3. A study in Somalia found that 97 percent of nursing students had been infibulated, mainly by traditional midwives; 40 percent of the students said they would infibulate their daughters, while 55 percent would only circumcise them. While the nursing school educational program ignores the topic of infibulation, medical students are taught about the medical complications of the procedure. Interestingly, most of the male medical students stated that their families would not approve of marriage to an uncircumcised woman, noting that it would be "the equivalent of marrying a prostitute" (Gall 1985).

attempt to regulate female morality. Infibulation creates the ultimate chastity belt, one forged out of the woman's own flesh (Morgan and Steinem 1980). An infibulated woman is a guaranteed virgin most of the time and is therefore marriageable. Excision, by removing the sensitive clitoral area, is thought to attenuate sexual desires in a woman, who, freed from personal lust, can concentrate solely on pleasing her husband. In many African cultures, women whose genitals have not been modified are regarded as lustful, odd, and unworthy of being a wife and mother. The Arabic word *tahur* refers to purity, cleanliness, and circumcision; the uncircumcised woman is thought to be unclean and to have an offensive smell that emanates from her clitoris. The notion of "enclosedness" is important symbolically in many African cultures, and infibulation is one means of expressing this notion. "In that infibulation purifies, smooths, and makes clean the outer surface of the womb, the enclosure of the home of childbirth, it socializes or culturalizes a woman's fertility. Through occlusion of the vaginal orifice, her womb, both literally and figuratively, becomes a social space: enclosed, impervious, virtually impenetrable" (Boddy 1982, p. 696). The rituals are perpetuated because marriage and motherhood are the only viable social roles for women. Attempts to abolish the operations often meet with vigorous protests from the women who have endured them and from the midwives who perform them for income.

Female genital modification is primarily practiced by African non-Muslims and Muslims. Although Muslims outside of Africa and the majority within Africa steadfastly deny that the procedure is sanctioned by Islam, there is a literature of scholarly debate about it (Abu-Salieh 1994). Those in favor of it claim that it is consistent with Islamic principles in that it helps females to be shy, virtuous, and less likely to be shameless and to give in to their sexual instincts.

African immigrants to Europe and, more recently, to the United States, have caused a stir because of their desire to continue the procedure (Burstyn 1996). European interest was heightened in France in 1982 when a young Malian girl died as a result of a poorly done excision; the *excisuse* fled to Africa, but the girl's parents were charged with criminal negligence. Another Malian child in Paris was barely saved by French physicians. Her father had performed a clitoridectomy with a pocketknife; he brought her to a hospital after she bled sporadically for several days. French police charged the father with performing an illegal operation, but a Malian laborers' group protested. They argued that female circumcision is a customary procedure in their culture, just as male circumcision is customary in many Western cultures. Reporters in England discovered in 1982 that some wealthy African families were bringing their young girls to private surgeons in London to be circumcised. The practice was denounced in a series of articles in English newspapers and magazines. A BBC television program on the topic was so vivid that only a curtailed version was televised. The CIRP (Circumcision Information and Resource Pages)Web site (www.cirp.org/pages/female/) is a highly recommended resource.

The First Congress on Genital Mutilation of Girls in Europe and the Western World was held in London in 1992. It concluded that "any form of genital mutilation or genital surgery to the girl child is a violation of her basic human rights and must be abolished." The procedure has been banned in most European countries but, in England, where the practice continues, there have been no prosecutions. In Italy, a compromise of sorts permits only symbolic excisions—a light cut to produce a drop of blood—to respect "tradition" without injuring the child. Many African countries have also banned the procedure, but enforcement is lacking. In Egypt, physicians are allowed to perform only partial excisions but not in government clinics. In the United States a "Federal Prohibition of Female Genital Mutilation" bill was passed in 1995.

In February 2009, the *Independent*, a national British newspaper, published a lengthy article about campaigns to end genital modification (e.g., the Amazonian Initiative Movement in Sierra Leone "tries to protect young girls from the knife"). Hirsi Ali, a feminist who has renounced Islam, moved to England from the Netherlands after threats to her life. She has been a staunch advocate of forbidding genital operations on both girls and boys. In her autobiography, *Infidel* (2007), she notes that excision of women is cruel and painful and sets girls up for a lifetime of suffering. An innovative program in Spain produces women's bathing suits with hygienic protectors that feature the picture of a rusty razor blade in the crotch area in order to increase awareness of female genital modification.

Debate about clitoridectomy is not new to England. In the 1860s, Sir Isaac Baker Brown, president of the Medical Society of London, was an ardent advocate of the procedure. He believed that female masturbation gave rise to a series of diseases beginning with hysteria and eventually leading to spinal irritation, epileptoid fits, cataleptic fits, true epileptic fits, idiocy, mania, and death. Brown honestly felt that these conditions might be cured by removing the cause of peripheral nervous excitement, namely, "the clitoris and nymphae." Brown's book on the topic, *The Curability of Certain Forms of Insanity, Epilepsy, Catalepsy, and Hysteria in Females*, was published in 1866. A reviewer for the *Church Times* recommended the book highly and urged clergymen to bring their epileptic female parishioners, especially the poor ones, to medical attention in order that they might undergo the operation.

In 1867 the Obstetrical Society of London held a heated debate on Brown's procedure. It was labeled quackery, and he was portrayed as an unscrupulous profiteer. Brown was stripped of his fellowship in the Obstetrical Society and was expelled from membership (Fleming 1960).

Clinical Cases of Genital Self-mutilation in Women

The female genitalia are the object of many intrusions (e.g., intercourse, abortion, insertion of foreign bodies during masturbation, surgical procedures, and childbirth). However, psychopathological nonsuicidal self-injury (NSSI) of the genitalia is rarely reported. Few publications on the topic exist in the literature.

Unexplained vaginal bleeding of two years' duration was the admitting complaint of a 19-year-old unwed mother. The bleeding began six weeks after the birth of her daughter. Over a two-year period, she received three dilation and curettage operations, conization of the cervix, and multiple cauterizations. Because these procedures failed to control the bleeding and because the patient pleaded relentlessly for a hysterectomy, she was hospitalized for a thorough evaluation. When asked about self-injury, she stated that she "might do something like that in my sleep, something I couldn't control." She agreed to have a dye (gentian violet) painted on her vaginal wall that night. The next morning, she was bleeding profusely from her vagina; the dye was present on her fingernails and hands. A psychiatrist diagnosed her as having a histrionic personality disorder on the basis of her whining and childlike speech, her *belle indifference* to the bleeding, her seductive and histrionic behavior during the interview, her multiple surgeries, and a history of multiple sexual partners with little emotional involvement (Goldfield and Glick 1970).

French and Nelson (1972) reported the case of a 38-year-old epileptic housewife who was hospitalized for intractable overeating and self-induced vomiting. Her husband bragged about her girlish figure, but she considered herself fat. She regularly induced vomiting to keep from gaining weight. Her husband reported finding "buckets of moldy old puke hidden around the place." The woman felt isolated in her rural community and in her marriage. Although her epilepsy was well controlled, she had lost her driver's license. As her nervousness and vomiting increased, she was slowly extruded from family membership. Following a marital argument, she slashed her genital area with a razor blade; the cuts were superficial. French and Nelson noted that because her husband's interest in her was largely sexual, "she cut the only part of her he was interested in."

Simpson (1973) reported on a 22-year-old woman whose birth was the result of an unwanted and bitterly resented pregnancy. She received little attention from her parents, who were deeply involved in church work and who often quarreled over the wife's abhorrence of intercourse. At the age of 12 she masturbated by putting pencils in her vagina but soon stopped for fear "of doing damage." At the age of 15 she vomited after a boy put his arm around her. After leaving school she was hospitalized three times for abdominal pains, urinary problems, heavy bleeding during her periods, and intermenstrual bleeding. Fearing pregnancy after intercourse one day, she put a needle in her vagina to produce bleeding. As a result, a dilation and curettage had to be performed. Shortly afterward, she cut her wrists.

The next few years were marked by numerous hospitalizations for such problems as fainting, fever of unknown origin, wrist cutting, drug overdose, swallowing metal objects, smashing windows, inserting objects into her vagina and rectum, slashing her breasts, self-strangulation, cutting her vagina with a kitchen knife, severe dieting, compulsive overeating, and vomiting. She admitted that she planned her self-cutting carefully, that she enjoyed the anticipation, and that no pain accompanied the cuts. She was fascinated at the sight of her blood and felt that "something evil and tense within her [was] leaking away." A variety of treatments, including electroshock and many different types of medications, proved unsuccessful. Simpson noted that genital NSSI in women is a rare event, that a specific syndrome had not yet been established, and that no consistently helpful management advice could be offered. He concluded by wondering whether the female genital mutilation scene in Ingmar Bergman's film *Cries and Whispers* would inspire imitations. (The film was released in 1972–73; I have found no published or anecdotal reports implicating it in any self-harm attempts.) The 2009 Cannes Film Festival showed the Danish filmmaker Lara Von Trier's *Antichrist*, which contains a graphic scene of female vaginal cutting.

Standage et al. (1974) reported the case of a 20-year-old woman who had schizophrenia. She placed numerous objects in her vagina and ears in response to hallucinatory commands (her cervix and vaginal vault were lacerated by pieces of glass, plastic, a pin, and a pen top). She felt that people were reading her mind and that men were following her and threatening to assault her sexually. Her NSSI decreased as her psychosis abated; treatment included major tranquilizers and electroshock therapy.

In 1975 Goldney and Simpson described two women, aged 33 and 28 years, whose major symptoms were severe eating disorders and hysterical personality characteristics. Their "mutilation" consisted of repeatedly shaving off their pubic hair; this was interpreted by their psychiatrists as "a rejection of adult femininity."

Another patient, a 39-year-old housewife, had three "alleged" spontaneous abortions. She carried two pregnancies to term but was hospitalized during each of them for at least five months because of vaginal bleeding. Three weeks following the delivery of her second child, she was hospitalized for vaginal bleeding. Her husband caught her attempting to hide a blood-covered metal comb, but she talked him out of informing hospital staff. Following a hysterectomy the patient developed anorexia and occasional vomiting. Goldney and Simpson felt that "her difficulty in accepting the feminine role [normal sexual relations had never been established in her marriage] culminated in its rejection by genital self-mutilation and enforced hysterectomy" (p. 437). They proposed the term *Caenis syndrome* to describe the clinical triad of female genital NSSI, dysorexia, and hysterical personality.[4]

A 23-year-old woman sought help at a hospital emergency room for bleeding after she had inserted a razor blade into her vagina. She had a history of repeated sexual abuse by her relatives and foster parents, two brief chaotic marriages, prostitution, and polysubstance dependency. She was hospitalized with diagnoses of major depression and borderline personality disorder and after two weeks inserted another razor blade in her vagina (Alao et al. 1999).

A 26-year-old woman entered a partial hospitalization program for treatment of depression and almost fatal suicide attempts. After five years of treatment, she disclosed her childhood sexual abuse, adolescent rape, and severe symptoms of dissociative episodes including total loss of memory for ten months during her adolescence. She admitted to recurrent cutting of her vagina with razor blades and a surgical scalpel and of even partially sewing up her vaginal orifice to protect herself from further sexual abuse (Waugaman 1999).

Clinical Cases of Self-castration

Castration refers to the cutting off of the penis and or testicles. The first case in the medical literature dates back to 1882–83 (Warrington). A 29-year-old single farmer and stonemason named Isaac Brooks, claimed that several neighbors attacked him, cut his scrotum with a knife, and pressed out his left testicle. A physician replaced the organ and the patient recovered; his assailants were sentenced to ten years of penal servitude. Two years later, Brooks claimed he was attacked

4. As described in book 12 of Ovid's *Metamorphoses*, Caenis was a beautiful girl whom many men desired although she rejected all thoughts of marriage. One day, the god of the sea raped her while she was walking on a private beach. The god Neptune was pleased and thought she was too, so he offered to give her anything she wanted. Caenis said she wanted to become a man. Her wish was granted.

again by several men who severely gashed open his scrotum. The physician who previously treated him was called, and the patient confessed that he had inflicted both wounds. He died within a year; while on his deathbed he signed a confession that freed his neighbors from jail. Warrington noted that it was not uncommon for insane persons to mutilate their genitals. According to him, such patients often followed a similar course. They were neurotic and therefore unable to cope with sexual desires. This strain increased their nervous weakness, and their condition soon escalated to paranoia, impulsivity, and hallucinations, which directed them to do things they opposed. Their struggles led them to hypochondriasis, brooding, and irritability. Finally, in obedience to the Holy Scriptures, they cut off the offending member and then accused others of tampering with them.

Adam (1883) described an 18-year-old farm servant who had been dull and moody for several months. He went into the field one night with a penknife and "completely and cleanly removed the whole of his penis" because he had masturbated and felt it was his duty to follow the biblical injunction that "if thy right hand offend thee cut it off." He was hospitalized because of violent behavior, his belief that people were plotting against him, his refusal to eat food for fear his mother was poisoning him, and his assertion that he was Paul the Apostle. His mother attributed his self-castration to confusion resulting from his strenuous activity in putting out a farm fire the previous week. He had been unable to sleep and kept vigil at the family farm in case someone should set it on fire. He took to reading the Bible and Salvation Army publications. He became depressed and taciturn and then experienced an excited, exalted, and religiously exhilarated period. When his wound healed, his mental state returned to normal.

In 1884 two lively articles on male genital self-mutilation appeared in midwestern American medical journals. Galt reported on a small-town saloonkeeper whose wife accused him of being "no good, for your penis is no account." In a frenzy, he took a huge penknife and gashed his breast, sliced open his neck, and cut off his penis. "The man's stump of a penis reminded one of a bloody chicken's neck after its head is wrung off. It was a clean cut; a surgeon's knife could not have performed a better amputation" (p. 226). The patient recovered rapidly. His wife filed for divorce. Galt concluded: "Bereft of his money, his wife and his penis the patient will probably for the remainder of his life spend his time either in lamenting his attempt or cursing his failure to perfect the job" (p. 228).

Whiting (1884) described a 30-year-old marble cutter whose wife left him because of his excessive desire for intercourse. After she left, "his nights were spent in horrid dreams and frequent emissions and his days were one longing desire to be with some women" (p. 298). He resorted to masturbation but was so disgusted with himself that he cut open his scrotum and squeezed out his left testicle (as a child his right testicle had been surgically removed after being injured in a fall). The patient recovered and returned to his wife, but "the castration did not have the desired effect. He enjoyed the connubial felicities as of yore and was quite brutish. She only lived with him two weeks after he was out of bed—then for solace fled to parts unknown" (p. 300).

In 1901 Stroch reported the case of a 27-year-old florist who complained of chronic despondency, nervousness, poor memory, and testicular pain. He was a social recluse who never associated with women. Devoid of strong sexual feelings, he never masturbated. He attributed his misery and lack of success to the condition of his sexual organs. One night, to relieve his testicular pain and free himself from the unhappy influence of his genitals, he "seized the scrotum and testicles in his left hand, and with a razor cut from above downward, with a sawing motion, severing successively all the structures. . . . The pain was not very great. . . . To the remark that he might have amputated the penis in his haste, he laughingly replied that he was careful not to do that" (p. 270). His testicles, wrapped in a handkerchief, accompanied him to the hospital. Close inspection revealed them to be free from disease.

In the first three decades of the twentieth century the theme of castration was discussed in great detail in the psychoanalytic literature. Although actual castration was not commonly encountered, the fear of castration (with the subsequent formation of a psychological "castration complex") was thought to play a vital role in both normal childhood development and later psychopathology. Castration fears were thought to lead to suicide, desire for surgical removal of body parts, fantasies that one's genitalia had been cut, delusions of being emasculated by enemies, and actual self-removal of the genitals to cure masturbation or to protect against perverse sexual cravings.

According to Freud and the early psychoanalysts, the male castration complex is a form of self-punishment intended to relieve guilt over incestuous oedipal desires arising in childhood. Additionally, a boy supposedly desires to castrate his father because the father retains possession of the boy's mother. This desire may grow into a wish to castrate his brothers and all other males so that the boy will assume world power. Because such desires obviously can never be fulfilled, they are repressed, and they are eventually inverted so that self-castration becomes a feared punishment for these desires.

Karl Abraham, Ernest Jones, and other early analysts developed the notion that women as well as men develop a castration complex. Upon discovering that they lack a penis, little girls supposedly develop fantasies of having been "robbed" of their penis and of being left with only a gaping wound. Thus, their castration complex develops, marked by hatred toward and envy of men (because they possess a penis) and by the hope of receiving a child from the father (the child being a substitute for the penis that was taken from them). The castration complex is revived in later life by menstruation and defloration. This hatred and envy of men may be manifested by vaginismus, by dismissal of the importance of the penis (the supposed origin of the concept of an immaculate conception), and by frigidity.

In a series of somewhat rambling psychoanalytic articles with multiple references, Lewis (1927, 1928, 1931) coined the term *Eshmun complex* to describe the psychodynamics of patients who mutilated themselves by actual or symbolic castration as an expression of "the incest mechanism in action."[5] Lewis presented many case reports of psychotic patients who demonstrated this complex, although in many instances the presence of an "incest mechanism" is not apparent to me. A typical case is that of a 28-year-old man who had cut out his left testicle seven years earlier for unknown reasons. Three months before the current hospitalization, he attempted to remove his remaining testicle as a cure for chronic masturbation. His wound healed, but he lost his job. He began to have religious hallucinations, prayed incessantly, and cried a lot. In the hospital he was coquettish. He adopted feminine mannerisms, imitated the sufferings of Christ, and cut out his right testicle with a piece of glass because he wanted to be a priest. A follow-up examination nine years later revealed him to have an effeminate voice and eccentric clothing. He demonstrated frequent silly smiles, said that his castration was God's will, admitted to personal communication with God, and was convinced that he really was a priest.

Other cases of the so-called Eshmun complex include the following:

- A 25-year-old man with chronic schizophrenia was destructive and uncooperative, and he sat in one spot for long periods of time repeating profane phrases. He said he was the devil, and he was usually silly and incoherent. He bit off his lower lip and gouged out both of his testicles with his fingernails for no apparent reason.
- A 30-year-old schizophrenic naval officer thought that his shipmates had accused him of perverted sexual practices. He heard voices that told him to do odd things and left him bewildered and confused; while in such a state

5. Eshmun was a handsome Phoenician nature deity. To avoid being seduced by the mother-goddess, Astronae, he castrated himself and was then transported to the heavens, where he became the moon deity. Thus, Eshmun's self-castration was done to avoid incest; following the act, he became associated with neutral and feminine activities (the moon with its monthly cycles).

he cut off his genitals with a razor. Lewis interpreted the mutilation as a punishment for incestuous desires because the patient's father had left home when the patient was 8 years old, leaving him "wholly in possession of his mother without competition."

- A 28-year-old man who had been depressed for three years was hospital-ized for serious blood loss after a self-castration attempt. He said that voices "told me they could make me take out my testicles and if I didn't do it they would make me lose my voice." He had long struggled with homosexual desires and said that he attempted castration to humiliate himself and to expiate some of his sins. During adolescence he had made a previous castration attempt following homosexual experiences: "I thought I was a terrible person. . . . it seemed that it might prevent me from indulging in sodomy" (p. 183).

Women, too, could manifest the Eshmun complex. A 39-year-old single school-teacher developed a homosexual attachment to a nurse while in the hospital. She muttered to herself that she came from heaven and Jesus Christ was her father. She heard voices, claimed that electrical impulses passed through the walls and into her body, and destroyed property in periods of excitement. At the age of 50, she felt that her body was alive but her brain was dead. She tried to rip out her womb, pull out her teeth, tear out her umbilicus, and scratch her eyes with her fingers and a nail file.

Lewis considered the castration reaction to be "the basic theme in all life." He related it closely to suicide, noting that "one who dies, dies a temporal death, while the castrate dies eternally since his germ plasm has perished" (p. 197). The relationship between suicide and self-mutilation received widespread attention because of Karl Menninger's popular *Man against Himself* (1938). He theorized that "the suicidal impulse may be concentrated upon a part as a substitute for the whole" (p. 231). Menninger noted that psychotic men who feel guilty about sexual sins related to women, homosexuality, or masturbation "do the obvious thing of ridding themselves of the guilty part of their body" (p. 270). Because of con-scious or unconscious homosexual impulses, castration not only accomplishes self-punishment but also converts the castrate "into a passive, penis-less indi-vidual, anatomically comparable with the female" (p. 270). Thus, while castration appears to be an act of atonement for homosexual wishes, in reality it allows a man to become closer to these wishes; it makes him incapable of the active role while predisposing him even more to the passive role.

In 1933, Bradley presented a case report to his colleagues at the Saint Louis

Medical Society. The patient was a 61-year-old lifelong "sexual pervert" with hyperactive sexuality. He first had sexual intercourse at the age of 9. He admitted to frequent sexual acts with cattle, sheep, and hogs and to chronic masturbation during his marriages. At the age of 40, remorseful about his hypersexuality, he went to the barn, sharpened his knife, and cut out both testicles. This did not curb his sexual appetite, however, and he married for the third time. He contracted gonorrhea, and, again feeling remorseful, cut off half of his penis with a pocketknife. Bradley was unable to present the patient to the medical group, however, noting: "Unfortunately, I am unable to show the patient tonight. He is a prisoner, charged with attempting to rape a girl 10 years old. When I asked him why he did such a thing and stated that it would have done him no good, he said he thought it might do the little girl some good" (p. 134).

For a decade genital self-injury was not written about in the medical literature. Then, in 1948, Beilin and Gruenberg reported, primarily from a urological perspective, on psychotic patients in state mental hospitals.

- A 52-year-old man who had hebephrenic schizophrenia and tuberculosis tied a string around his penis, causing swelling of the organ and extensive tissue destruction. He was confused, incoherent, disoriented, weak, and debilitated and was unable to recall the act or the reason for it. He died three months later.
- A 19-year-old man who had excited catatonia, the son of a Baptist minister, was guilty of committing numerous sexual acts with children. After the court recommended castration, the patient cut off his testicles with a razor blade. While in the hospital he attempted to gouge out his eyes. He died three months later.
- A 24-year-old schizophrenic man amputated his testicle with a buckle because he was fearful of the electroshock treatments he was receiving. The patient wrapped his excised testicle in tissue paper on which he had written, "Exhibit A, one meatball."
- A 48-year-old man who had severe organic brain disease avulsed the left half of his scrotum. He was totally disoriented and unable to provide any information.

Hemphill, in 1951, reported the case of a 66-year-old man who had a history of depression. He cut his wrist with a razor, amputated his penis and one testicle, and felt enormous mental relief. Throughout his life he was plagued by feelings of guilt about being closely bound to his mother, about an incestuous affair with a female cousin, and about his promiscuous sexual behavior. After becoming impotent due to diabetes he felt that his genitals "had let me down and were now no good to me—that I should get rid of the organs." He regarded them as independent sources of temptation that controlled and misled him. He did not regret his actions and claimed that they gained him moral tranquility, because he could now live "a proper life" with his cousin. Hemphill concluded that several conditions appear to be necessary before genital self-mutilation can occur, namely, "an abnormal attitude toward the genitals; a tendency to regard them as being capable of exercising an independent influence over the organism as a whole and therefore inviting the possibility of rejecting the genitals in order to avoid sin or danger . . . an abnormal integration of the concept of the body or of the body image . . . [and] a strong motive consciously understood, such as incest or fear of the destruction of the body as a whole by physical illness" (p. 294).

In 1953 Kenyon and Hyman published several case reports. A Japanese college student became mentally disturbed because of low grades. He amputated all of his genitals with a butcher's knife. A 38-year-old depressed man with chronic alcoholism "in the kitchen of his home and in the presence of his alcoholic wife, placed his genitalia on the table and completely amputated them with one stroke of an ordinary bread knife" (p. 207). Bleeding profusely, he walked to a nearby police station, shook the specimen in his hand, and proclaimed "his act and his heroism" to the precinct captain. He was diagnosed as schizophrenic, spoke incoherently about his act, about his cowardice and courage, about his loss of sex, and his desire to become a woman.

Three cases from Australia were published by Lennon in 1963. In one, a 60-year-old psychotically depressed man felt guilty over alleged sexual misdemeanors in his younger years and cut off both testicles with a razor blade. In another, a 28-year-old schizophrenic man whose illness was characterized by inadequacy, passivity, reclusiveness, and mystical ruminations amputated his penis for fear of becoming a homosexual. A third case, that of a 42-year-old well-educated man, provided details of self-castration performed during a manic episode. He had a stormy marriage that he attributed to his overly demanding sexual attitude. His wife filed for a divorce. A day before the divorce became final, the patient was severely manic. He saw a letter about his brother's change of address to a street with an odd-sounding name. His mother wrote of the address, "This may look funny, but it isn't." The patient dwelled on the word "funny" and eventually concluded that it would be "funny" to cut off his penis. He used a rubber band for a ligature and cut off his penis with a razor. Although it was painful, he felt happy and cheerful. He drove to work after throwing his penis on the car floor. As he recovered from his mania in the hospital, he maintained a bland complacency about his amputation and jocosely stated that "I knew my divorce was coming up, and I would have no further use for it." The patient's lack of remorse and his complacency led Lennon to believe that the castration had provided a satisfactory solution to an unconscious conflict. Lennon concluded that "by amputating his penis, the symbol of his manhood, he had made himself acceptable to his wife, in so far as he could not now be accounted a man; in addition he had gotten rid of the organ he believed responsible for his marital disharmony, and had in some way contributed a peace offering towards a future reunion" (p. 81).

In 1963, Blacker and Wong published a study of four men with psychosis or borderline disorder who mutilated their genitals. In this widely quoted paper the authors identified six commonalities among the patients: (1) They came from disturbed homes in which the father was often absent and the mother was dominant. (2) Their self-castration was a culmination of a long, intense sexual confusion that resulted in a gradual disassociation of their alien genital organs from their body scheme. (3) Their relationships with women were submissive and masochistic and indicated a desire for an infantile relationship with a mother figure. Castration removed the threat of genital sexuality from such a relationship. (4) Their self-mutilation served to relieve depression and "could be considered an attenuated suicide, a compromise that averted total annihilation of the organism" (p. 175). (5) They had a confused sexual identity as manifested by strong feminine identifications. (6) They repudiated their male genitals. Unclear as to whether they were male or female, they attempted to resolve the issue in a primitive way.

Typical of the cases is a man whose childhood was characterized by poverty and deprivation. His nervous father was a religious fanatic and a bully. The patient's mother saw him with an erection when he was a child and said, "Shame, little boys who play with themselves have to have part of it come off." This incident made him reluctant to be a boy. He said that "nothing like this could happen to a girl because girls are safer." He began to prick his scrotum and penis with pins and often pulled his breasts in the hope of enlarging them. He eventually married and had a responsible job. At the age of 32, he cut his urethra to make himself "more like a woman." His wife later divorced him, and he married a motherly woman. After five years, he drank alcohol heavily and developed intense desires to have female breasts, suckle children, and destroy his penis. At the age of 49, he became sexually involved with a 65-year-old man. In a state of depression, he got drunk and felt a savage desire to get rid of his penis. "I resented the penis because I had been born wrong and then blamed for it." He placed his penis on a wood block and chopped it off with a hatchet. He was disoriented and had both visual and auditory hallucinations upon hospitalization. His condition cleared rapidly, and after two weeks he returned to work.

Kushner (1967) focused on the significance of religious delusions in the self-castration of two paranoid schizophrenic men. The first patient was hospitalized at the age of 26 because of auditory hallucinations, ideas of reference, incongruity of affect, and religious preoccupations. Upon discharge he preached in public, carried a religious sign after shaving his head, and almost died while meditating in the hills during winter. His search for spiritual purification alternated with profound guilt following episodes of drunkenness, aggression, masturbation, and promiscuity. At the age of 32 he cut off both testicles "as a freewill offering to God" and arrived at the hospital carrying them in a box. Five years later, following the death of his father, the patient drank alcohol heavily and had his first homosexual experience. He felt disgusted and turned to the Bible, where he was impressed by Matthew 19:12: "and there be eunuchs who have made themselves eunuchs for the Kingdom of Heaven's sake." He purchased a block of wood and a razor and waited until he felt sexual desire. He then cut off his penis, threw it into a fire, and watched it burn. He sought help, stating, "Even if I do get certified [as legally insane] and in the eyes of the world I am mad, it is far better for me to have cleansed myself" (p. 295).

The second patient was a shy, withdrawn man with an excellent work record. He was constantly afraid that people would consider him a homosexual because of his gentleness. At the age of 35 he suddenly developed deep religious feelings. His work deteriorated as his religious preoccupation increased. He was hospitalized and received electroshock treatment. He dwelled on the Bible and on outer space and decided that he must renounce "the sex life of the world." Influenced by Matthew 19:12, he castrated himself with a razor in the belief that this act of purification would qualify him to serve as the pilot who would carry the godly to outer space.

Kushner noted that anxiety over homosexual tendencies caused patients such as these to strive for purity and salvation; religion was the medium they chose to obtain relief from guilt. Because society tolerates such wide differences in religious thought, Kushner stated that it may be difficult to distinguish a religious belief from a delusion. In both patients, however, religious ideas about sin and redemption were extended into delusions that were supported by a concrete interpretation of biblical references.

Hahn and Hahn (1967) reported the case of a 20-year-old schizophrenic Korean man who amputated his penis with a razor following his first sexual experience, intercourse with a prostitute. He had always failed in his desperate attempts to gain his mother's love, was angry and hostile toward her, and unconsciously identified the prostitute with her; he sacrificed his penis out of guilt and depression.

In 1973, Goldfield and Glick reported the case of a 22-year-old high school graduate with a yearlong history of schizophrenia. He complained of feeling "machinelike" and thought that he was Leonardo da Vinci. He spent fifteen hours a day painting and slept only three or four hours. He laughed to himself and talked unintelligibly. Then "the voice of God" told him to castrate himself with a razor. He proceeded to remove his testicles from the scrotal sac. Although he felt an urge to cut off his penis, he did not because the voice of God became silent. In a bland and emotionless state he drove himself to a friend's house.

Anumonye (1973) was the first to report self-amputation of the penis in Africa. Two Nigerian patients castrated themselves after receiving promotions (one to an important chieftaincy, the other to a better position at work). Neither had manifested premorbid psychopathology. Their elevation to a higher, more responsible social status triggered a brief psychotic episode, which resolved rapidly. Their lack of remorse, however, suggested that the castration had resolved some unconscious conflict.

In 1974, Engelman et al. reported the case of a 26-year-old schizophrenic man who cut off the tip of his penis with a razor. His agitated, psychotic condition had been precipitated by acute drug and alcohol use. He had a history of repeated failures in traditional male roles, and his rejection of his masculinity was intermingled with strong guilt and a need for self-punishment. He regretted his actions, however, and desired to have the tip of his penis reattached surgically.

The following unpublished case from 1976 was supplied to me by Dr. Wolfgang Jilek of Vancouver, British Columbia. A 31-year-old Mennonite had a history of chronic schizophrenia and many hospitalizations. He sat on a bucket of ice, took pain-killing pills, and removed both of his testicles with a razor blade because he believed that people were torturing him through his testicles. A voice repeatedly told him to "squeeze them till they burst." He frequently had thoughts of blinding himself by staring at the flame of a welding torch or by sticking pencils in his eyes. Dr. Jilek believed that the patient's self-castration was a substitute for self-blinding.

In 1977, Evins et al. described a 25-year-old man with paranoid schizophrenia who removed both testicles with a razor blade. He then cut the base of his penis in an abortive attempt at amputation. He had auditory hallucinations; his mother's voice told him that he could not enter the kingdom of heaven unless he cut off his penis and testicles.

In 1979, Greilsheimer and Groves described a 23-year-old unemployed Catholic man (a twin) who had been reared by a nervous and extremely religious mother. At the age of 18, he decided to become a priest but was refused admission to a seminary. He became psychotic and was hospitalized for paranoid schizophrenia. At the age of 23, he suffered nightmares and terrors, became withdrawn, and read the Bible incessantly. When both his dog and an injured bird that he had rescued died, he became acutely psychotic. He stated that his penis and his aunt's clitoris "were standing out at each other." On the first anniversary of his twin sister's marriage (of which the patient did not approve), he cut off his penis with a razor blade in obedience to Matthew 18:7–9. The act was sudden and painless and was followed by a sense of immediate relief.

Kalin (1979) described a young man who feared that his compulsive masturbation was destroying his body and nervous system. At the age of 21, he asked a surgeon to perform a total orchiectomy to save him from his "hyperaggressiveness." He stated, "I'm no homosexual or transsexual. I still want a hugging and kissing relationship with a woman." After being rejected for the castration, he injected himself with chemicals to lower his testosterone level. He hoped this would decrease his sexual fantasies and enhance his well-being. He was hospitalized when an abscess formed, and he was diagnosed as having schizophrenia, gender identity problems, and possible temporal lobe epilepsy. He later briefly received a nonfeminizing antiandrogen hormone. Unable to find a physician willing to continue his hormone treatment, he cut off his testicles. Two months later, he operated on himself again and tried for eight hours to denervate his adrenal glands; he had to stop because of great pain in attempting to retract his liver. He was unresponsive to medication and unable to form a working alliance with a psychotherapist.

Suk and Son (1980) reported on four Korean men with schizophrenia who castrated themselves. All four were lower-social-class single men who had impoverished childhoods and were depressed before their self-castration. They identified with their mothers, had confused sexual identities, and had difficulty with the male role. Three revealed homosexual wishes.

Pabis et al. (1980) described a man who had spent ten years in a class for emotionally disturbed children. At the age of 17, he was diagnosed with psychotic depression. He withdrew from social activities and believed that masturbation drained his brain of "nuclear material." He sought out prostitutes to perform sadomasochistic acts and served as a homosexual prostitute. At the age of 29, he waded into the ocean and cut off his scrotum and testicles with a kitchen knife. He brought his testicles home and handed them to his mother. He felt that his mother had "half died" at his birth; by presenting her with his testicles, he intended to give back to her the life she had given him at birth. After the castration his anxiety, depression, and many of his delusions diminished. He expressed no regrets and was especially happy at the loss of some facial hair.

Clark (1981) presented the case of a middle-aged man who was hospitalized several times for depression. He reported periods of "overexuberance," drank alcohol heavily, felt guilty over his sexual interest in prepubertal girls, and considered suicide. After weeks of desperate deliberation on the biblical texts about plucking out one's eye and about becoming a eunuch for heaven's sake, he decided to castrate himself. He was refused admission to a mental hospital and then cut off his testicles. He benefited from psychotherapy after his self-castration and published several books before he died of natural causes fifteen years later.

In 1981, Hall et al. reported the case of a young man whose family lived in a sparsely inhabited rural island. As an adolescent he had periods of intense interest in Buddhism and reincarnation along with heavy marijuana use. Because of his "sinful" sexual thoughts he felt unworthy of dating. At the age of 22, he became suspicious and thought that he was disliked by his colleagues at work because of his "terrible" thoughts and dark skin color. When the family cat jumped into his lap, he became sexually stimulated and attempted intercourse with the animal. Feeling guilty and hopeless, he believed that God would forgive him only if he atoned for his behavior. Voices commanded him to amputate his hand and penis. Hungry and sleep deprived, he chopped off his right hand and the tip of his penis. He received the diagnosis of paranoid schizophrenia with a superimposed depression.

Rada and James (1982) published a thoughtful report on six men whose genital NSSI involved inserting objects into their urethra. All were inmates in a hospital for the criminally insane. None had ever been psychotic. The number of urethral mutilations per patient varied from one to twenty-six. Most occurred during the daytime, frequently when the inmate was in seclusion.

The group was characterized by poor sexual and social adjustment, female identification (three were bisexual), chaotic home environments during childhood, and extensive involvement with the criminal justice system. Five had a history of fire setting, while the sixth had "accidentally" burned his face before his first urethral insertion. Five had a history of self-cutting before their current acts; they also swallowed razor blades, open pins, or cleaning solution before or during the acts of urethral insertion. Two were adult head bangers.

The most common motive for their NSSI was to secure transfer to a different unit. The authors noted that the inmates experienced a buildup of tension, anger, and dysphoria before their NSSI. The acts were painless, but most inmates experienced pain later. Within minutes, news of a urethral insertion spread throughout the institution and gained a special reputation and identity for the inserter. The contagious nature of the acts was clear; each person had a personal relationship with at least one other inserter, and many of the acts were temporally related.

The staff response to the acts was typically focused on the patients' manipulativeness. Repulsed by the acts, many staff members stated that state money would be saved if the physician let the inmates cut off their penises. The staff's need to ventilate contributed to the rapid spread of news about the acts throughout the institution. After staff agreed not to talk about the acts, new incidents of self-mutilation did not occur in other units. Three of the inmates stopped their mutilative behavior immediately after being transferred.

In 1983, Thompson and Abraham reported two cases of castration after paternal death. In the first case, a 24-year-old single man with no prior psychiatric history attempted to circumcise himself with a pair of scissors. Depressed after the death of his father one week previously, he said that "this might lift him out of his depression." The second case was that of a 37-year-old unemployed single man who was hospitalized for loss of blood after he had cut out one testicle and part of the other. He said he had led a religious movement during a previous incarnation in eighteenth-century Russia, was persecuted, and had castrated himself with a red-hot poker. He received the diagnosis of acute psychotic episode in reaction to the death of his father three days earlier. He was treated surgically and his mental state improved.

Thompson and Abraham speculated that genital self-mutilation after paternal death might indicate an unresolved oedipal complex. The bereavement might intensify previous guilt, and the son might then mutilate his genitals as a self-imposed punishment. The patient's psychiatrists were unaware that his remarks about self-castration with a red-hot poker in eighteenth-century Russia were a reference to the Skoptsi sect. This appears to be the only report of self-castration influenced by knowledge of the Skoptsi.

A case on which I consulted in 1984 involved a 35-year-old man who had chronic schizophrenia and mild mental retardation. He had lived with a chronic schizophrenic woman for six years; she had recently been hospitalized for an exacerbation of her condition. He had a high sex drive and felt frustrated because his companion had developed a "phobia" to sex and refused his sexual advances. He masturbated three to five times daily, sometimes so violently that blood came out of his penis. Feeling lonely during his woman friend's hospitalization, he heard the voice of the devil, who told him to cut off his genitals. He got drunk and the devil said, "Now you can't control yourself. Go ahead and cut it off." He secured his penis with a barbecue fork and cut it off. He was brought to the hospital and said he would now get along better with his woman friend because he would no longer be bothered by his penis. He had no regrets for what he had done but felt "a little embarrassed." For several days the voice of the devil told him to complete the job by cutting off his testicles, but the voice gradually diminished. The patient planned to live peacefully with his woman friend, to rejoin the Pentecostal church, and to be reborn in the Holy Spirit.

Schweitzer (1990) reported on two cases of self-castration in psychotic men, one of whom had previously amputated his hand. The author proposed the name Klingsor syndrome for cases of self-castration, but the name has not been adopted. (Klingsor is a character in Wagner's opera *Parsifal*; he castrated himself in a vain effort to join the brotherhood of the Teutonic Grail Knights.) In 2001, Myers and Nguyen reported a case in which self-castration was the first sign of incipient schizophrenia; in 2002 Duggal et al. reported on the acute onset of schizophrenia following self-castration. In 2008, Ristic et al. reported on two brothers with religious psychotic experiences and sexual guilt who mutilated their genitals. Ajape et al. (2010) reported the case of a Nigerian student who removed one of his testicles while severely depressed; he had made two suicide attempts in the three months prior to this event. For a psychodynamic study of psychosis and male genital mutilation see Fisch (1987).

Self-castration in the Absence of Psychosis

The literature on self-castration traditionally emphasized its invariable association with psychosis. Then, in 1954, Esman reported on a man whose self-castration was a nonpsychotic, isolated, impulsive act. Other cases of nonpsychotic self-castration have since appeared in the medical literature. Most fall into the general diagnostic category of gender identity disorders, the most common being transsexualism. Male transsexuals have masculine genital organs but perceive themselves to be really female. For them, self-castration is often a procedure to correct a flaw of nature and to fulfill a longstanding wish to live as a female. A single case report documents self-castration in a transsexual man who was also schizophrenic (Mellon et al. 1989).

The patient described by Esman never had any homosexual contacts and regarded homosexuality as unnatural. When he was 19 years old a man suggested that he might earn a lot of money as a female impersonator. He tried on women's clothing but felt unattractive. He developed problems with alcohol and at the age of 44 he said, "I want to be loved. I want to be more like a girl. I want to have my penis and scrotum cut off, have my testicles pushed up into my abdomen. . . . I want to wear my pretty dresses with lace fringes. . . . I want to be more of a child, not just a girl" (p. 80). Several months later, while drunk, he cut out his testicles with a razor blade. He was neither significantly depressed nor delusional but rather told his story coherently, logically, and fluently. Esman interpreted the castration to be the isolated, impulsive act of a person who had a schizoid personality structure and sought "a dependent, narcissistic oral relationship with a mother figure." Because he felt even the possibility of genital sexuality would threaten this sort of relationship, he castrated himself.

In 1956, Cleveland reported on men whose self-castration appeared to be "deliberate and purposeful behavior, not the random self-mutilation of a frenzied patient." An example was a man who was treated cruelly in an orphanage. The matrons threatened bed wetters with castration, and girls were treated preferentially. He envied girls and longed to be one. He injured his scrotum accidentally and felt he would be better off without such a painful appendage. When he divorced his first wife, he attempted castration but stopped because the pain was too great. At the age of 25, following a second divorce, he deeply gashed his scrotum; he was depressed over failure to gain custody of his children. At the age of 29, he felt that his problems would be resolved if he lost his disturbing sexual drive, so he carefully excised his scrotum and testicles. He was not psychotic, although he reacted to the castration with bland unconcern. The patient wrote a clear self-analysis of his mutilation and related it to his dependency, insecurity, and envy of girls.

Schneider et al. (1965) published an in-depth study of a man who experienced marked cyclic changes in sexuality although intensive examination revealed no endocrinological abnormalities. As an infant, he had been diagnosed with bilateral cryptorchidism. He had vague feelings of uneasiness about his role as a boy. He quit high school because of the ridicule he received over his large breasts. After an emergency appendectomy at the age of 23, he became increasingly feminized; his breasts grew even larger, his voice rose, his facial hair stopped growing, and his body fat assumed a feminine distribution. This process continued for about two years until suddenly, for no apparent reason, he started to remasculinize. The eight-month period of remasculinization was trying to the patient, and he felt more comfortable when he then began to refeminize. He took to dressing and passing as a woman. Upset when the remasculinization process started again, he carefully amputated both testicles. Following this, he experienced a short cycle of feminization followed by masculinization. He was hospitalized after he attempted to amputate his penis. Six months after discharge from the hospital he meticulously cut off his penis.

Lowry and Kolivakis (1971) reported the case of a 35-year-old hospital attendant who cut off his testicles, burned them, and flushed them down the toilet. He stated that he had lost about fifty cubic centimeters of blood during the castration and that this was "the usual amount lost by a woman during menstruation." Since the age of 6, the patient had wanted to be a girl. He had been preoccupied with a desire for a sex-change operation since adolescence, when he began to cross-dress openly. He claimed that he always felt disgusted by his sexual organs, that the cross-dressing was not sexually exciting, and that he had never masturbated. In the army, he was regarded as a homosexual although he denied any homosexual interest. Over the years, he was arrested several times for cross-dressing. He got a job as a practical nurse. To prepare himself for castration, he obtained a position in the urology department, where he familiarized himself with the surgical instruments and procedure. The self-castration was not preceded by any important psychological or social stress, and he was not psychotic. He was admitted to the psychiatric ward, where he dressed bizarrely as a female, with an ill-fitting wig and false breasts. His request for a surgical penectomy and construction of a vagina was deferred, but he was placed on estrogen. Over the next four years, he engaged in psychotherapy, relentlessly established his feminine identity, and even was accepted for membership in a women's church group.

Perhaps the most widely quoted study on genital self-surgery in relation to transsexualism is that by Money and DePriest (1976). An artist-farmer, inspired by his study of Jungian psychology, developed a complicated theory about the "lost bisexual secret of the urethral orgasm," which he derived from mythical, artistic, and literary symbols. He cut an opening in his penis at the penoscrotal angle designed to allow a "host penis" to reach his urethra. He thought that the intromission of a man's penis into this opening would prevent death. He likened his condition to that of Australian aborigines who practiced subincision, and he wondered if they too experienced the ecstasy of urethral orgasm. At the age of 63, he was found wandering the streets in a fugue state, naked and disoriented.

Another case involved a 45-year-old paranoid man who had a delusional belief that while his external genitals were clearly those of a male, his internal sexual organs were female and that his vagina shared a common outlet with his rectum. He asserted that an ileostomy would keep his "vagina" cleared of feces. A year earlier, he had cut off his penis with shears. To be sure that his penis would not be sutured back in place, he flushed it down the toilet. He believed so strongly in his "rectal vagina" that he attempted to become pregnant by inserting sperm into his rectum. During a ten-year follow-up it became clear that he could not cope with sex-reassignment surgery nor could he live in the female role as a transvestite. He continued to live as a male but had constant fantasies of living as a female.

A third case was that of a 51-year-old man who cut off his testicles using ice packs and a clamp marketed for the castration of farm animals. He believed that castration would allow him to feel like the girl he longed to be. Since adolescence, he had had a persistent compulsion to dress as a woman and to live as a female. As a form of self-therapy, he had married and reared three sons. As much as he desired to be a "girl," he was deeply dependent on his wife's companionship. He removed his testicles but spared his penis, thus achieving some resolution of his conflicts.

Money and DePriest noted that in the first two patients the transsexual compulsion was embedded in a delusional system, while in the third it was manifested as an idée fixe. The patients obtained no erotic pleasure from their self-surgery and would gladly have accepted the services of a surgeon.

Some patients who are perturbed by the slowness of the evaluation for sex reassignment surgery may cut off their testicles to convince clinic staff of their seriousness; others may do so because of their inability to pay for the surgery (Haberman and Michael 1979; Krieger et al. 1982). These patients tend to remove their testicles neatly, with little tissue damage; usually they have studied the anatomy of the area in detail and have long-term goals for their self-surgery. In contrast, a psychotic person who castrates himself tends to act impulsively, to lacerate the area, and may mutilate his penis as well as his testicles with a fair amount of blood loss.

Cases of self-castration in nonpsychotic and non-gender-dysphoric men have been reported. Eke and Elenwo (1999) published the case of a twenty-six-year-old Nigerian man who castrated his penis and both testicles. He claimed that his "master," a man that he knew, had performed the operation, but the police could not corroborate this. No motive for the castration was established. Tsao et al. (2009) described a patient whose mother threatened to "cut that thing off" as a method of stopping his bed-wetting. At age 17 he stuck needles into his penis, a practice that he continued throughout his life because it relieved feelings of loneliness and emptiness and sometimes resulted in orgasmic sexual arousal. He abused substances and his wife of 10 years left him for another man. At age 49 he cut off the right side of the tip of his penis for no apparent reason. His mental status examination was within normal limits. A month later, while watching a football game on television, he put his penis on a cutting board and sliced through the entire shaft. Psychological testing and mental status examination were negative, and he was diagnosed with borderline personality disorder. Remorse over his behavior "seemed superficial." Interestingly, he had cut off his nipples with scissors at age 18 because "they stuck out so much"; at age 45 he had bilateral breast reduction surgery. Male breast self-injury is rare; Coons (1992) reported bilateral breast amputation by a nonpsychotic man who had a schizotypal personality disorder. Female breast amputation is also rare (Coons et al. 1986).

An odd case involves a Chinese man who castrated himself in a desire to stop having painful erections. The authors felt that he had a variant of body dysmorphic disorder involving an internal body image (Leung et al. 1996). Patel et al. (2007) reported an exceedingly rare case of self-castration in a man with prion disease which caused fatal neurodegenerative changes in the brain. There are three reports of men who castrated themselves because they said that they wanted to die. A 72-year-old man with a normal mental status was so angered by disputes among his children related to property and finances that he castrated himself to get them to stop arguing (Tharoor 2007). He believed that the source of life was related to his penis. Three Chinese men severed their penises as a way of killing themselves but were dismayed and surprised that they remained alive (Yang and Bullard 1993). Conacher et al. (1991) reported the case of a nonpsychotic man who justified his attempt to commit suicide by mutilating his penis as a rational action. Finally, a 24-year-old nonpsychotic man castrated himself in an attempt to attain Moksha, spiritual salvation via liberation from the cycle of death and rebirth and all the suffering of worldly existence (Bhatia and Aurora 2001).

Comments on Genital Mutilation

The majority of deviant male genital self-mutilators tend to be psychotic at the time of the act (the most frequent diagnoses are schizophrenia and major depression), and they have an average age of 32 years. Alcohol ingestion before the act may be a contributing factor in about 25 percent of cases. (Also see Bromberg and Schilder's 1933 article on castration and dismembering motives in alcoholic hallucinosis.) Removal of the testicles is somewhat more common than removal of the penis, which, in turn, is more common than removal of both organs. There is no correlation between a specific diagnosis and the genital organ selected for mutilation. The most common reasons provided by patients for their self-mutilation are: the wish to be or delusions of being female; concerns about homosexuality;

relief of physical pain or somatic illness; guilt over sexual urges such as incest; religiosity; command hallucinations; and punishment for failures in the male role.

Nonpsychotic self-mutilators are, as noted, likely to be men with character disorders who act impulsively or transsexuals who have premeditated their actions. The genital mutilations of transsexuals are usually well planned and neatly done. While many psychotic persons castrate themselves impulsively and with little regard to surgical technique, transsexuals typically have studied the procedure and perform it in a controlled fashion with a minimum of unnecessary trauma.

The literature on deviant female genital self-mutilation is too limited to allow for any definitive comments. The claim that a specific syndrome exists, in which female genital self-mutilation and an eating disorder are present, is only partially true. The fact is that females with an eating disorder comprise a high-risk group for *all* forms of self-mutilation.

Certainly the male genitalia are more suited for drastic mutilation than are the female genitalia. Men have a greater tendency to localize their sexual feelings to their protruding genitals, while females tend to have a more diffuse sexuality. Male genital mutilation involves a greater sacrifice than female mutilation in that successful removal of the penis, for example, eliminates the possibility of sexual functioning. Castration allows men to overcome heterosexual and homosexual urges, to gratify feminine longings, and to atone for sexual guilt. Female genital mutilation is more limited in its effects. Men can emulate women anatomically by removing their penis and testicles, but women, even if they want to, cannot emulate men by cutting tissue. For cultural and hormonal reasons, men tend to be more aggressive than women, and because the phallus is an intrusive organ, one might anticipate a higher frequency of male genital mutilation. Left to their own devices, men are more apt than women to mutilate their genitals under culturally accepted conditions as well as during times of mental illness.

From a global and historical perspective, women, even when mentally ill, do not often voluntarily mutilate their genitals. In comparison with culturally accepted male genital mutilative practices, female practices pose clear-cut, serious physical problems to women who undergo them. Cultural explanations and rationalizations for the practices are few, and most can be linked ultimately with social control. The practices seem to stem from men's need to dominate women and to regulate what is perceived to be the rapacious female sexual appetite. In contrast, male practices have diverse explanations and rationalizations ranging from the vulgar and utilitarian to noble and profound sentiments associated with religion and amity.

PART THREE

INSIGHT AND TREATMENT

In the previous chapters, I have presented an overwhelming array of cultural and clinical information on deliberate self-harm. This section is devoted to pulling the material together and making sense of it all. The first step in accomplishing this task involves providing a classification of self-harm behaviors into those that are culturally sanctioned and those that are pathological.

Culturally sanctioned practices, such as body piercing and tattooing, have become enormously popular but may be faddish for most people, a minor "walk on the wild side" or an act of rebellion or an attempt to be noticed as an individual with a personal identity in a world where our existence is increasingly defined by computer-generated numbers, passwords, and PIN codes. Culturally sanctioned rituals, however, have a deeper meaning that is often associated with the elemental human experience of healing, spirituality, and social orderliness. An understanding of these beneficial associations allows for a broader perspective on self-harm and can provide us with the equanimity needed to interact with self-injurers.

I divide pathological self-harm into four types: major, stereotypic, compulsive, and impulsive. This classification is atheoretically based on observed behaviors. It is clinically useful because each type is associated with specific mental disorders.

New methods of assessing and evaluating self-injury, beyond the usual clinical observation, are presented, as are data on its prevalence and the influence of the media and the Internet. Among the various models that attempt to explain the origins and maintenance of NSSI, the psychodynamic is given its due not so much because it is therapeutically useful for larger numbers of patients but rather because it offers evocative insights unobtainable by other approaches. The up-to-date approaches are the four function model, which focuses on differing types of reinforcement behavior, and interpersonal models. In these models, instances of NSSI are examined as "harmful behaviors," rather than symptoms of mental illness. Since much NSSI begins in late childhood/early adolescence, the role of problematic child development is discussed. The complicated biological findings related to NSSI are presented, a promising but still poorly understood field of inquiry.

Our ultimate goal is to prevent and to successfully cure or, at least, to adequately treat self-injurers. The chapter on treatment covers the major psychological and biological approaches. It offers a unique take on why some self-injurers seem to stir up negative feelings in therapists, and it includes Deb Martinson's important "Bill of Rights for People Who Self-harm."

I conclude this section with personal reflections that end with a message of hope. Sometimes it is easy to forget that, despite all our clever understandings and laborious therapeutic machinations, hope and circumstances carry the day.

CHAPTER NINE

Understanding Self-injury

What Is Self-Injury?

To understand self-injury, we need to define it. Life is filled with real and potential self-injury. Police officers, firefighters, soldiers, race car drivers, football and hockey players, skydivers, and scientists who swim among sharks all put themselves in harm's way. People who have lung disease and smoke heavily, people who have diabetes and do not keep to their diets, people who do not take prescribed medications or refuse to continue with unending dialysis treatments, people who consistently overeat, all are injuring themselves. However, for our purposes, *self-injury is the deliberate, direct alteration or destruction of healthy body tissue without an intent to die.* This construct excludes excessive dieting, pathological anorexia, acts committed with an intent to die, overdoses or ingesting objects and substances, body sculpting by drugs or weightlifting, risky behaviors, and cosmetic surgery (a topic for another book). Self-injury and self-harm are general terms that include both nonsuicidal self-injury (NSSI; cutting, burning, etc.), self-mutilation (amputation, castration, etc.), and body-modification practices and rituals (penis cutting, tongue piercing, etc.).

Why Do People Self-injure?

Most acts of self-injury counterintuitively provide relief from distressing situations and from deeply troubling emotions, thoughts, and behaviors. The relief is usually short-lived, but in some cases of major self-mutilation, such as castration or amputation of a limb, the relief may be permanent because a conscious problem or unconscious conflict is resolved, albeit at a great price. Also, self-injury may at times be a proverbial "cry for help" or an attempt to influence others (e.g., a lover, a therapist, or prison personnel). In addition to providing relief, self-injurious acts may "tap into" the ancient human potential for healing, for spiritual gain, and for providing social and personal order.

The Relationship between Self-Injury and Suicide

In short, self-injurers do not want to die but rather want to live free from trouble-some emotions, thoughts, and behaviors. People who really want to die commit suicide. Suicide is an exit into death, an act of escape, and a desire to end all feelings, but self-injury is a morbid act of regeneration, a return to a state of normalcy, and a seeking to feel better.

The longer explanation is that the concept of suicidality is complicated (Nock and Favazza 2009). Many people at various times in their lives may have suicidal ideas or passive thoughts of death and dying. Suicidal plans may be vague or may be concrete and well developed. People may engage in suicide attempts but do not expect to die (Nock and Kessler 2006). People may make preparations to commit suicide but not carry out the act (Posner et al. 2007) or may develop cold feet and stop at the last minute (an aborted suicide attempt) (Barber et al. 1998), or someone may prevent them from attempting suicide (an interrupted suicide attempt). People may make suicidal threats and gestures to communicate with others but with no intent of carrying out the act, just as some self-injurers do. Self-injury, by definition, excludes an intent to die but self-injurers may have passive thoughts of dying or even some thought of making a suicidal attempt or gesture. In most cases, an astute clinician can validly access a person's intent to die, but there is much variability in what people really mean regarding suicidality (Silverman et al. 2007a, 2007b).

Although Graff and Mallin (1967) described the typical wrist cutter as a woman who feels relief after the act but "does not commit suicide," and Pao (1969) distinguished "delicate self-cutting" from suicide attempts, it was Simpson (1976) who first boldly declared that "self-mutilation is an act of antisuicide, for the cutting is used as a direct reliable and rapidly effective way of coming back to life from a dead unreal preceding state." In 1979, Ross and McKay noted that self-mutilation was counterintentional to suicide and cannot be understood in terms of explanations of suicide. In 1983, Pattison and Kahan presented a deliberate self-harm syndrome that excluded suicidality. The publication of the first edition of *Bodies under Siege* (1987) and Walsh and Rosen's *Self-mutilation* (1988) solidified the understanding that self-mutilation is distinct from suicide; two major reviews upheld this distinction (Tantam and Whittaker 1992; Winchel and Stanley 1991).

It may seem odd that the concept of self-injury does not include swallowing objects (glass, nails, etc.), self-poisoning, or drug overdose (the British literature still does not make this distinction). The best explanation for this is offered by

Walsh and Rosen (1988): "In the case of ingesting pills or poison, the harm caused is uncertain, ambiguous, unpredictable, and basically invisible. In the case of self-laceration the degree of self-harm is clear, unambiguous, predictable as to course, and highly visible. In addition, the self-laceration often results in sustained or permanent visible disfigurements to the body, which is not the case with overdose. In these various ways, therefore, these two forms of self-harm are quite different; the danger in combining them in a single category is that these important differences (including their clinical implications) are overlooked" (p. 32).

It is important to note that in Favazza and Conterio's study (1989), 59 percent of female habitual self-injurers had overdosed on drugs and half had overdosed at least four times. A third of the subjects expected to be dead within five years. The overdoses resulted from depression and demoralization over an inability to control their self-injury, and their scars and burn marks caused them to lead socially isolated lives. In addition, suicidality is common in many mental disorders, such as schizophrenia, depression, and borderline personality disorder. People who have these disorders also may engage in self-injury. A fifteen-year follow-up study of severely ill psychiatric inpatients revealed that most of those who had serious suicidal intent but did *not* commit suicide had histories of impulsivity, manipulative suicide attempts, and NSSI (Dingman and McGlashan 1988). Accidental death during NSSI, such as cutting a major artery, can theoretically occur, but I am unaware of any cases.

The Classification of Self-injurious Behaviors

A spectrum of behaviors directly and deliberately alter or destroy healthy body tissue. I have developed a classification that, from a psychiatric perspective, is clinically useful. Current psychological research takes the view that NSSI is a harmful behavior serving four functions that relieve negative (aversive) interpersonal and intrapersonal affective and social situations and experiences. In my classification, at one end are culturally sanctioned behaviors that fall into the category of body modification. At the other end are deviant behaviors that are the products of mental illness and are termed pathological (Favazza 1989a). The classification is as follows:

Culturally Sanctioned Body Modification
— Rituals
— Practices

Pathological Self-injury
— Major
— Stereotypic
— Compulsive
— Impulsive
    Episodic
    Repetitive

Why Is It Important to Know about Culturally Sanctioned Body Modification?

Knowing about culturally sanctioned body modification adds a perspective to help us better understand pathological self-injury, which traditionally was regarded as horrific, senseless, and somehow related to suicidality. Self-injurers were considered difficult to understand, and they engendered a host of negative feelings in people who cared for them and in therapists, who often felt hopeless, betrayed, furious, and sad.

By examining body modification rituals in many cultures, one can see that piercing, damaging, and cutting the body was often associated with healing, spirituality, and social order. Body modification has been practiced for millennia because people have believed that it made their lives better. Seen in this light, pathological self-injury may be beneficial beyond the relief of symptoms. Body modification rituals, as it turns out, serve many of the same purposes as pathological self-injury.

Body Modification Rituals versus Body Modification Practices

Cultural *rituals* are meaningful activities that are repeated in a consistent manner over at least several generations and reflect the tradition, symbolism, and beliefs of a society. They affect the individual participant but, because they are woven into the fabric of social life, they also affect the entire community. The Sun Dance of the Plains Indians exemplifies a body modification ritual. Urged on by tribal members at a yearly ceremony, spiritually and physically elite young braves gazed at the sun and struggled until the skewers that were inserted under the muscles of their chest and back broke free. Relieved of the bonds of the flesh and invigorated by the rays of the sun that passed into their staring eyes, the participants received a vision of how to better their lives and the lives of their tribe members.

Because of their persistence and the "deep" meanings attributed to them by societies, self-mutilative rituals inform us about basic elements of social life. Examination of the rituals reveals that they serve an elemental purpose, namely, the correction or prevention of destabilizing conditions that threaten people and communities. A few examples of destabilizing conditions are diseases; angry gods, spirits, and ancestors; failure of boys and girls to accept adult responsibilities when they mature; conflicts of all sorts (for example, male-female, intergenerational, interclass, intertribal); loosening of clear social role distinctions; loss of group identity and distinctiveness; immoral or sinful behaviors; ecological disasters. Self-mutilative rituals (and some practices) serve to prevent the onset of these conditions and to correct or "cure" them if they occur. The rituals work because people believe that they promote healing, spirituality, and social order.

Cultural *practices* imply activities that may be faddish and that often hold little underlying significance, although there are some exceptions. The piercing of earlobes or noses to accommodate jewelry is an example of such practice. Male circumcision is a practice when performed by Gentiles and a ritual when performed by Jews.

Body Modification Rituals That Can Promote Healing, Spirituality, and Social Order

In regard to *healing*, animals are aided only by their instincts in a struggle for survival and the avoidance of pain, but human beings are able to transcend instinct and to devise strategies to heal wounds, disease, and pain. Before science existed, body modification rituals were one strategy to deal with threats to survival, and some of these rituals have been present from the earliest days of human existence. Many examples of healing associated with body modification rituals have been presented in previous chapters. These include the Hamadsha, Muslim healers in Morocco, who slash open their heads for the sake of ill persons, who dip bits of bread or sugar cubes into the blood and then eat them; it is thought that a therapeutic power rests in the healers' blood; "the island of menstruating men," in Papua New Guinea, where it is believed that women are healthy because of their monthly menstrual bleeding, and to maintain their health, strength, and attractiveness, men mimic the natural cycle of female self-purification by inducing periodic nasal hemorrhages; the South African tribes that used to remove one testicle to prevent sickness and cut off their fingertips to treat illnesses: the trephination of skulls performed originally to alleviate headaches by allowing evil spirits to exit the sick person's head; the healing of people through contact with the spirit world by shamans, who, to become healers, must be cured of an initiating sickness—the curing process is horrific and involves dismemberment, scraping away of flesh, substitution of viscera, and renewal of blood during trance and dream states.

In regard to *spirituality*, the establishment and maintenance of the right relationship with spirits to avoid disaster and to promote prosperity in this world and the next has long been a major motivation for human activities. Self-mutilative ritual sacrifice and atonement are especially pleasing to spirits and, according to some mystics, are capable of helping humans achieve special states of ecstasy and insight. Priests devoted to the great mother goddess Cybele castrated themselves to demonstrate their mourning and identification with Attis, who had castrated himself, died, and was resurrected. The Eastern Orthodox Skoptsi sect practiced self-castration to avoid sinful sexual intercourse and to reclaim the pure state of Adam and Eve before the Fall. By their wounds, the Old Testament Suffering Servant and the New Testament Jesus gave holiness and salvation to humankind. Alone to the alone, the Christian desert fathers punished their bodies to achieve redemption, and for centuries the church canonized as saints persons who zealously mortified their flesh. Some Hindus pierce their bodies to make themselves more pleasing to the god Murugan. Shiva lingam stones representing the self-castrated phallus of Shiva are among the holiest Hindu objects of veneration. Indian sadhus (holy men) engage in prodigious acts of mortification, such as sticking pins all over their bodies or stretching their penises with weights or hanging from flesh hooks, to achieve spirituality. The Olmecs, Aztecs, and Mayans anointed sacred idols with blood from the penis as a sign of devotion and penitence.

In regard to *social order*, chaos is the greatest threat to the stability of the universe. Without social order, men and women would not know how to behave properly, and many men in various cultures believe that uncontrolled female sexuality would then run riot, turning things topsy-turvy. Without order, boys and girls would not accept the responsibilities of adulthood when they came of age. People would be unable to distinguish tribal members from foes, leaders from followers, married women from unmarried ones. The alteration or destruction of body tissue helps to establish control of things and to preserve the social order. As noted, in some African countries, female sexuality is controlled by a surgical procedure on their genitals; in China, it was done by breaking the bones in women's feet so they could not stray. Scarification patterns not only enhance beauty but also may indicate social status; for Tiv females in Nigeria they depict genealogical descent. A number of tribes cut off specific fingers to indicate a clan badge

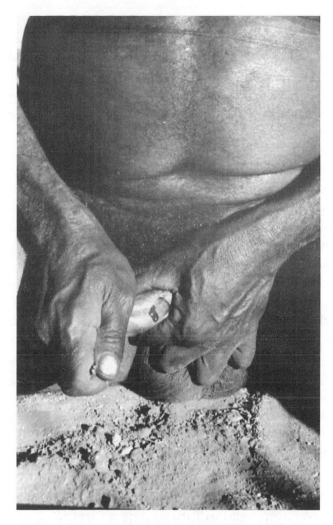

Fully initiated aboriginal tribesmen in central Australia have a
subincision, by which the penile urethra is converted into an
open channel. Here, a man is using the subincision site as a
convenient source of ceremonial blood by pricking the erect
member with a thorn. (See Cawte 1974; photo courtesy of
Dr. John Cawte)

or sort of surname; a widow cuts off a finger upon remarriage. The Flathead Indians molded the skulls of their children to produce a clearly identifiable head
shape. Circumcision of male infants has been a distinctive sign of Jewish identity
for millennia. Young men of the Abidji tribe slice open their abdomens the day

after tribal members meet to reconcile divisive issues; the healing of the wounds symbolizes the social healing that has taken place within the entire community. The mutilative process is so important that the primary Indo-European cosmological myth tells about the sacrifice and mutilation of the Primordial Being from whose dismembered body parts the universe was created and the world was formed, as were the flora and the fauna and human beings, and thus everything was ordered properly.

In coming-of-age initiation rituals, adolescents acquire new social roles and status necessary for the orderly preservation of communal life (see Brown 1963; Cohen 1964; Gluckman 1962; Turner 1969; van Gennep 1909; Whiting et al. 1947). The rituals are painful and often brutal: teeth may be knocked loose, the nasal septum pierced, the penis mutilated, and large areas of skin scarified, so as to heighten the drama and significance of the ritual, focus attention on the adolescents, and allow them to demonstrate their inner strength. They also are a warning that the social group has great power and will not tolerate revolt against authority; children are transformed into adults when they overcome their fear and allow themselves to be subjected to pain and mutilation. The intense emotions of the ritual tend to foster bonding between the adolescent participants and the adults and induce a peak emotional experience that "has the potential to mature consciousness by wasting the innocence of childhood and giving birth to the heightened self-awareness and greater consciousness of adulthood" (Morinis 1985). Adolescents agree to surrender part of their autonomy, and to voluntarily endure pain and body modification as a visible notice of relinquishing childish ways. It is the price that must be paid to partake of adult communal life.

How Does an Understanding of Body Modification Rituals Affect Clinical Care?

An understanding of the beneficial effects of body modification rituals allows clinicians to approach self-injurers with a more positive mind-set. Behaviors that damage the body to achieve higher goals have been present since the earliest days of humankind and are embedded in the experience of what it is to be human. They are not alien to the human condition, and they may "to a greater or lesser degree remain unarticulated in most of us. That is, such patterns already exist in muted intensities within the patient's social field. . . . The history of these images reaches at least as far back as Passion of the Cross and has prevailed among some of the most respected members of our culture" (Podvoll 1969). People may unconsciously tap into the inherited wisdom gleaned from body modification rituals, although any discussion of how this might occur would be as speculative as the notion that our brains are hardwired for belief in a god, an entity, or a purpose that transcends mortal existence and provides meaning to our lives.

Body Modification Practices

Body modification processes, such as tattoos, body piercing, and earlobe piercing to accommodate jewelry, are behaviors that may be faddish and that often hold little underlying or deep significance, although there are some exceptions (e.g., a piercing or a tattoo that serves to mark the control or reclamation of one's body after an attack or a rape). This being said, body modification practices have become enormously popular around the world. Decades ago, Fakir Musafar was among the first to attach a deeper meaning to some practices when he promoted the notion of "modern primitivism" and of "body play." The best information on these is found in *Modern Primitives* (Vale and Juno 1985) and, in a highly intellectualized form, in Featherstone's edited edition of *Body and Society* (2000). Modern primitives are persons in the body modification community who, feeling powerless in today's personally restricted society of computers and passive television watching, assert to control what they do have power over, namely, their bodies. Without trampling on the rights of others, they desire a return to primitive ways of experiencing a world and a recognition of what the novelist D. H. Lawrence called humankind's "blood nature." Vale and Juno make the point that body modifications "bear witness to personal pain endured which cannot be simulated. . . . Pain is a uniquely personal experience. . . . Virtually every experience in the world today from touring Disneyland to trekking on photo safaris in Africa, has already been registered in the brain through *images* from a movie or TV *program*. We are programmed, but for what? And where does image end and reality begin? . . . *All* sensual experiences function to free us from 'normal' restraints, to awaken our deadened bodies to life. . . . Our most inestimable resource, the unfettered imagination, continues to be grounded in the only truly precious possession we can ever have and know, and which is *ours* to do with what we will: *the human body*" (pp. 4–5).

Fakir Musafar outlined seven categories of body play:

1. Contortion (e.g., yoga exercises, temporary foot binding, cupping [applying a partial vacuum created in a cup by heat or by suction to draw up the underlying tissues and create blood stasis], etc.)
2. Constriction (e.g., corsets, tight rubber clothing and belts, body presses, etc.)

3. Deprivation (e.g., fasting, sleep deprivation, sense isolation in boxes, cages, helmets, body bags, etc.)
4. Encumberment (e.g., manacles, heavy chains, etc.)
5. Fire (e.g., moxibustion [burning mugwort on the skin], steam/heat baths and boxes, electric currents [constant and shocks], etc.)
6. Penetration (e.g., flagellation, piercing, tattooing, bed of nails, etc.)
7. Suspension (e.g. suspended by multiple hooks, "witches' cradle" [standing in a metal swing while blindfolded and wearing ear-plugs], hanging on a cross, etc.)

According to Fakir, body play is fun in both erotic and nonerotic ways and sometimes leads to the experience of spiritual and ecstatic states. "To *not* have encumberments, to *not* have holes in your body, to *not* have tattoos may be debilitating—this is something that people have to consider. They may not be getting the most out of life because they *don't* do these things. People may be missing beautiful, rich experiences because of cultural bias and conceit" (Vale and Juno 1985, p. 14).

While Fakir finds a higher purpose in body play, some people engage in it for adulation, for show business (see Gregor's 1998 *Circus of the Scars*), for relief from boredom, for a touch of "danger" and fear, for the novelty of doing something most people are not willing to try, for erotic thrills (Favazza 1991), and for just plain fun. Body modification takes the center stage in "performance art," during which artists pierce, brand, and execute the acts of body modification on willing performers before an audience. A well-known performance artist, Ron Athey, ritually cuts performers and rubs paper on bleeding wounds to produce unique pieces of art. Athey, who was reared by his evangelical aunts to become a preacher, uses martyr symbols and the stigmata in his performances. He says that his art is about "redemption from self-destruction and suicide" (Breslauer 1994).

There are performers (not illusionists or tricksters) who are capable of amazing physical acts. A European named Mirin Dajo (1912–48) was hypnotized by a colleague. Then a third member of the team stuck a sword all the way through Dajo's back until it exited through the chest on the other side of his body. The sword had a blunted tip so as not to cut internal organs. Obviously, the placement of the sword was crucial. X-rays show that the sword did, indeed, go through Dajo's body. A well-known photograph shows him jogging with a sword stuck completely through his abdomen.

The most spectacular group performers are Sufi (a branch of Islam) male dervishes who belong to an order known as Tariqa Casnazaniyyah ("the way that

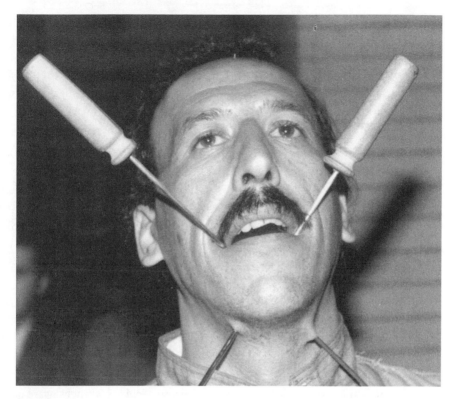

A member of a Sufi Islamic sect known for inserting skewers and spikes into their bodies without experiencing pain or blood loss. Group members regard such acts as a manifestation of spirituality. (Photo courtesy of Jamal Hussein, Paramann Programme Laboratories)

is known by no one"). Among the feats they perform are the insertion of skewers and spikes into the body (face, neck, arms, breast, abdomen), the hammering of knives into skull, and the swallowing of glass shards and razor blades. They consider these acts to be miracles (no pain is felt, no blood is shed, and the wounds heal) that are demonstrated to win converts. A group of physicists and physicians in Jordan (Paramann Programme Laboratories) has been studying the group (Al-Dargazelli 1993–94; Hussein et al. 1993) to find a way for all human beings to access the ability to control pain and heal wounds. They report that the feats can be performed not only in a religious context but also in the most sterile environment. Measurements of the dervishes' brain wave (EEG) activity failed to show any systematic changes either during or after the demonstrations. This finding is interesting because American and German researchers found changes (onset of alpha waves and increased theta waves) in two subjects who allowed spikes and needles to be inserted into their bodies (Green and Green 1977; Larbig 1982). Because these changes are associated with meditative and trance states, the absence of EEG changes in the Tariqa group suggests that the dervishes do not perform during an altered state of consciousness. The Paramann Programme group's scientific credibility, unfortunately, becomes suspect when they state their belief that the dervishes' abilities were spontaneously transmitted to them during an initiation ceremony when ritualistically shaking the hand of a Califa (an especially distinguished dervish) and reciting a brief religious vow. The dervishes' abilities are thought to derive from the prophet Muhammad.

A modern American named Tim Cridland, whose stage name is "The Torture King," is able to perform spectacular feats without recourse to supernatural explanations or mystical mumbo-jumbo. He studies films and videos closely and is impressed that fakirs and dervishes know exactly where to pierce for maximum penetration with minimal damage. He learned how to pass a skewer through his biceps and then perfected a procedure for placing a skewer in his mouth that exits near his neck. It is now part of his act. He has told me that he "never takes a blind stab in the dark." He studies each piercing in great detail and notes that "I have no intention of putting myself in an emergency room." He dislikes pain and bleeding; he is able to control both through self-hypnosis. He is acutely aware of what he is doing during a piercing; "I don't want to hit an artery or harm myself." He denies any masochistic pleasure from his performances. He has mastered the ability to change the experience of pain into "just another type of sensation as though someone were touching me." He can achieve this state of self-hypnosis rapidly and with little effort. He is currently attempting to learn more about a fakir piercing in which a small sword is inserted through the neck from side to side, going behind the windpipe and in front of the spine. He has high admiration for the Sufi piercers and speculates that their knowledge was gained "at the expense of a number of lives."

For the majority of persons who engage in body modification, there is no link with pathological self-injury. For some, however it may serve as sublimation or controlled substitute while for others it may serve as a stepping-stone (e.g., the controlled behavior of body modification may make it easier to slip into deviant self-injury). In specifically questioning students in his certified school for body modification practices, Fakir found that a majority had formerly been cutters. In my clinical observations a minority of cutters had engaged in body modification.

The Classification of Pathological Self-injury

Pathological self-injury—self-mutilation and NSSI—is classified into several types: Major, Stereotype, Compulsive, and Impulsive (which may be episodic or repetitive). It is a descriptive classification based on the observation of behaviors without any theoretical implications about causation and is subject to change with increased knowledge, especially of biological markers and mechanisms. Its main advantage is that it is comprehensive and useful clinically. Each type of self-injury, for example, is usually more prevalent in certain mental disorders either as a central diagnostic or an associated feature.

Major Self-injury

Major self-injury, or self-mutilation, refers to *infrequent behaviors such as eye enucleation, castration, and amputation of body parts that result in the destruction of significant body tissue.* They tend to be messy and to occur suddenly with a great deal of tissue damage and bleeding; an exception is carefully planned transsexual self-castration. These acts are not essential symptoms of a specific disorder but rather are associated features. They are most commonly associated with psychosis, acute intoxication, and transsexualism. In a literature review of major self-mutilation, 75 percent of cases involved a psychotic illness, mainly some form of schizophrenia; of these, about half occurred during a first, acute psychotic episode (Large et al. 2009).

Psychosis is a mental state that involves a loss of contact with reality as manifested by hallucinations (stimuli that exist only in one's mind such as voices, visions, strange smells or tastes); illusions (misperception of real events); delusions (false beliefs about persecution, grandiosity, eroticism, body functioning / sensations / physical appearance); ideas of reference (thoughts that stimuli—a radio show or a newspaper article or an airplane flying overhead, for example— have a singular personal meaning); feeling that people can read one's mind or that one can broadcast thoughts to others; disordered thought processes; disorganized or bizarre behavior; unintelligible speech; and poor social interaction. Any of these symptoms may be intense or minimal, and may be episodic or fairly constant (such as fixed delusions). Not all of the symptoms have to be present to determine that a person is psychotic. They signify a major breakdown in brain functioning.

People who are psychotic are usually diagnosed as having brief psychotic disorder, schizophrenia, schizoaffective disorder, major depression, bipolar mania or depression, and drug (alcohol, cocaine, amphetamine, psychedelic, etc.) intoxication. Less-common diagnoses include brain damage, brain tumor, Alzheimer's and Parkinson's diseases, electrolyte (blood levels of sodium, calcium, phosphorus, magnesium) imbalance, certain vitamin deficiencies, malaria, syphilis, encephalitis, and some personality disorders.

Some people who are psychotic may be amazingly indifferent to their self-mutilation, while others may offer explanations that defy understanding (e.g., to enhance general well-being). Among the most common reasons for self-mutilation from cases previously described in earlier chapters are:

- Concrete interpretations of biblical texts about tearing out an offending eye, cutting off an offending hand, and becoming a eunuch for the Kingdom of Heaven's sake.
- Identification with Christ, who suffered and was tortured.
- Atonement, purification, and punishment for real or imaginary sins.
- Commands from god or other heavenly beings.
- Demonic possession and commands.
- Fear of giving in to homosexual urges.
- Control of troubling hypersexuality.
- Repudiation of one's genital organs.
- The appeasement of paranoid persecutors.
- Obsession with amputation (other than that found in body integrity identity disorder).
- Elimination of a body organ perceived to be painful or dangerous to others.
- Belief by men that they are really women and who castrate themselves out of desperation because they have been refused gender reassignment surgery, cannot afford the surgery, or are frustrated by the long preoperative process.

Acts of major self-mutilation are tragedies. An enucleated eye is inevitably lost and amputated body parts often cannot be reattached surgically. The calmness that many patients exhibit after self-mutilation suggests that the behavior may resolve unconscious conflicts. In many instances, alas, the resolution is only temporary, and the self-harm behavior may return with a vengeance. (An exception is that of some transsexuals whose self-castration may resolve certain psychological difficulties and make it more likely that professional surgical, medical, and psychological help will be made available to complete the process of changing gender.) The calmness may also reflect realistic resignation: what's done is done. When there is a clearing of consciousness in individuals whose actions were performed during a state of intoxication, the realization of their loss may be exquisitely sobering.

Stereotypic Self-injury

Stereotypic self-mutilation or NSSI consists of behaviors such as *head banging* (the highest reported rate was 5,400 times an hour); eye *pressing and gouging; biting* lips, tongues, cheeks, and fingers; *orifice digging; arm hitting; face and head slapping*, and *tooth extraction*. These acts may be monotonously repetitive and even have a rhythmic pattern. It is usually impossible to ascertain any symbolic meaning, thought content, or associated affect with the behaviors. The acts are more likely than those in other types of self-injury to occur in the presence of onlookers. Stereotypic self-injurers seem to be driven by a primarily biological imperative to harm themselves shamelessly and without guile.

Stereotypic self-injury is highly prevalent in institutionalized people who have mental retardation, but not all self-injury in this population is stereotypic, nor are specific personality types or behaviors uniquely associated with mental retardation. Mental retardation is a general term, has many different etiologies, and may be seen as the final common pathway of various pathological processes that affect the functioning of the central nervous system. People who have severe or profound mental retardation (about 5% of cases) are at particular risk for self-injury.

Among the disorders, many of which are genetic, in which stereotypic self-injury is prevalent are autism; de Lange syndrome (rare; profound mental retardation; see Murphy 1985); Retts disorder (rare, profound mental retardation occurring only in females); diseases associated with hereditary neuropathies (neuropathy refers to various types of limb pain and extreme sensitivity to touch) such as acanthosis, insensitivity to pain, and type I tyrosinemia (Gadoth and Mass 2004); and Lesch-Nyhan syndrome, an inborn error of purine metabolism and a model disorder for studying self-injury with awesomely rapid biting off of oral tissue and fingers (Baumeister and Frye 1985; Christie et al. 1982; Jankovic 1988; Nyhan 1976). Few people are aware that a third of people who have Tourette's syndrome, well known for its association with motor and vocal tics, also display stereotypic self-injury (Robertson et al. 1989). The first report, in 1885, described a 24-year-old man: "His mouth opens wide; when it closes again one can hear the teeth of both jaws gnashing violently. Quite often the tongue is caught between them and abruptly seized and lacerated; moreover it is all covered with scars." Occasionally stereotypic self-injury is encountered in acute psychosis, schizophrenia, and amphetamine abuse. It is also seen in young children with neonatal brachial plexus injury as they mature and experience limb pain (the brachial plexus is a group of nerve fibers that run from the cervical and thoracic spine through the neck, armpit, and arm) (McCann et al. 2002), as well as in adults who have sustained traumatic injury to their brachial plexus (Procacci and Maresca 1990).

Among the many explanations that have been offered for stereotypic self-mutilation in general are a way to obtain attention, an autoerotic response to understimulation, an expression of frustration, a way to deal with pain, an attempt to heighten a proprioceptive sense of self, and a turning inward of anger and aggression. Head banging specifically has been seen as an attempt to re-experience the comfort to hearing a mother's heartbeat. (See Collins 1965; de Lissovoy 1961; Frances and Gale 1975.)

Compulsive Self-injury

Compulsive self-injury encompasses repetitive acts, such as severe skin scratching, nail biting, and trichotillomania, or pulling out hair (Swedo and Rapoport 1991). The acts, which may be purposeful or may evolve into unthinking bad habits, result not in pleasure but in a brief relief from anxiety. Some persons deliberately create skin lesions to assume the sick role and receive medical attention. Persons who focus on a specific anatomical spot, often on the face, that is normal but is perceived to be ugly or deformed are diagnosed with body dysmorphic disorder. As noted in chapter 7, the most serious form of compulsive NSSI is skin digging to eliminate what are delusionally perceived to be parasites.

Impulsive Self-injury

Impulsive NSSI consists of acts such as skin-cutting and burning, pin sticking, interfering with wound healing, and smashing hand or foot bones. It is impulsive because people cannot resist the impulse, drive, or temptation to self-injure, often feel mounting tension or arousal before the act of self-injury, and then feel relief, pleasure, or gratification after it; two-thirds feel better immediately and, of these, a third still feel better for a few hours while only 18 percent still feel better for a few days. This short lived beneficial effect means that another act of NSSI may occur if the tension and arousal return. I have written widely on impulsive NSSI (see Favazza and Conterio 1989; Favazza and Rosenthal 1990, 1993; and Favazza and Simeon 1995; in addition, see Herpertz et al. 1997).

Impulsive NSSI is not an official diagnosis in psychiatry's *Diagnostic and Statistical Manual of Mental Disorders* and is listed as a diagnostic criterion only for borderline personality disorder and trichotillomania (which, as noted, I consider to be usually compulsive). In fact, it is also encountered as an episodic behavior in numerous disorders including generalized anxiety; posttraumatic stress; acute stress (Pitman 1990); anxiety due to a general medical condition (thyroid disorder, hypoglycemia, cardiac conditions, adrenocortical disorder [Rajathurai et al. 1983], epilepsy, pheochomocytoma, vestibular dysfunctions, benign intracranial hypertension [Ballard 1989], etc.); substance induced anxiety (exposure to or withdrawal from stimulants, cocaine, inhalents, hallucinogens, etc.); somatization and pain disorders; factitious disorder; dissociative identity (multiple personality) and depersonalization disorders; anorexia and bulimia nervosa; kleptomania; histrionic, antisocial, schizoid, and schizotypal personality disorder; dysthymia; major depression; bipolar disorder; delusional disorder; schizophrenia; and obsessive-compulsive disorder (Primeau and Fontaine 1987).

The reasons given by persons for engaging in impulsive NSSI are too numerous to list, but these, some of which have already been noted, are among the most frequent:

- Relief from anxiety (by far the most common; "It's like popping a balloon.").
- Terminating depersonalization episodes (emotional deadness; diminished normal sensations; altered sense of time; estrangement from the environment; feel like an automaton [Favazza and Dos Santos 1985]).
- Sense of security and uniqueness ("If I am emotionless and empty, the pain and blood is always there for me"; "I cut myself because I need to be special. Take it away from me and I'm like everyone else.").
- Establishing self-control (racing thoughts; swirling emotions).
- Influencing others (attempt to evoke a caring response or guilt in others; to get attention, a communication of despair).
- Pressure from multiple personalities (one alter ego inflicts pain on another alter). See Bliss 1980; Putnam et al. 1986.
- Relief from depression (self-punishment for forbidden fantasies or perceived or real misdeeds, guilt, feeling emotionally "dead").
- Revenge (the body as a proxy for powerful or dead persons who were abusive).
- Sexuality (usually to diminish unwanted sexual feelings but also, in a sado masochistic setting, to enhance sexual feelings).
- Magically forestalling or lessening "uncontrolled" menstrual bleeding.
- Venting anger (when it is inappropriate or unwise to express anger outwardly).

- Dealing with traumatic events and flashbacks (reclaiming one's body; marking significant events).
- Self-stimulation and euphoria (especially among prisoners in isolation cells).
- Thrill seeking.
- Relief from alienation ("A dose of the good things—loving, hugging— would provide relief from a profound sense of alienation from the rest of the world, but it's simpler to reach for a razor blade.").
- Expression of autonomy (in controlling and repressive environments).
- Establishing an identity (a unique person; a mark of group membership).
- Dealing with psychosis (appeasing paranoid persecutors; obeying "voices" to make them go away).

Borderline personality is the most common disorder in which impulsive NSSI is encountered. Many of the just listed reasons for engaging in this behavior apply to borderlines whose illness is characterized by fears of abandonment; short-lived episodes of dissociation, depersonalization, psychotic-like symptoms, anxiety, irritability, and depression; intense and rocky relationships; a vacillating self-image and sense of self; rapidly fluctuating emotions; chronic feelings of emptiness; intense and inappropriate anger; suicidal behaviors; and impulsive acts such as binge eating, abusing drugs, and going on spending sprees. Their lives are often tumultuous and filled with real and imaginary crises that result in discontinuities such as failed marriages, lost jobs, and incomplete educational experiences. Many, but not all, borderlines are reared in unpleasant circumstances (family conflicts, sexual and physical abuse, neglect, and early parental loss or separation). NSSI ends the depersonalization and mounting anxiety, provides solace, stabilizes emotional swings, and so forth. The popular film *Fatal Attraction*, in which the heroine (or villain, depending on one's perspective) cuts herself, is a fairly accurate portrayal of someone who had borderline personality disorder. Deborah, the main character in the popular autobiographical novel *I Never Promised You a Rose Garden* (Greenberg 1981) vividly remembered a childhood operation for urethral tumor and the use of probes and needles "as if the entire reality of her body were concentrated in the secret evil inside that forbidden place." As she grew aware of her father's incestuous feelings, she became a compulsive eater, painlessly cut and bruised herself, hurled her body against walls, and mentally constructed a fanciful world with strange gods who sent her omens and made demands on her. Her psychoanalyst diagnosed schizophrenia, but in a review of the case Murray (1993) felt that "perhaps" the correct diagnoses were posttraumatic and dissociative disorders. Most psychiatrists today would add borderline personality disorder. All this being said, it is *inappropriate for clinicians to automatically diagnose cutters and burners as having borderline personality disorder.*

Repetitive NSSI Syndrome

Episodic NSSI becomes repetitive when the behavior becomes an overwhelming preoccupation in those persons who may adopt an identity as a "cutter" or "burner," who describe themselves as addicted to their self-harm, and whose NSSI seems to assume an autonomous course. No set number of NSSI episodes marks the switch from episodic to repetitive. In some persons the switch may occur between the fifth and tenth episode; in others between the tenth and twentieth. Unlike episodic NSSI, which is best considered a symptom or associated feature of a mental disorder, such as borderline personality disorder (BPD) or generalized anxiety disorder, the repetitive type is best considered a separate disorder of impulse control that I call repetitive NSSI syndrome. This syndrome usually begins in early adolescence and persists for decades, during which the self-harm periodically heats up and cools down and may coexist with other impulsive behaviors, such as eating disorders, alcohol and substance abuse, and kleptomania (stealing unnecessary objects). Persons who develop this syndrome tend to be female (about a three to two ratio) and are at high risk for overdoses due to demoralization over their inability to control their NSSI. Multiple scars result in great social morbidity. An interest in plastic surgery to reduce scars is one indication that the syndrome is abating (Favazza 1992; Favazza and Rosenthal 1990, 1993).

The historical recognition of this syndrome began many decades ago when researchers proposed various syndromes such as wrist cutting (Graff and Mallin 1967) and delicate self-cutting (Pao 1969). Two epidemiological studies did not support a specific syndrome but both were flawed because they regarded cutting solely as a suicide attempt and examined only isolated cutting episodes severe enough to require a police report or hospital treatment (Clendenin and Murphy 1971; Weissman 1975). In England, Morgan (1979) first used the phrase "nonfatal, deliberate self-harm" to describe behavior in which suicide was clearly not intended, but he included drug overdoses in his construct. In Denmark, Bille-Brahe (1982) identified two groups of suicide attempters: one group engaged in single, acute attempts, while the other engaged in lower lethality repetitive attempts. These ideas stimulated Pattison and Kahan (1983; Kahan and Pattison 1984) to develop the concept of a deliberate self-harm syndrome that marks the beginning of modern interest in self-injury. A "prototype" model of the syndrome, derived from analysis of fifty-six published reports, was characterized by multiple episodes and types of low lethality self-harm, onset in late adolescence, and duration of many years. Anxiety, despair, anger, and cognitive restriction were prominent symptoms. Predisposing factors included lack of social support, male homosexuality, drug and alcohol abuse, and suicidal ideation in women. Overdoses were excluded, as were bona fide suicide attempts. The syndrome occurred more frequently but not necessarily or exclusively in borderline and histrionic persons. They classified the deliberate self-harm syndrome as a disorder of impulse control.

I have refined this prototype model to identify the repetitive NSSI syndrome. Data collected on 240 female, habitual self-mutilators, for example, described a typical subject as "a 28-year-old Caucasian who first deliberately harmed herself at age 14. Skin cutting is her usual practice, but she has used other methods such as skin burning and self-hitting, and she has injured herself on at least fifty occasions. Her decision to self-injure is impulsive and results in temporary relief from symptoms such as racing thoughts, depersonalization, and marked anxiety. She now has or has had an eating disorder, and may be concerned about her drinking. She has been a heavy utilizer of medical and mental health services, although treatment generally has been unsatisfactory. In desperation over her inability to control her self-harm behavior, this typical subject has attempted suicide by drug overdose" (Favazza and Conterio 1989).

People who have this syndrome usually use multiple methods of self-injury. Some may brood about harming themselves for hours and even days and may go through a ritualistic sequence of behaviors, such as tracing areas of their skin and placing their self-harm paraphernalia in a special order. Self-harm acts are usually performed in private. Even seemingly bizarre behaviors such as drinking one's blood or saving it in small vials are not associated with psychosis. People who have this disorder often describe it as an "addiction" and may avidly seek professional help. Some people demonstrate traits found in the personality disorders during the course of the disorder, but these traits may subside or disappear when the syndrome remits. People who have the syndrome frequently have problems with eating and may develop or have a history of anorexia and/or bulimia nervosa. Some people may have a history of, or may develop, episodic alcohol abuse and/or kleptomania. When an eating disorder or alcohol abuse develops, NSSI often diminishes but sometimes returns as the eating disorder or alcohol abuse abates. In some persons, these impulsive behaviors occur simultaneously.

The syndrome usually begins in late childhood or early adolescence. It waxes and wanes and may become chronic. In many patients, the disorder lasts ten to fifteen years, although isolated episodes of NSSI may persist. Significant predisposing factors, as noted, appear to be physical and/or sexual abuse in childhood, an early history of surgical procedures or illness, impulsivity (Lacey and Evans 1986), parental alcoholism or depression, and residence in a total-care institution. Other factors include a proneness to accidents, perfectionistic tendencies, dissatisfaction with body shape or sexual organs, poor problem-solving skills, a depressive outlook on life, limited strategies for dealing with stress and with sexual feelings, and an inability to tolerate and express feelings. The most common precipitants are real or perceived rejection and situations that produce feelings of helplessness, anger, or guilt.

Evans and Lacey (1992) studied fifty women attending an alcohol treatment unit. These women demonstrated other impulsive behavior: one-quarter cut themselves deliberately, 16 percent had an eating disorder, half described impulsive physical violence, and half acknowledged a period of promiscuity. Fichter et al. (1994) reported on thirty-two "multi-impulsive bulimics." Among their impulsive behaviors were NSSI (75%), shoplifting (78%), alcohol dependence (34%), drug abuse (22%), and sexual promiscuity (53%).

These findings are consistent with those of Favazza and Conterio (1989) that about half of repetitive self-injurers develop or have a history of anorexia, bulimia, or both and that about 20 percent develop or have a history of episodic alcohol abuse. There is no fixed sequence, and one of the three self-harm behaviors usually predominates at any time. Patients claim that alcohol abuse is the easiest behavior to overcome and that NSSI is the hardest.

An objection to the identification of a repetitive NSSI syndrome is that impulsivity and self-harm are key elements in an already existing diagnosis, especially BPD. In a comparison of self-injuring and non-self-injuring personality disordered individuals, Simeon et al. (1992) found that all the subjects had higher than normal impulsivity; the self-injurers also had greater aggression, "which when combined with poor impulse control takes the form of self-mutilation rather than less aggressive impulsive behaviors assessed by the Schedule for Interviewing Borderlines such as gambling, promiscuity, over-eating, and oversleeping." Thus, NSSI may be a marker for more severe borderline pathology, or self-injury might best be viewed as a distinct Axis I impulse control disorder. Both interpretations may be correct. NSSI is one of eight diagnostic criteria for BPD but by itself is neither necessary nor sufficient to establish a diagnosis. Its presence may indicate a more severe form of the disorder. When the behavior becomes repetitive, it may develop into the repetitive NSSI syndrome.

Many Axis I disorders coexist with BPD; Gunderson and Zanarini (1987) listed panic disorder, substance abuse, gender identity disorders, factitious disorders, disorders of impulse control, attention deficit disorder, and eating disorders. Concurrent depression is also frequently cited. Because the criteria for BPD include symptoms of all the disorders listed above, the existence of a concurrent disorder often depends on the quantity of the symptoms in question. Occasional binge eating or shoplifting episodes, for example, are consonant with the construct of BPD, but a pattern of frequent, uncontrolled, repetitive episodes warrants the additional diagnoses of bulimia nervosa and kleptomania.

An identical argument can be made for NSSI. People who have the syndrome demonstrate a pattern of uncontrolled and repetitive NSSI in response to disturbing psychological symptoms or environmental events, are captive to their preoccupation with acts of self-harm, experience cravings to self-harm and withdrawal symptoms when prevented from indulging their cravings (just as pathological gamblers do if unable to gamble), and may assume an identity as a cutter. These people should not to be confused with those who episodically cut their wrists. In addition, some people experience a remission from the syndrome, and they no longer demonstrate a full-fledged personality disorder. The situation is analogous to that of an alcoholic person whose "personality disorder" disappears after prolonged sobriety. The diagnosis of a personality disorder such as BPD has traditionally been a life sentence, but there is mounting evidence that some people grow out of the disorder. I have encountered serious, chronic self-injurers who have told me that one morning they awoke, decided that they would no longer cut themselves, and, in fact, honored this decision.

In England, Tantam and Whittaker (1992) reviewed these issues and favored the concept of a separate "diagnostic category of repeated, deliberate self-harm, sui generis, which could also include other compulsive and self-destructive behaviors." A special advantage of this concept is that it would then be possible to study the effect of repeated self-harm on relationships and emotions: "whether, in other words personality abnormality may be consequent on, rather than antecedent to, repeated self-harm."

Clinical Case: Repetitive Self-mutilation

An articulate 31-year-old farmworker sought me out because of my interest in self-injury. He wanted to discuss his experiences and to learn about his prognosis.

He had an uneventful childhood but preferred to stay at home rather than to seek out playmates. Despite contracting mononucleosis, he had a high score on the national college entrance examination and was accepted by a prestigious local college. He decided to attend a state college, however, because he wanted to assert his independence. During two years in college, he was discontented with his tendency to avoid intimate relationships. After a hike in the woods during a snowstorm, he decided to break down the defensive shell he had erected around himself.

He got a job in a large city and took night college courses. Although he made a few friends, he still felt isolated and was disappointed with his life. He then experienced an episode of mounting tension: "It was like looking down a tunnel into nothing. Then I saw red streaks and black fire. And then I carved my arm with a razor blade and the pressure went away."

He read anthropological books about shamanism and hallucinogens as a way to gain insight and healing. He took LSD a few times and gained some insights about himself, but as a result of one trip he began to dwell on his childhood faults. Once again he felt a mounting tension, and he relieved it by cutting the skin on his chest and stomach. He sought professional help but could not convince the psychiatrist that he had no suicidal intent.

He became involved with the drug subculture and used phencyclidine (PCP) and intravenous heroin for four months. He lost his job and cut himself on the chest several more times "to relieve the pressure." He again sought psychiatric help but rejected his diagnosis as a suicide-prone schizophrenic. He developed a close relationship with a woman who supported herself by part-time prostitution.

After voluntarily participating in a drug rehabilitation program, he moved in with his parents, stopped cutting his skin and using drugs, and took a civil service job, which he held for eight years. He then moved into an apartment and secretly cut his chest again—twelve times over a two-year period. Each episode was similar: he would introspect about his life, become angry with himself for his past mistakes and for his inability to do better, experience intense pressure, and then cut himself for relief. During this period he reentered the drug subculture.

Then, he stated, "All of a sudden I came into focus, without being able to explain such a change." He stopped taking drugs and cutting himself. He dated, developed self-confidence, and began to meet new people and establish friendships. He took college courses again and got married. His wife had a large financial debt, and he worked two jobs to pay it off. To stay awake at work, he used amphetamines, but he did not cut himself. His wife filed for divorce. The patient's last cutting episode occurred on the day he signed the divorce papers. He experienced depersonalization and enormous pressure. Relief came after he slashed his chest, stomach, and arm. He contemplated suicide but decided against it.

Although deeply hurt by his wife's departure, he continued working two jobs and paid off her debt. He made numerous friends, "dabbled" in occasional drug use, and drank alcohol ("more than I should have"). A friend invited him to work on his farm in the Midwest, and he accepted. After working on the farm for more than a year, he said that he was content, experienced no stress, drank beer for relaxation, and had no desire to take drugs or cut himself. He recognized that he had a bad attitude toward women but hoped that he could "work on the problem." He planned to buy some farmland of his own.

CHAPTER TEN

The Assessment, Psychology, and Biology of Self-injury

This chapter examines the assessment and evaluation of self-injury, its prevalence in community and clinical samples, the role of the media and the Internet, psychoanalytic/dynamic theories, psychosocial models, the role of child development and abuse, and biological findings.

Assessment and Evaluation of Pathological Self-injury

Major self-injury is usually a singular act and self-evident except for castration, which may be hidden. The *motivation* and *circumstances* of the act should be determined as should be the patient's *current mental status*. Agitation, psychosis, and bizarre appearance often signal an impending second act, while resignation and calmness are favorable prognostic signs. A diagnosis of the mental disorder in which the self-injury is an associated feature must be made.

Stereotypic self-injury also is usually self-evident. The *frequency* and, *most important*, the *circumstances that precede* the behaviors must be determined as well as their *consequences* (e.g., Do they result in increased attention or in relief from stressful or confusing activities or situations, or are they habitual, seemingly unprovoked acts?). Does the patient seem to be in pain from medical conditions such as constipation, otitis, or finger infection? Many patients cannot communicate intelligibly, so the clinician must rely on informants (parents, teachers, attendants, etc.). The *Motivation Assessment Scale* (MAS) contains sixteen questions that identify attention, escape (relief), tangible, and automatic reinforcement functions that might be controlling the behaviors. The *Functional Assessment Interview* (FAI) has eleven sections—sleep patterns, mealtime routines, interpersonal contacts, medical status, etc.—that provide a comprehensive review. In one assessment technique, *Functional Analysis* (FA), the clinician observes or interacts with the patient for fifteen minutes daily under contrived conditions (e.g., social disapproval, academic demand, unstructured play, and the patient alone in a room). This allows the clinician to evaluate the various reinforcement functions that might be influencing the self-harm behaviors. See Luiselli (2009) for references and information about the MAS, FAI, and FA.

The telltale signs of compulsive-self-injury—scratched skin, missing hair, damaged fingernails—are easily observable. Check for delusions of parasitosis. Be sure that the self-injury is not focused on one perceived abnormality which could indicate body dysmorphic disorder which has a high rate of suicidality. Although not used very often, the *Structured Clinical Interview for Obsessive-Compulsive Spectrum Disorders* (SCID-OCSD) provides useful information about compulsive self-injury (du Toit et al. 2001).

Impulsive self-injury is the most difficult type to assess and evaluate. It is important to determine the *frequency*—episodic or repetitive—of the behavior, the *age of onset, course* of the behavior, the *methods* used (typically cutting and burning), and any true *intent to die*. Determine the *location* (bathroom, bedroom, kitchen, etc.) where the behavior occurs, and the patient's state of mind (*thoughts and emotions*) just before most acts of self-injury and the *degree of relief*, if any, afterward. Find out about patients' social networks, social morbidity, feelings about their *scars*, and *areas of the body* that have been injured.

I recommend reading Klonsky and Weinberg (2009) for an excellent description of and the appropriate references pertaining to assessment instruments that deal with nonsuicidal self-injury (NSSI). The *Suicide Attempt Self-Injury Interview* (SASII) contains thirty-one structured questions about NSSI both with and without an intent to die. It is comprehensive and well worth the time it takes to administer. Because it explores each act of self-injury in some depth, a short form is available for repetitive self-injurers. The *Self-Injurious Thoughts and Behaviors Interview* (SITBI) is an easy to administer, useful, non-time-consuming tool that comes in a long (169 items) and a short (72 items) form. Another brief but useful instrument is the *Inventory of Statements about Self-Injury* (ISAS), which uncovers motivations for NSSI; among the functions it measures are affect regulation, self-punishment, interpersonal influence, and peer bonding. Although many other instruments can be used to assess NSSI, the three above-mentioned are probably the most useful.

Episodic NSSI is an associated feature of many disorders (only in BPD and trichotillomania is it a criterion) and a *diagnosis* must be made. Repetitive NSSI in the context of the repetitive NSSI syndrome can be diagnosed as an *impulse control disorder not elsewhere classified*.

The Prevalence of Pathological Self-injury

Prevalence here refers to the number or percentage of self-injurers in a population. After a thorough review of the literature, I believe that only a few meaningful statements can be made (see Rodham and Hawton [2009] for a list, with appropriate references, of epidemiological studies).

- Major self-injury is rare. Most clinicians with a larger practice will encounter only a handful of cases during a career.
- Stereotypic self-injury is encountered in about 10 to 20 percent of persons who have mental retardation (Griffin et al. 1985; Oliver et al. 1989; Schroeder et al. 1978). It reaches 100 percent in Lesch-Nyhan and about 30 percent in Tourette's syndrome.
- The percentage of females who engage in NSSI is slightly higher than that of males.
- Up to 80 percent of persons who have a diagnosis of borderline personality disorder commit at least one act of NSSI (typically cutting or burning).
- Among people who currently commit or have committed acts of NSSI, the average age of onset is 12–14.
- About 15 percent of high school and college students have committed at least one act of NSSI.
- The prevalence of NSSI seems to be increasing and probably affects about one percent of the total population over a lifetime.

Considering all the studies that have been done, there is not much meaningful clinical information about the prevalence of self-injury. A number of factors inform my somewhat pessimistic view. Most studies from the United Kingdom, Australia, and New Zealand cannot be accurately compared with American studies because they include self poisoning and overdoses—fairly common behaviors—as well as other failed suicide attempts as NSSI. In many studies NSSI is not clearly defined nor is intent to die determined. One act of NSSI technically allows a person to be counted as a lifetime self injurer but this may not be a clinically relevant finding.

Although not a prevalence study, Nock et al. (2009) reported on the "real-time" thoughts of NSSI among thirty adolescents and young adults with a history of recent self-injury. The subjects carried a personal digital assistant (a type of recording device) for fourteen days and were instructed to enter information about NSSI thoughts or acts when the device beeped (at midday and in the evening) as well as whenever they experienced a self-destructive thought or behavior. The entries provided information about what the subjects were doing when they experienced NSSI thoughts or behaviors, who they were with, what led to the thoughts, and what they were feeling. The subjects reported an average of five NSSI thoughts per week, most often of moderate intensity and short duration (one to thirty minutes), and one to six episodes of NSSI per week. "Thoughts of NSSI rarely were accompanied by suicidal thoughts—highlighting the distinction between these different forms of self-injurious thoughts and behaviors—but co-occurred with thoughts of alcohol/drug abuse and binging/purging approximately 15% to 20% of the time." Encouragement by other people to engage in NSSI, while not common, almost doubled the odds that NSSI would occur. Similarly, feelings such as numbness and rejection greatly increased the odds of NSSI behavior, although they were present during a minority of NSSI thoughts. NSSI was reportedly performed for intrapersonal reinforcement 85 to 90 percent of the time, and for interpersonal reinforcement only 15 to 20 percent of the time. Results showed that NSSI helped persons to regulate distressing emotions and distracted them from unwanted negative thoughts. This is a significant study but, as the authors point out, the sample size was small and some of the antecedent and consequent events maintaining the subjects' NSSI may occur outside of their conscious awareness.

One of the largest and most publicized recent studies demonstrates both provocative findings and the difficulties of conducting research on NSSI. College students at Cornell and Princeton Universities were randomly invited to participate in an Internet survey of NSSI. Only 37 percent of the 8,300 invited to participate responded and 182 reports were eliminated (missing data) leaving a sample size of 2,875 cases. Of these, 490 (17%) admitted over their lifetime to having engaged in NSSI; 118 (25.4%) engaged in one act; 154 (33.2%) in 2–5 acts; 72 (15.5%) in 6–10 acts; 45 (9.7%) in 11–20 acts; and 75 (15.2%) in more than 20 acts. The average age of onset of NSSI in the sample was age 15 to 16 years. Of the 372 persons who engaged in two or more acts of NSSI, 179 (79.8%) stopped this behavior after five years of starting, and 71 (40%) after one year of starting. The twelve-month prevalence rate was 7.3 percent, and 9.7 percent of subjects had not self-injured in the past year. Overall, 53.3 percent of persons who engaged in any NSSI reported physical (12%), sexual (20%), or emotional (44%) abuse. Of all self-injurers, 75.9 percent reported having considered or attempted suicide, had elevated levels of distress in their past month, and/or had a "characteristic" of an eating disorder. The percentage of the just mentioned problems increased from a baseline in no-self-injury subjects to those who admitted to just one act of NSSI and really escalated in those with more than one act of NSSI.

How can these results be understood? Questionnaire studies (I have done some myself) are quick but "lazy" in comparison to interview studies. How did the fact that 63 percent of students declined to participate affect the study? What types of NSSI were reported? By far, the most common was severe skin scratching or pinching (51.6%), followed by banging and punching objects to the point of bruising or bleeding (37.6%), skin cutting (33.7%), and self-punching or banging with bruising or bleeding (24.5%). The highest percent of skin scratching or pinching is a surprise finding. Typically the focus in other studies and in clinical practice is on cutting and burning. Does the commission of one act of severe skin scratching at the age of 16 years mean that for the rest of their lives these persons should be counted as a self-injurer, or does this simply inflate the "lifetime" prevalence rate of 17 percent found in this study (this high rate was highlighted both in a Cornell University press release and in numerous online and print publications). Are the rates of physical, sexual, and (especially) emotional abuse "real" or "perceived," and does the perception of abuses make them real anyway? What exactly is a "characteristic" of an eating disorder?

In my commentary on the study (Favazza 2006), in which I admittedly did not correctly interpret the odds ratio used in the study's multivariate analysis, I stated that it was difficult to believe that a single act of NSSI—the most common being severe skin scratching/pinching and banging/punching objects—had predictive potential. In nonclinical populations, for example, it is not uncommon for frustrated male adolescents to punch a wall and for young girls to scratch their skin. I noted that, for me, skin cutting and burning were more salient acts of NSSI, and that, even with cutting, I pay little attention to persons who report one impulsive or compulsive act of NSSI done years ago. I would, however, be concerned if a patient had recently engaged in NSSI. My biggest worry would be that the behavior was the beginning of a pattern that must be stopped to avoid progression to repetitive NSSI and development of the repetitive NSSI syndrome.

In response to my commentary, Whitlock et al. suggested the single incident NSSI may be a manifestation of subclinical emotional disorders. They may be correct, but it's a bit of a stretch. More pertinently they wrote, "Ultimately, we make no claims about whether single SIB incidents predict clinical pathology. All of the self-injurious respondents in this survey were functioning at a high enough level to obtain and maintain admission to competitive universities. That so many of the self-injurious students had never sought therapy for any reason and, if they did, were not likely to disclose self-injurious behavior suggests that they may be qualitatively different than patients in clinical settings. Indeed, our finding that the vast majority (74.6%) of self-injurious students report ceasing the behavior within five years of starting (40% cease within one year of starting) suggests that few suffer from the more serious long term psychiatric problems associated with the Deliberate Self-Harm Syndrome—although the extent to which this cessation indicates resolution of underlying distress or pathology likely to manifest in other

ways is unknown. Our data also suggest that many of these students are at elevated risk for suicide-related behavior and other risk behaviors, even if for a short
period of time."

My somewhat lengthy discussion of this study is meant to point out the difficulties associated with conducting research on NSSI. I applaud Whitlock and
her colleagues, who are among the current leaders in studying NSSI. and I look
forward to their follow-up studies (although it may prove difficult to track down
students after graduation) and other research in this area. In fact, the next section
of this chapter relies heavily on their work.

The Role of the Media and the Internet in NSSI

A paper that I published with Karen Conterio in 1989 provided data on female
habitual self-injurers, mostly cutters. Only 6 percent knew someone who had
self-injured, while 3 percent had read about it. The others stumbled onto the behavior ("The event just happened"). Interestingly, this sample of convenience was
drawn from persons who were watching one of the first daytime television shows
on the topic. Since then, however, the tables have turned and the overwhelming
majority of self-injurers now report that they were turned on to NSSI because of
stories in newspapers and magazines, television shows, movies, and the Internet.
In 2005, Rideout et al. reported that persons from 8 to 18 years old are exposed
to more than eight hours a day of media messages.

Among the various theories used to explain the effects of media and the Internet on NSSI are convergence, emergent norm, social learning, disinhibition, and
script; in simple terms these theories provide for an introduction to and the
spread of new-to-the-viewer NSSI behaviors, the normalizing of these behaviors,
and priming—(through the creation of "scripts") which slowly prepare a young
viewer to try or to adopt behaviors that had never been considered (Whitlock
et al. 2009). Virtual communities with an interest in NSSI form on the Internet,
and through shared postings members may affect offline behavior such as imitating NSSI behaviors or creating new ones. Whitlock et al. (2006; 2007) found
more than five hundred self-injury Internet message boards in 2006 on which
members "seek and provide support and information. . . . They also exchange
and share strategies for ceasing the behavior, finding help, avoiding detection,
treating severe wounds, and even injuring in new or different ways." The variety
of message boards is bewildering (I even found one for Christian eunuchs!). Self-
injurers also communicate through blogs, sites such as Facebook, Twitter, and
personal pages with photo galleries, short stories, and original poems ("border-

line" poetry is a literary genre unto itself). Some sites are overseen by Web administrators, who may intervene when postings are thought to be noxious, while on other sites most anything goes. The most common themes that I have discerned from examining many sites is that NSSI is abnormal and that controlling it means enduring frustrations, being misunderstood, and a need for bravery. Less common themes are that NSSI is a normal way to deal with anxiety, depression, and past maltreatment, and that it sometimes is a pleasant, unique experience. Persons who post photos of their wounds or provide detailed information about them are almost always told to stop it because they are seeking attention.

From 1966 to 2005, Whitlock et al. (2009) identified forty-seven movies with unambiguous NSSI scenes or characters and 89 songs with NSSI references. Twenty movies and fifty songs appeared between 2000 and 2005, a clear upward trend. The typical movie character was a white, middle- or upper-class female cutter with an age range from the teens to the 30s. Most had an overt or implied mental illness and received no treatment for their NSSI. A third attempted or completed suicide. There were 435 news stories about NSSI from 1991 to 1995, 1441 from 1996 to 2000, and 1750 from 2001 to 2005. This degree of exposure undoubtedly has contributed to the absolute and relative rise of NSSI behaviors, especially cutting. Among the many reasons for the increased public and professional interest in NSSI since the early 1990s are Karen Conterio's ongoing appearances on television and radio shows, my numerous (more than three hundred) presentations to psychiatric and medical groups, wide press coverage of the publication of the original edition of *Bodies under Siege* in 1987, revelations of NSSI by well-known personalities (Morton's 1992 biography described Princess Diana's cutting episodes, and 1993 actor and then–teen idol Johnny Depp displayed the scars on his forearm for a major magazine article; he said that his body was like a journal and that he cut himself to mark special times in his life), and the explosion of the body modification movement.

Psychodynamic Theories of Self-injury

Psychodynamic theories about self-injury use concepts that include symbolism, the unconscious mind, repression, sublimation, mental defense mechanisms, libido, ego-superego-id, transference and countertransference, and psychic energy. Although most psychiatrists and psychologists do not use these concepts very much nowadays, psychoanalytical/dynamic case studies provide many useful insights into NSSI (Hartman and Powander 1987). Two old concepts, however, have been discredited. The first is the all self-injury somehow relates to self-castration (early psychoanalysis was phallocentric). The second is that self-injury is a form of "focal suicide" and that it is a substitute for suicide; only in a few cases does major self-mutilation forestall suicide.

In everyday life it is possible to obtain some respite from moderately heightened levels of tension and anxiety through such methods as increased physical activity, massage, orgasm, meditation, and muscle relaxation exercises. But when tension and anxiety reach pathological levels, none of these methods has much effect. An act of NSSI, however, may be efficacious. One explanation for this effect relates to the problematic theory of "psychic energy." Briefly stated, this theory holds that the mind-brain system operates best within a certain range of tension levels. If the level gets too high, the mind-brain system will operate automatically to divest itself of "quantities of excitation." As noted, when tense patients cut themselves, they in fact often describe the results in words such as "It's like lancing a boil" or "It's like popping a balloon." The implied metaphor is clear: in cutting their skin they provide an opening through which the tension and badness in their bodies can rapidly escape. What does leave the body is blood, a precious substance that throughout human history has been associated with the cure of illness, preservation of health, salvation, and resolution of social conflict. Many cutters like to watch the blood drip from their wounds; a scene sometimes reminiscent of Jesus on the cross with his blood spurting out. It seems likely that the outward flow of tension following self-cutting is linked with the flow of blood, with all its symbolic connotations. The term *bad blood*, for example, is used to indicate inimical relationships, especially among close friends and family members. Cutters may feel relief because they have eliminated some "bad blood," thus symbolically decreasing the tension arising from impaired relationships. Some self-injurers burn their skin. This does not draw blood but the procedure is efficacious because badness and tension slowly leak out of their bodies in the serous fluid caused by the burn. In fact, a fluid-filled blister serves as a safety valve that can be "popped" when needed.

Another mechanism through which NSSI may exert therapeutic effects is the cathartic release of anger. As stated by one patient, "Often I can feel the pressure build up internally until NSSI can create a cathartic reaction. It is as if I need to purge myself in some medieval ritual." Many cutters are angry with themselves for not living up to their expectations, for causing misery for others, or for being "no good." They may be angry with their parents and other important people in their lives or with institutions such as mental hospitals, schools, or prisons that have failed them. Often they are angry with their fate and with the unjust universe. By wounding their bodies, such persons provide an outlet for their anger.

Certainly NSSI is a safer outlet than the direct expression of anger toward parents and important people who might retaliate. As an expression of anger against institutions, private self-mutilation is not as effective as writing letters to newspapers, picketing, public fasting, or immolation by fire on a busy thoroughfare, but it is some sort of action and is preferable at a personal level to passivity and resignation.

Kernberg (1987) feels that self-mutilators develop "feelings of resentment, rage, and impotence in an effort to control an important person (including the therapist), and that the experience of NSSI is the relieving enactment of revenge." The expression of anger is important in another formulation: abused children may mutilate themselves to punish the original perpetrators of the abuse in effigy, using their own skins as a symbol for the offending persons. Rarely, the intense anger will be directed outward as well as inward, but social forces "conduce women to inhibit the direct expression of violent feelings against the offending parties, whereas men who feel violated tend more readily to become aggressive" (Stone 1987). Girls at a repressive correctional institution carved their skin as a demonstration of autonomy; the authorities at the institution tightly controlled the girls' lives but were relatively helpless in stopping the carving (Ross and McKay 1979).

NSSI in some cases, however, may be "the product of introjects which are excessively cathected with primitive aggression. . . . The primitive self carries out the functions and activities that have been modeled and acted out in reality by a very disturbed parental figure" (Figueroa 1988). Aggression is a plastic drive that seeks expression when a person is frustrated. Early childhood self-attack, for example, results when aggression is forced inward because its expression outward is blocked by a child's physical disability, external restrictions on physical expression, physical distance from the object of aggression, or fears of loss of love, of punishment, and of destroying the love object (Cain 1961). Anna Freud (1946, p. 56) referred to turning-against-the-self as an early defense mechanism that is "as old as the instincts themselves, or at least as old as the conflict between instinctual impulses and any hindrance which they may encounter on their way to gratification." In a regressive slide from object to self, an object of hate may be incorporated or introjected so that the internalized representation becomes the target of aggression. Adult self-injurers report lifetime histories of greater aggression than do non-self-injuring personality-disordered controls, and there is a direct correlation between the frequency of NSSI and chronic anger (Simeon et al. 1992).

The pathological condition in which a person experiences an alteration in the perception or experience of one's mind and body is known as a depersonalization disorder. Mild depersonalization episodes are common in young adults but are not associated with significant impairment or NSSI. Severe episodes, however, are frightening. Depersonalized individuals may feel that their bodies are unreal, that time and the environment have mysteriously changed, and that they are becoming insane. As noted by Nemiah (1985), "It is a curious paradox that, even though the patient complains of being emotionally dead and estranged, he is capable of being emotionally upset by that very sense of loss. Indeed, all the manifestations of depersonalization are acutely unpleasant and not only motivate the patient to seek medical help but often drive him to vigorous activity or to inducing intense sensations in himself in order to break through the prison walls of his sense of unreality" (p. 955). NSSI, especially skin cutting, is usually effective in ending an episode of depersonalization (Coons and Milstein 1990). As stated by a patient, "I'd rather die than face being unreal. You go through life doing things automatically, like a machine. And then at the end of the day you try to match events with an emotion and try to experience them as a whole being. It's all right to hurt yourself because it proves you are real." Sometimes it is the pain, but more often the sight of blood that seems to be effective in restoring a sense of reality. Asch (1971) described a sequence of events in a group of adolescent girls, who when threatened by rejection, experienced depersonalization that was relieved by wrist cutting. In the words of one girl: "There was too much white, white nurses, white doctors, white sheets, white walls. It was such a relief to cut and see the red blood flow" (p. 632). The presence of blood not only interrupts the monotony of depersonalization but also indicates that the cutter is, indeed, alive and that the body's border of skin is intact and in place.

The skin encloses and maintains the body, and the "skin ego" maintains and encloses the psyche. Infants first internalize their mothers through skin contact. The skin "is one of the most primitive channels for preverbal communication, where nonverbalized affects may be somatically experienced and observed. Through her handling of the child the mother's skin may convey the full range of emotions from tenderness and warmth and love to disgust and hate" (Gaddini 1982, p. 315). There is supposedly an initial merging of the mother and the infant. Eventually infants establish their own sense of self, but a maternal core remains within them (the internalized mother). If the skin ego of infants is impaired because of diffuse instinctual anxiety, as adults they may use the physical pain of NSSI to repair their outer shell. If the skin ego is impaired because of unsatisfactory early nurturing, the adult may attack the internalized mother by NSSI. Self-cutters demonstrate unresolved issues dealing "with the very first assault on their bodies, the site of which is the skin" (Hibbard 1994).

Persons who have clinical depression think poorly of themselves and believe their symptoms to be the just deserts of bad thoughts or deeds. They cannot escape harsh self-judgment but can hope for some relief by paying for their "crimes," just as criminals may be reconciled with society by suffering in a penitentiary. If depressed persons imagine themselves to have committed heinous crimes, they may sentence themselves to death by suicide. Of course, for less-serious "crimes" the sentence may be lighter and the punishment less great; for example, self-cutting or sticking needles into one's skin may suffice to bring the relief that follows paying for one's transgressions. As one patient said, "I feel that I have to be punished and after harming myself I feel relief. I never wanted to die. I just want my emotions to die." NSSI in these cases represents the workings of a harsh superego that functions as police officer, judge, jury, and jailer to enforce punishment on a criminal.

Feelings of badness and hostility may find relief in self-injury through the mechanism of localization. Rather than consider themselves totally bad, persons may localize the bad part to a specific organ, such as the eye; removal of the organ provides a method for removing the badness or demon as well.

For some people, NSSI serves to remedy perceived internal or external flaws. One patient stated, "I feel lonely and ugly and disfigured inside. Terribly imperfect. Which leads to feeling the need to correct something outwardly, so I cut off my hair. I think about death a lot." More drastic is the use of self-castration among men whose psychopathology centers on problems with gender identity, functioning in the male role, and sexual conflicts. Men who perceive themselves to be women may regard self-castration as a surgical remedy to correct a flaw in their anatomy. Other men may castrate themselves to fulfill a desire to be "like" a woman, to enhance or to establish a relationship with a woman (such as mother) by removing the threat of sexuality, and to resolve conflicts over homosexual desires.

Self-cutting of an exposed area of the body can be a most effective demonstration of desperation. "My self-harm began my senior year in high school. I watched a movie where a guy killed himself and was—strangely—moved by it. One of the girls in my class had tried to kill herself that night. She had taken pills to die but her favorite method was the blade. I began scraping myself with a key and by cutting the words 'HELL ME' on my arm. I was scared to death the next morning and told my teacher. She saw the words as 'HELP ME.' I purposely did *not* write that because it is too conventional. She helped me start seeing a psychologist." A possible explanation of this behavior has been proposed by Benjamin (1987): abused children learn that acknowledging inflicted pain often ends the perpetrator's attacks and may then result in nurturance. A pattern is established so that later in life persons faced with seemingly terrible problems inflict suffering on themselves through NSSI in the expectation that the problems will end and nurturance will follow: "The internal phenomenology of the self-mutilator is a replay of family history."

Sometimes NSSI can be a manipulative ploy to gain attention and to coerce others into providing a caring, mothering response (Kwawer 1980). As emotional blackmail, it often works. It is difficult enough to see strangers, much less family members or loved ones, cut and burn themselves without intervening. Especially as self-injurers escalate the frequency and intensity of their acts, observers become overwhelmed by guilt and acquiesce to their demands.

NSSI can be an attention getter in a negative way. It is an unappealing behavior; indiscriminate scars and burn marks are ugly and even frightening at times. The legend of Saint Lucy tells how she drove away an unwanted suitor by enucleating her eyes and sending them to him. Figueroa (1988) notes, "Especially when sexual abuse has occurred, the mutilation may be an attempt to turn away future sexual contact/abuse by ensuring that one is physically unattractive and, thus, undesirable."

In his book on symbolic wounds, Bettelheim (1955) addresses female adolescent self-mutilation. His theory is that girls in their transition to adult status may demonstrate an identification with their mother by symbolically creating a vagina (the cut skin) and menstruation (the bloody wound). Bettelheim was aware of tribal rites of passage; his theory is not as far-fetched as it would seem at first glance. Identification with the mother also is the major theme in a different formulation of NSSI: "The induced bleeding in the cutting is an attempt to undo the current separation by identifying with the bleeding woman (mother) symbolic of this mother-infant unit in the past" (Asch 1971).

The perturbations of sexual drives commingled with aggressive drives serve as the basis of several psychoanalytic theories. Biven (1977) writes about the excitable, elated, sexualized orgasmlike feelings associated with the behavior; and Daldin (1990) notes that "cutting the skin also represents a self-stimulating masturbatory (autoerotic) activity involving both the attempted expression of masturbatory sexual gratification as well as a punishment for the impulse to stimulate the self." Siomopoulos (1974) describes gaping cuts as producing little female genitalia, which may then be touched and manipulated uninhibitedly.

NSSI is a method to relieve emotional dysphoria, which is usually precipitated by issues of separation, loss, and failure (Liebenluft et al. 1987). The psychological mechanisms for this relief include reduction in guilt through self-punishment; the redirection of pain away from disturbing thoughts and feelings; cutting as a counter-stimulus; arousal and amplification of distantly and nebulously perceived conflicts so that they are clearer, more easily understood, and less frightening; and the amplification of pleasurable emotions (e.g., masochistic sexual practices) (Figueroa 1988).

NSSI prevents ego disintegration by helping reestablish control over racing thoughts, rapidly fluctuating emotions, and an unstable environment. "I didn't 'decide' on self-abuse. I just did it because it calmed me down. I would be so hurt and angry I'd feel like I was exploding. Better cut me than someone else. The pain gave me a focal point, then I'd put whatever was bothering me out of my mind." "Self-harm gives me a feeling of control when I cannot find control in the environment. It also makes me feel real. I enjoy it. It makes me feel better. Release from emotional pain. A form of security." Persons who feel a loss of control in other areas find that NSSI is a behavior over which they have total control. Only they can start it, and only they can stop it. Women who experience dyscontrol of bleeding during their menses may cut themselves not only to prove that they can at least control something but also to attempt to magically divert blood away from the vaginal area.

NSSI may be symptom reducing by providing stimulation (e.g., institutionalized children living in a sterile environment are prone to head banging and face slapping as a means of self-stimulation) (Collins 1965). Persons who have an antisocial personality disorder appear to have an inordinate need for excitement and stimulation. When locked in a prison cell or placed in a restrictive environment, they experience mounting tension because of stimulation hunger that is relieved by NSSI.

Impulsive NSSI may have religious symbolism: "I have carved a cross on my chest so many times that there is a raised red scar and have made cuts on my sides. I keep thinking of something said when they baptize babies in our church: 'Receive the sign of the cross on the forehead and chest that you have been redeemed by Christ the crucified.' I also think of the 'stripes' Christ received when I cut my side. I understand that Christ died for everyone but, somehow in my mind, not for me."

Self-mutilation may occur in response to hallucinations or paranoid fears. Voices may command psychotic persons to injure themselves, or visions may be interpreted to indicate that self-injury is necessary. When the hallucinations indicate that self-injury fulfills a higher destiny, such as God's will, people who are mentally ill may feel exalted because they have been chosen. When the voices are persecutory, the act of self-injury may be a gesture of appeasement (e.g., "I have hurt myself, therefore you no longer need to persecute me"). Hallucinations may range from continuous, pesky noises to extremely frightening visions (especially when drug induced); self-injury may represent a desperate attempt to distract attention away from the hallucinations or to end a frightening episode.

Among female habitual self-injurers, multiple scars are located on the arms (74%), legs (44%), abdomen (25%), head (23%), chest (18%), and genitals (8%) (Favazza and Conterio 1989). NSSI may be therapeutic because the symbolism associated with the formation of scar tissue indicates that healing has occurred. Thus, with a few strokes of a razor the cutter may unleash a symbolic process in which the sickness within is removed and the stage is set for healing as evidenced by a scar. The cutter, in effect, performs a primitive sort of self-surgery, complete with tangible evidence of healing. Scarring serves an additional purpose in that it can "mark" a hurtful occasion. Just as a significant event symbolically can be burned in one's memory, so too it literally can be burned into one's skin.

Psychological and Psychosocial Models of Self-injury

I have presented many examples of diagnostic categories, psychological states, and social situations that are associated with self-injury. Newly developed functional and interpersonal models offer a different framework for understanding exactly why self-injury occurs.

A focus on events that precede and immediately follow acts of self-injury allows for an understanding of the functions that these acts serve. Nock and Prinstein's four function model (FFM), is the major one used in this area (see Nock and Cha [2009] for a full discussion with references). It is based on the separate dimensions of positive and negative reinforcement, and on automatic and social contingencies.

The most commonly used function is *automatic negative reinforcement* (e.g., NSSI allows people to feel better; it reduces or eliminates negative states such as mounting anxiety or racing thoughts). A second function is *automatic positive reinforcement* (e.g., NSSI allows people to gain relief from emotional numbness, dreadful joylessness, or depersonalization, by generating feelings). A third function is *social positive reinforcement* (e.g., people engage in NSSI to get attention or to engender nurturing feelings toward them by others). The fourth function is *social negative reinforcement* (e.g., NSSI is used to drive people away and to make fewer demands). The development of this four-function model is mainly based on patients' self-reports, which may not always be accurate but, when considered from the totality of clinical experience, support the model. A few physiological and behavioral studies also support the model: compared with a control group, persons who have a recent history of NSSI have higher physiological arousal when stressed; adolescents who have a history of NSSI tend to chose maladaptive solutions in tests of problem-solving, such as selecting NSSI to get attention.

Most people deal with unpleasant emotions, thoughts, or situations without self-injury. So, why do some people choose NSSI? Nock and Cha (2009) provide four answers: (1) self-injurers report highly significant levels of self-criticism, and NSSI may be a way for them to punish themselves; (2) NSSI is natural (animals do it), quick, immediately effective, and readily available; (3) people pay attention to it more than, say, to crying or complaining; and (4) NSSI is modeled after peer behavior and media reports. These answers, however, are meaningful only when put into a larger context that includes predisposing biopsychosocial vulnerabilities (poor communication and problem-solving skills, low distress tolerance, high emotional reactivity, childhood maltreatment, etc.), stressful triggering events, and inadequate regulation of emotional experiences and social situations.

Another way to look at the vulnerabilities, triggering events, and reasons for engaging in self-injury is through the use of interpersonal models (see Prinstein et al. 2009 for a full discussion with references). Among the identified risk factors are poor childhood experiences with parents, siblings, peers, and others, as well as childhood maltreatment. These early disturbed relationships may portend problems with emotional regulation and with relationships later in life, feelings of social alienation, blurred interpersonal boundaries, and higher pain thresholds that result in NSSI in order to generate feelings. Conflicts with family, friends, romantic partners, and adult authority figures are interpersonal events that trigger NSSI. Two of the functions in the four-function model deal with NSSI as a method of dealing with interpersonal relationships by getting people's attention in order to obtain a nurturing response or by driving them away. NSSI certainly has the power to change self-injurers' social environments. In some cases, NSSI results in a reexamination of family dynamics with a consequent improved quality of relationships among family members. In other cases the re-examination, or failure to re-examine, may result in more hostile relationships. At times, self-injurers may attract other self-injurers as friends who mutually reinforce their deviant behaviors.

Child Development and Self-injury

Because much NSSI begins in late childhood / early adolescence, it seems obvious that problems in childhood development are significant as a vulnerability for self-injury. In my study of female, habitual self-mutilators 54 percent selected the adjective "miserable" to describe their childhood, 8 percent selected "happy," and the rest selected "average" (Favazza and Conterio 1989). Childhood abuse was noted by 62 percent of the subjects. Of these, 29 percent reported both sexual and physical abuse; 17 percent reported only sexual abuse; and 16 percent reported only physical abuse. The average age of onset of sexual abuse was 7 years, and the average duration was twenty-four months. The sexually abusive people most commonly listed were a family friend (43%), brother (25%), father (23%), uncle (13%), mother and stepfather (6% each), and grandfather (4%). The average age of onset of physical abuse was 6 years and the average duration was five years. The physically abusive people most commonly listed were mother (50%), father (45%), brother (16%), other (16%), stepfather (4%), and sister and uncle (3%). Patients' statements about childhood abuse should be accepted on face value, although recollections may become distorted over time and it is often impossible to verify the quantity and intensity of the abuse. Some sensitive persons may magnify the experiences of abuse, become fixated on them, and attribute their psychosocial and psychological problems as well as their NSSI to them. Other persons may repress and minimize the abuse. At any rate the actuality and the perceptions of abuse must be dealt with, although to facilitate the recall of repressed memories, in the hands of the wrong therapist, may have deleterious consequences (e.g., patients may produce false memories to please a therapist).

Yates (2009) summarized many studies in this area and provides relevant references. At the heart of the matter is the issue of child maltreatment such as neglect and physical, sexual, and emotional abuse (Carroll et al. 1980). Although it has not been well studied I expect that childhood maltreatment in the form of inconsistency or insensitive child rearing, childhood witnessing of domestic violence, and poor modeling as a result of severe poverty and mental illness / substance abuse in caregivers also may be significant. Child maltreatment has been associated with the development of a host of behavioral problems and mental illnesses. In the case of NSSI, the strongest association is with persisting abuse by a person known to the child, especially when force or penetration occurs during sexual abuse. NSSI may result from self-blame in incest victims (Shapiro 1987).

Maltreated children often develop a negative perspective on life and may consider themselves to be defective and unlovable, other persons as frightening or malevolent, and relationships as unstable and perilous. They may blame themselves for this maltreatment and punish themselves by self-injury, or, because they may avoid or mess up their relationships, may self-injure out of frustration. Maltreated children also may develop a dissociative coping style in which there is a split between thinking and feeling. When abuse occurs, for example, victims may "turn off" their feelings about the perpetrator and what is happening to them. During sexual abuse, for example, a child victim may blankly stare at the ceiling where the self hovers timelessly in space and is disconnected from the body. When carried into later life, this coping style may manifest itself as depersonalization in stressful times; cutting is the only regularly effective method of ending depersonalization. The experience of abuse often is a precursor of posttraumatic stress disorder, and NSSI may occur when the trauma is mentally relived. Maltreated children also demonstrate a deficiency in verbally processing and describing their experiences and emotions, which then are expressed through their behavior and their bodies, sometimes in the form of self-injury. Maltreated children may develop alterations in physiological areas such as the HPA (hypothalamic-pituitary-adrenal) axis, which mediates responses to stress and may influence NSSI (van der Kolk et al. 1991).

No one likes the idea of children being abused, but several issues need to be kept in mind. While about 50 to 60 percent of repetitive self-injurers have been abused, the majority of abused children do not self-injure. The timing of the abuse during child development, its duration, its intensity, and the perception of abuse may be crucial. One patient told me that he was a "human ashtray" as a child; his parents put out their lit cigarettes on his body, while another patient said that she was abused because her brother touched her breasts once. In one careful study, sexual abuse was *not* associated with an increased risk for NSSI but rather for suicide attempts (Nock and Kessler 2006), and in an analysis of multiple studies childhood sexual abuse did not have any great effect on NSSI (Klonsky and Moyer 2008). Various studies show a relationship between physical abuse and episodic NSSI and between sexual abuse and repetitive NSSI (Yates 2009); the necessity of PTSD symptoms for a significant relationship between sexual abuse and NSSI (Weierich and Nock 2008); the necessity of problems with expressing emotions for a significant relationship between physical/emotional abuse, but not sexual abuse, and NSSI (Gratz and Roemer 2008; Paivio and McCulloch 2004). Childhood maltreatment clearly plays a role in adolescent and adult NSSI, but a lot more work needs to be done to clarify the situation.

Negative experiences, other than maltreatment, include adult self-injury of organs that were intentionally injured or diseased during childhood (e.g., castration of a testicle previously affected by mumps or orchitis, or amputation of a limb in which a bone had been broken). In other instances, organs that were self-injured as a child become targets of attack later in life. Also, Rosenthal et al. (1972) found that sixteen of twenty-four female cutters had experienced surgery, hospitalization for serious illness, or lacerations before the age of 12 years. None of the twenty-four women in a control group of noncutting suicide attempters had such a history.

Biological Findings and Self-injury

The vast majority of biological studies of self-injury focus on impulsive NSSI, usually cutting, and on the role of chemicals that affect the transmission of impulses among the billions of neurons in the brain. This incredibly complex topic may, to make it somewhat understandable, lead to *simplistic statements* (e.g., if people are depressed and feel "low," then they have low serotonin levels; administering antidepressant drugs makes serotonin levels go up and therefore causes people's moods to go "up").

It must be understood that there are *a large number* of known neurotransmitter agents; for example, monoamines (serotonin, dopamine, norepinephrine, histamine, acetylcholine); amino acids (glutamate, GABA, glycine); neuropeptides (more than one hundred are known and include adrenocorticotrophin hormone, corticotrophin-releasing factor, beta-endorphin, leu-enkephalin, and met-enkephalin); prolactin, substances K and P, thyrotropin-releasing hormone, oxytocin; neurotrophins (NGF, BNDF, N-T-3, N-T-4); nitric oxide; carbon monoxide; hydrogen sulfide; endocannabinoids (anandamide, 2-AG, NADA, noladin ether, virodhamine); eicosanoids (omega-3 fatty acids, EPA, E-EPA, DHA); and neurosteroids. None of these agents affects a single neuronal function but rather affects multiple neural pathways, which, in turn, affect multiple behavioral and physiological processes. Each process is modulated by multiple neurotransmitter systems. Thus, studies on self-injury that focus on, say, dopamine or beta-endorphin present only a *partial picture* of what is happening in the brain (e.g., neuropeptides commonly affect monoamine transmitters). Neurotransmitters may be produced within the brain and/or other body sites (e.g., 80% of serotonin is found in the gastrointestinal tract primarily but also on blood platelets, and only 2% in the brain). Because brain serotonin cannot be measured, studies rely on *indirect* measures (that may or may not reflect what is transpiring in the brain) such as peripheral serotonin found on blood platelet cells or 5-HIAA (5-hydroxyindoleacetic acid), which is a metabolite of serotonin found in the cerebrospinal fluid or, even better, on another metabolite (5-hydroxytryptomine or 5-HT) whose activity is based on a reduced prolactin response to d-fenfluramine, a drug that specifically increase the production of 5-HT and also inhibits its reuptake. But even this test can be influenced in women by estrogen fluctuations during the menstrual cycle. There are similar problems with neuropeptides, such as the enkephalins (a major focus of current self-injury studies). Blood plasma levels do not necessarily reflect brain levels because enkephalins in the blood are unable to enter the brain (the blood-brain barrier) except for a tiny amount. Enkephalin levels in the cerebrospinal fluid can be measured, but this fluid is taken from the lumbar region of the spine and is physically distant from the higher forebrain sources of peptides; it also is subject to peptide production by spinal cord cells. Position emission topography (PET) scans may be the best answer.

It is evident from even this brief and partial overview that *any claims regarding the role of specific brain processes and self-injury are conjectural at this time.* Another major problem that must be addressed is the self-injury status of subjects in biological studies. One would not expect to unearth meaningful conclusions based on persons who have engaged in one act of NSSI years earlier, or even one recent act. Relevant findings might be discovered in persons who are repetitive self-injurers, but how many acts of NSSI, occurring over what period of time, puts a person into this category? Most biological studies use a cutoff point of two or more acts. Robust findings are much more likely to be found in more hardcore self-injurers with an extensive and ongoing history of NSSI.

All this being said, what biological findings *seem to be possibly meaningful, as I* interpret them? The largest and most consistent literature, dating from the 1970s, seems to implicate low levels of serotinergic function in the brain, using the fenfluramine challenge procedure, in impulsive aggression directed against both the self and others (Coccaro et al. 1989; Markowitz and Coccaro 1995). Although peripheral serotonin levels do not measure serotonin functioning in the brain, there is a literature that links it to impulsive aggression and self-injury (Joiner et al. 2005). Simeon et al. (1992) measured peripheral platelet serotonin in self-injuring and non-self-injuring persons who have personality disorders; the self-injuring group had significantly more personality psychopathology, greater lifetime aggression, more antisocial behavior, and lower levels of serotonin activity. A study of eighteen female adolescents concluded that low peripheral serotonin was a vulnerability factor for self-injury, especially in family contexts characterized by negativity and conflicts (Crowell et al. 2008). A German study, in which I participated, used psychometric instruments (Barratt Impulsiveness Scale, State-Trait

Anger Expression Inventory, etc.) and the fenfluramine challenge test (performed with regard to the menstrual cycle of female subjects) to measure serotonin functioning to psychiatric inpatients. Four groups were studied: fifty-four self-injurers (three or more acts of NSSI), thirty-three non-self-injuring but compulsive subjects, thirty-three patients with no impulsive behaviors, and forty-five nonclinical control subjects. Our results demonstrated that lower serotonin levels were correlated with NSSI and with impulsivity (Herpertz et al. 1997).

The role of enkephalins, opiumlike substances produced by the brain and various glands, in self-injury has been conjectured for several decades (see Sher and Stanley [2009] for a review and references). It is thought that because enkephalins suppress pain and produce a feeling of well-being self-injurers attempt to induce their production as a response to the painful stimulus of NSSI. Persons learn to associate NSSI with positive feelings, and whenever they are perturbed by unpleasant anxiety, emotions, or thoughts they cut or burn themselves in order to feel better (Konicki and Scholtz 1989). "As in opiate addiction, tolerance develops, requiring repetitive self-injurious behavior to prevent 'withdrawal'" (Russ 1992). The enkephalin response to the pain of NSSI is problematic because in the Favazza and Conterio (1989) study of 240 self-injurers, 64 percent experienced little or no pain, and only 10 percent felt great pain during the act of self-injury. A study of ten habitual cutters with BPD found markedly increased blood plasma levels of enkephalin. The highest levels correlated with the most recent and severe acts of cutting. The levels returned to normal as the patients' condition improved. All the patients stated that their acts of cutting were *painless* and provided temporary relief from dysphoria, tension, or depersonalization (Coid et al. 1983).

A number of studies have found high levels of plasma enkephalins in persons who self-injure, while other studies have found higher levels in cerebrospinal fluid. What is really needed is a measurement of enkephalin activity in the brain itself. The only method of doing this to date is by using position emission tomography (PET) ligand activation scans, in which a chemical (the ligand) binds to opiodergic receptor sites in the brain that can then be measured. A recent study has shown that this complicated technology can, indeed, measure opiodergic activity in the brain (Boecker et al. 2008). Ten trained male athletes were tested before and after a strenuous two-hour run. The results showed both increased levels of euphoria (the "runner's high") and of opioidergic activity in prefrontal cortex and limbic/paralimbic brain structures, areas that play a key role in emotional processing. Because all the athletes had previously experienced the "runner's high" many times, and because attaining euphoria is associated with reward, the authors expected to but did not find changes in the brain's nucleus accumbens, a major structure for reward processing with known opioid-dopamine processing. This is a puzzling nonfinding. But we now know that *strenuous activity* results in increased opiodergic activity in special areas of the brain. Continuously banging one's head, as seen in stereotypic self-injury, might increase opiodergic brain activity, but can an act of cutting that is usually painless do the same?

The role of the neurotransmitter dopamine in self-injury is unclear, although it interacts with serotonergic and other neurotransmitter systems. It has been implicated in the stereotypic self-injury (biting off finger tips and oral tissue) found in the rare Lesch-Nyhan syndrome (Gillman and Sandyk 1985). This genetic disorder of purine metabolism is caused by an enzyme (HGPRT) deficiency that causes uric acid to accumulate in all body fluids, resulting in severe gout, kidney problems, mental retardation, involuntary writhing, and repetitive limb movements. The self-injurious behavior may be a result from reduced dopamine activity: HGPRT deficiency may interfere with dopamine synthesis. Drug-induced stereotypic behaviors, such as skin picking secondary to amphetamine abuse, may be mediated by dopamine dysfunction (Van Putten and Shaffer 1990).

The genetics of NSSI have not been addressed. In an interesting case report six of nine children in a family were self-cutters; the effect of genetics versus child rearing and other family factors was impossible to determine in this case. However, one child who was adopted out at birth and had no biological-family contact also was a cutter (Lim and Seng 1985).

The ability to perceive pain may be a factor in NSSI. Using a standard painful stimulus test (placing a hand in cold water), borderlines who said they experienced pain during acts of self-mutilation were compared with those who said they did not experience pain. The pain ratings in response to the test were consistent with reports of pain during self-mutilation. Additionally, those who reported no pain during self-mutilation reported an improvement in mood following the cold water test. The no pain group "seemed" to have an earlier onset of self-injurious behavior and, perhaps, a more chronic course, with more lifetime episodes (Russ et al. 1992). The authors concluded that subtypes of self-mutilating borderline patients might be differentiated according to their perception of pain, mood improvement after self-harm, age of onset, and severity of childhood abuse.

One might speculate that some patients who seem to actively seek surgical operations and painful medical diagnostic tests have a low sensitivity to pain. Such patients are not uncommon; they seem to relish being operated on and may go from hospital to hospital with fantastic and often convincing symptoms. This condition, sometimes called mania operativa, is a polysurgical addiction that may be associated with alcoholism, drug dependency, NSSI, hypochondriasis, and psychopathic personality, A study (Hunter and Kennard 1982) presented eight cases in which patients with mania operativa underwent unnecessary limb amputation as a result of their masterful display of symptoms. Less dramatic but probably more common are patients who sporadically trick dentists and physicians into performing minor surgical procedures.

In a psychophysiological study, male self-mutilators and control groups used guided imagery of a self-mutilative act while measurements of arousal and tension reduction were recorded. The subjects were presented with scripts that described the setting at the onset of the act, then events that led up to the act, then the self-mutilative act itself, and, finally, reactions to the act. While the subjects were imagining this sequence of events, their heart and respiratory rates, skin resistance level, and finger blood volume and pulse amplitude were measured. Results supported the often reported clinical observation that self-mutilation successfully reduces tension and thus reinforces and maintains itself as a coping behavior. A significant finding is that "participants reported continued negative feelings despite reduced psychophysiological arousal." This result suggests that it is the alteration of psychophysiological arousal that may operate to reinforce and maintain the behavior, not the psychological response (Haines et al. 1995). This lag interval between the physiological and psychological response to an act of self-mutilation could possibly be a target for a therapeutic medication and cognitive-behavioral intervention.

In the second edition of *Bodies under Siege* (1996), I asserted, based on clinical observations, that self-injurers are deficient in their ability to tolerate intense distress and that they use NSSI to reduce or eliminate this unpleasant experience. In 2008, Nock and Mendes published the first objective behavioral study of distress tolerance among self-injurers. They examined sixty-two adolescents and young adults with a history of self-injury and thirty non-injurious control subjects. About half of the subjects were currently receiving psychological and/or psychopharmacological treatment, and 76 percent had at least one current psychiatric disorder. A well-studied Distress Tolerance Test—a series of frustrating tasks involving the correct placement of stimulus playing cards—was administered to the subjects while their levels of physiological arousal was measured by changes in their sweat glands (skin conductance levels), known to be reliably related with psychopathological states. Compared with the controls, subjects did indeed demonstrate greater levels of physiological arousal (especially in those whose NSSI served "to get rid of bad feelings") as well as poorer distress tolerance. As part of the same study a novel performance-based task called the Social

Problem-Solving Skills test was administered in which subjects were assessed on their responses to eight problematic social scenarios. The self-injuring group chose significantly more negative solutions and their ability to perform adaptive solutions was rated much lower than that of the controls. The authors rightly point out that these findings support treatments, such as dialectical behavior therapy, that help self-injuring patients learn to deal better with emotional distress and to develop good problem-solving skills.

Certainly the unique biological discovery regarding self-injury is the discovery of the neurological basis of body integrity identity disorder by Vilayanur Ramachendran (Colapinto 2009; McGeoch et al. 2009). Persons who have this disorder report a compulsion from early childhood to have a healthy limb amputated. "They could draw a line at the exact spot where they want the amputation to occur (and) attached little or no erotic significance to the condition. Furthermore, none rejected the limb as 'not belonging' to them. . . . Instead they said that the limb *over*-belonged to them: it felt intrusive." From his work with patients with phantom limb pain, Ramachendran discovered that the pains did not originate in the limb stump but rather are produced in the sensory cortex of the brain, where neurons related to the stump had been displaced by neurons for the face. He found a complex relationship involving the sensory cortex, the frontal lobe's motor cortex, and the right superior parietal lobule (an area that integrates touch, visual, and nerve signals from muscles, joints, and tendons, to create a body image). Memories of these signals remain in the brain's neural circuits after the loss of a limb but cannot be processed because the body image map has been rearranged, resulting in phantom pain. Patients with body-integrity identify disorder also have deficits, probably congenital, in their right parietal lobule. They have normal sensations in their unwanted limbs, but their body image map cannot receive or process any stimuli because the pertinent neurons have been displaced to other sections of the brain, resulting in emotional distress. This theory seems to be true because, in experiments using magnetoencephalography scans, the right superior parietal lobule can be activated by stimuli everywhere on the patient's body except the area below the unwanted limb's amputation line. This discovery has replaced psychological theories about BIID and has therapeutic implications that are discussed in the next chapter.

CHAPTER ELEVEN

Treatment

Even though pathological self-injury may provide temporary relief from a host of ills, it is not a joyous activity. Self-injurers, deep down, feel miserable about their behavior, and one goal of my work has been to give public voice to their laments. The behavior is also tough on those who naturally care for them (parents, siblings, friends, spouses, children) and those who provide professional care. People who are alcoholic, abuse drugs, or self-injure are exasperating to deal with. Their promises are usually worthless and their crises never ending. Yes, they are "sick" and part of their sickness is the abrogation of personal responsibility, but we cannot help but feel upset when we are called in the middle of the night to tend to an alcoholic person on yet another bender or a cutter intent on feeling bloody better.

Self-injurers have a difficult life. There is significant physical morbidity when an irreplaceable body part is destroyed. Repetitive self-injurers often require medical attention for their cuts and burns. Hair pullers, skin scratchers, and others who interfere with wound healing may endure repeated infections. Many will make bona fide suicide attempts in desperation over their inability to control their behavior. Social morbidity also may be great. In addition to disfiguring scars, most repetitive self-injurers usually feel empty inside, misunderstood by all, a burden to others, and scared when close to anyone.

Put simply, no one loves self-mutilators. Their very presence seems to threaten the sense of mental and physical integrity of those around them. Although self-injurers nowadays are treated better in emergency rooms, they still sometimes falsely admit to a suicide attempt to facilitate a warmer reception. Even experienced psychotherapists are hard-pressed to maintain equanimity with repetitive self-injurers. Publications about psychotherapy with these patients often contain lengthy discussions of countertransference. Frances (1987) neatly summed up the situation: "Of all disturbing patient behaviors, self-mutilation is the most difficult to understand and treat. . . . The typical clinician (myself included) treating a patient who self-mutilates is often left feeling a combination of helpless, horrified, guilty, furious, betrayed, disgusted, and sad."

Frances's remarkable litany of adjectives reflects the extraordinary power of the self-injurious act. Although suicide is shocking, the grief of mourners may be assuaged by a host of convenient rationalizations, such as "It is all part of God's great plan"; and at least the victim is dead. But self-injury is horrific in its seeming senselessness, and the victim is very much alive and able to haunt us in the flesh.

The power of self-injury to perturb even seasoned therapists seems to derive from more than what are generally considered to be the sources of countertransference. Additionally, self-injury challenges our equanimity because its bloody tendrils reach out to touch the Sacred. In the scenario of the travelers to the Holy Temple (chapter 2), I tried to portray a sense of the Sacred. It is a scary place, so scary that all the trappings of organized religion may be defenses against the true religious experience of the Sacred. Through the mechanism of transubstantiation, the Sacred becomes palatable; a wafer of grain is digested more easily than the liver of a Man-God, and a sip of red wine is less likely to stick in one's throat than His blood. The release of symbolic sacrificial energy during the act of self-injury contributes to its unsettling potential as does the symbolic connection to ritual timelessness as described by Turner (1968). In sum, even though deviant self-injurers are not luminal beings whose acts have no real transcendency, even though their use of religious symbolism is based on private rather than public delusions, they open a window onto the turbulent, bloody space of the Sacred. It is a space that truly great shamans can visit briefly, although the voyage is dangerous and fearful. So can adepts of Tantric Buddhism who have achieved the great liberation through hearing in the bardo meditations. For most of us, however, it is a space in the cosmos and in ourselves that remains hidden. When self-mutilators draw us to this space, we resist and feel "helpless, horrified, guilty, furious, betrayed, disgusted, and sad." Our feelings are hurt when self-injurers reject our care and clever interpretations, feelings that may even turn to "hate" (Winnicott 1949).

The reason for this lengthy discourse is that the treatment of self-mutilation demands more equanimity on the part of the therapist than in dealing with other patients. The general clinical wisdom is that two repetitive self-injurers are the maximum that one therapist should deal with intensively at any one time. I have, more or less, come to grips with my feelings and will describe in this chapter the therapeutic strategies that I employ to help my patients and maintain my sanity. I am at a loss to explain my composure when dealing with self-mutilators (however, I find it almost impossible to deal with severely burned patients or young quadriplegics without feeling emotionally overwhelmed). Perhaps it is a result of my long reading on the topic followed by emotionally "safe" research. By the time I first provided serious clinical care, I was well prepared. A major factor certainly was my good fortune in having several patients who served as my teachers. I still continue to learn from patients but try to avoid generalizing "insights" from one patient to others.

I think it important, before any discussion about treatment, to present the following document written by self-injurers advocate Deb Martinson (and strongly endorsed by me) in 1998. She is a pioneer on the use of the Internet in providing information and help for self-injurers.

THE BILL OF RIGHTS FOR PEOPLE WHO SELF-HARM

Preamble

An estimated 1 percent of Americans use physical self-harm as a way of coping with stress; the rate of self-injury in other industrial nations is probably similar. Still, self-injury remains a taboo subject, a behavior that is considered freakish or outlandish and is highly stigmatized by medical professionals and the lay public alike. Self-harm, also called self-injury, self-inflicted violence, or self-mutilation, can be defined as self-inflicted physical harm severe enough to cause tissue damage or leave visible marks that do not fade within a few hours. Acts done for purposes of suicide or for ritual, sexual, or ornamentation purposes are not considered self-injury. This document refers to what is commonly known as moderate or superficial self-injury, particularly repetitive SI; these guidelines do not hold for cases of major self-mutilation (i.e., castration, eye enucleation, or amputation).

Because of the stigma and lack of readily available information about self-harm, people who resort to this method of coping often receive treatment from physicians (particularly in emergency rooms) and mental-health professionals that can actually make their lives worse instead of better. Based on hundreds of negative experiences reported by people who self-harm, the following Bill of Rights is an attempt to provide information to medical and mental-health personnel. The goal of this project is to enable them to more clearly understand the emotions that underlie self-injury and to respond to self-injurious behavior in a way that protects the patient as well as the practitioner.

The Bill of Rights for People Who Self-harm

1. The right to caring, humane medical treatment.
Self-injurers should receive the same level and quality of care that a person presenting with an identical but accidental injury would receive. Procedures should be done as gently as they would be for others. If stitches are required, local anesthesia should be used. Treatment of accidental injury and self-inflicted injury should be identical.

2. The right to participate fully in decisions about emergency psychiatric treatment (so long as no one's life is in immediate danger).

When a person presents at the emergency room with a self-inflicted injury, his or her opinion about the need for a psychological assessment should be considered. If the person is not in obvious distress and is not suicidal, he or she should not be subjected to an arduous psych evaluation. Doctors should be trained to assess suicidality/homicidality and should realize that although referral for outpatient follow-up may be advisable, hospitalization for self-injurious behavior alone is rarely warranted.

3. The right to body privacy.

Visual examinations to determine the extent and frequency of self-inflicted injury should be performed only when absolutely necessary and done in a way that maintains the patient's dignity. Many who SI have been abused; the humiliation of a strip-search is likely to increase the amount and intensity of future self-injury while making the person subject to the searches look for better ways to hide the marks.

4. The right to have the feelings behind the SI validated.

Self-injury doesn't occur in a vacuum. The person who self-injures usually does so in response to distressing feelings, and those feelings should be recognized and validated. Although the care provider might not understand why a particular situation is extremely upsetting, she or he can at least understand that it *is* distressing and respect the self-injurer's right to be upset about it.

5. The right to disclose to whom they choose only what they choose.

No care provider should disclose to others that injuries are self-inflicted without obtaining the permission of the person involved. Exceptions can be made in the case of team-based hospital treatment or other medical care providers when the information that the injuries were self-inflicted is essential knowledge for proper medical care. Patients should be notified when others are told about their SI and as always, gossiping about any patient is unprofessional.

6. The right to choose what coping mechanisms they will use.

No person should be forced to choose between self-injury and treatment. Outpatient therapists should never demand that clients sign a no-harm contract; instead, client and provider should develop a plan for dealing with self-injurious impulses and acts during the treatment. No client should feel that he or she must lie about SI or be kicked out of outpatient therapy. Exceptions to this may be made in hospital or ER treatment, when hospital legal policies may require a contract.

7. The right to have care providers who do not allow their feelings about SI to distort the therapy.

Those who work with clients who self-injure should keep their own fear, revulsion, anger, and anxiety out of the therapeutic setting. This is crucial for basic medical care of self-inflicted wounds but holds for therapists as well. A person who is struggling with self-injury has enough baggage without taking on the prejudices and biases of their care providers.

8. The right to have the role SI has played as a coping mechanism validated.

No one should be shamed, admonished, or chastised for having self-injured. Self-injury works as a coping mechanism, sometimes for people who have no other way to cope. They may use SI as a last-ditch effort to avoid suicide. The self-injurer should be taught to honor the positive things that self-injury has done for him/her as well as to recognize that the negatives of SI far outweigh those positives and that it is possible to learn methods of coping that aren't as destructive and life-interfering.

9. The right not to be automatically considered a dangerous person simply because of self-inflicted injury.

No one should be put in restraints or locked in a treatment room in an emergency room solely because his or her injuries are self-inflicted. No one should ever be involuntarily committed simply because of SI; physicians should make the decision to commit based on the presence of psychosis, suicidality, or homicidality.

10. The right to have self-injury regarded as an attempt to communicate, not manipulate.

Most people who hurt themselves are trying to express things they can say in no other way. Although sometimes these attempts to communicate seem manipulative, treating them as manipulation only makes the situation worse. Providers should respect the communicative function of SI and assume it is not manipulative behavior until there is clear evidence to the contrary.

Biological Treatments

The prescribing of medications has overtaken psychiatry, and there is good evidence that they can be helpful in treating illnesses such as panic disorder, major depression, bipolar disorder, schizophrenia, and so on. Unfortunately, the biological processes that predispose, create, or maintain the many different types of self-injurious behaviors are still unclear. Sandman (2009) wrote a thorough and well-referenced chapter on the psychopharmacologic treatment of self-injury to which I refer readers. He notes that although many studies report modest or minimal efficacy, there are undoubtedly an unknown number of studies (and, I would add, clinical experiences) of never-reported negative trials and effects. He concludes that "there is no agreed-on pharmacological treatment for NSSI."

This being said, I will report what medications I prescribe and for which kinds of patients. Major self-injury takes place rapidly and usually on just one occasion.

When I am called, the deed has already been done but the patient is at high immediate risk for a second assault and must be treated quickly with antipsychotic medication and a benzodiazepine. I prescribe the newer atypical antipsychotics such as Abilify, Geodon, Invega, and Saphris (aripiprazole, ziprasidone, paliperidone, and asenapine, respectively) because of their favorable side-effect profile. This combination may not be enough in the presence of agitation and obvious signs of a desire to enucleate an eye or to self-castrate, so the temporary use of physical restraints may be necessary. Prevention is better than treatment, so I will increase the use of antipsychotic medication in psychiatric patients who present warning signs such as a high preoccupation with religion and reading the Bible, a sudden change in appearance (cutting off hair, wearing strange clothes), or even the slightest hint that they are contemplating self-injury (see Sweeny and Zamecnik 1981).

The treatment of stereotypic self-injury can be difficult because often the patients are unable to articulate what might be bothering them. The first thing I do is check for infections, especially in the urogenital tract and the ear; an antibiotic may slow down the rate of self-injury. Patients who gnaw at their hands or fingers may be trying to eliminate pain, and I have had occasional success by simply prescribing analgesics. The biggest problem in deciding what psychoactive medication to use is that some patients respond to some medications some of the time. This conclusion reflects not only my clinical experience but also published studies. The use of multiple medications is often the rule rather than the exception.

I usually try to decrease impulsivity by using serotonergic medication (SSRIs) in moderate doses, such as Prozac (fluoxetine) or citalopram (Martin 2005). It is possible that some patients also are depressed, often a difficult determination, so an SSRI may be helpful in this regard (as may lithium compounds). I then may add a mood stabilizer with dopamine-blocking activity, such as an atypical antipsychotic, and/or Depakote (divalproex, valproate), Tegretol (carbamazapine) (the former is associated with weight gain and the latter with drug interactions), and Lamictal (lamotrazine), which are also antiepileptics: people who are mentally retarded have a high rate of epilepsy, which may contribute to self-injury. I then might add Inderal (propanolol), a beta-blocker with antianxiety effects, or clonidine, a drug used widely for aggressive, hyperactive children. What about naltrexone and naloxone, medications that bind to opioid receptors in the brain so that persons do not experience the usual effects after taking morphine, heroine, or opium? They also block the effects of opioids, such as the enkephalins, that are produced in the brain and produce a sense of well-being. Theoretically, if self-injurers harm themselves to feel good due to enkephalin release, the medications will prevent this response and the persons will stop the self-injury. Their use in stereotypic self-injury has shown mixed results: sometimes they work, sometimes (at a high dose) they increase the rate of self-injury, and, most of the time, they don't work at all. I have not had much success using them, but it's worth a try. That leaves the benzodiazepines, such as Klonopin, Ativan, Xanax (clonazepam, lorazepam, alprazolam), safe medications that work rapidly to reduce anxiety and have sedative effects. Sooner or later, they often become part of the drug regimen; I have never encountered worsening or disinhibition of self-injury with these medications.

The literature is filled with mostly case reports and some open-label, chart review, and a few blind studies hailing the efficacy of the just listed medications. It really comes down to hit or miss. One, or even a few, swallows do not make a summer, and one, or even a few, case reports do not signify reliable or definitive treatment. A novel study that has caught my attention involves injecting botulinum toxin (Botox) into the masseter cheek muscles that close the jaws during chewing to prevent a patient who has Lesch-Nyhan syndrome from biting off tongue and mouth tissue. The drug temporarily weakens the masseter muscles, and the authors suggest that it also may affect muscle sensory feedback loops as well as inhibit the actions of the glutamate neurotransmitter (Dabrowski et al. 2005).

Compulsive self-injurers do not often seek psychiatric help—they see dermatologists and family physicians—so the literature on the use of medication is limited. SSRIs, lithium, or one of the older tricyclic drugs, clomipramine, occasionally helps (Christenson et al. 1991; Swedo et al. 1993; Winchel 1992). The newest treatment uses N-acetylcysteine, an amino acid that increases the major excitatory neurotransmitter, glutamate, in the nucleus accumbens (the "reward" or "pleasure" center of the brain). In a well-designed double-blind, placebo-controlled study of 50 persons who had trichotillomania, 56 percent of those who received the drug were "much or very much improved" after twelve weeks, in comparison to only 16 percent of those who received a placebo (Grant et al. 2009). This one study needs to be replicated. If the drug works well, it could usher in a new era in the treatment of compulsive self-injury. As for delusional parasitosis, one review found limited evidence for the efficacy of antipsychotic medication (Lepping et al. 2008), while another case based review found that atypical antipsychotic medication resulted in a 70 percent partial or full remission (Freudenmann and Lepping 2008). In any case, the atypical antipsychotics should be given a try.

The pharmacologic treatment of impulsive self-injurers is often based on studies of borderline patients and on studies of impulsive aggression. In clinical practice, the medications that are most widely used are SSRIs and mood stabilizers.
In acute cases when NSSI is very active (e.g., cutting several times a week, a need
for deeper cuts to get a response), high doses of an SSRI may provide relief from
uncontrolled impulsivity (a benzodiazepine, such as clonazepam, often is needed
both for sleep and to keep patients from becoming too "wired"). These high doses
seem to become less effective after a month or two, so the dose should then be
lowered. The most commonly used mood stabilizers, given to possibly help with
emotional dysregulation and to prevent the brief, "mini-psychotic" episodes that
patients who have borderline or hysteric disorder may experience, are atypical
antipsychotics. Lamictal (lamotrigine) can be helpful with mood swings that are
primarily depressive in nature. Lithium should be avoided because it is lethal in
small doses in case of an overdose. For patients who have posttraumatic stress disorder, a beta-blocker such as Inderal (propranolol) may help. In one study, urges
to self-injure, high levels of tension, and dissociative symptoms in 12 females
with borderline personality disorder were markedly reduced within an hour of
taking clonidine (Philipsen et al. 2004). The opioid blockers naltrexone and naloxone occasionally work for actively repetitive self-injurers, but their efficacy
may be proportional to the enthusiasm expressed by the psychiatrist prescribing
them. The use of medications to treat impulsive NSSI sometimes makes it easier
for patients to engage in the more helpful treatment of psychotherapy and/or
to deal with life until healing takes place as a result of new or improved relationships, childbirth, employment, spiritual growth, and environmental changes.

Other biological treatments for NSSI exist, but they are not used very often.
Reducing or eliminating caffeine use should be encouraged because caffeine can
worsen tension and anxiety. Electroconvulsive therapy (ECT) was effective in four
cases of severe self-injury: a psychotic man who had mental retardation (Bates
and Smeltzer 1982); a child who had autism and mental retardation (Wachtel et
al. 2009); a treatment-resistant schizophrenic man (Dean 2001); and a psychotically depressed man who had bipolar disorder (Arora et al. 2008). In general,
people are frightened of psychosurgery as a treatment for mental illness because
it destroys brain tissue. Stories abound about the pathetic side effects of the old,
crude procedures, such as prefrontal lobotomies (e.g., a patient who became a
campus celebrity at a state hospital because of her incessant cutting provoked the
staff into performing a lobotomy; it ended her cutting and "she afterwards busied
herself cutting out paper dolls") (Burnham 1969). Refined, new techniques, such
as limbic leucotomy, have proven successful for severe obsessive-compulsive

disorder and NSSI (Price et al. 2001), and there are several reports of some success in decreasing stereotypic NSSI (Amandan and Wigg 2004; Fountas et al.
2007), but they are being supplanted by nondestructive deep brain stimulation
(Anderson and Lenz 2009).

Deep brain stimulation involves drilling open a hole in the skull and implanting a brain stimulator which emits electrical impulses. Depending on where the
stimulator is placed, therapeutic efficacy has been shown for Parkinson disease,
chronic pain, and disabling muscular contractions. It is thought to work by decreasing excitatory neurotransmissions and, in effect, creating a brain lesion. It
has been used in stereotypic self-injury and case reports demonstrate efficacy when
placed in the hypothalamus for a brain injured woman, and when placed in the
globus pallidus in a Lesch-Nyhan patient (Kuhn et al. 2008; Taira et al. 2003).
Deep brain stimulation was approved for psychiatric use (severe, untreatable
obsessive-compulsive disorder) in 2009 in both the United States and Europe.
We can expect that it will be tried in a variety of mental illnesses and, perhaps,
even self-injuring behaviors.

Repetitive magnetic stimulation noninvasively excites neurons in the brain
and there are some indications that it is helpful for depression and for auditory
hallucinations. It is not as precise as deep brain stimulation but with improved
technology it may be able to reach specific areas deep in the brain. There is an
outside chance that it may have a major impact on the treatment of mental illness
and NSSI.

Finally, I should mention a low-technology but promising therapy for people
who have BIID and seek limb amputation. The treatment, which uses only a mirror, evolved from dealing with people who have phantom limb pain. The theory
is that these patients often had preamputation cramping or clenching spasms
while their limb was immobilized in a sling or cast, often for months. Presumably, because it was impossible to move the immobilized limb, a sort of "learned
paralysis" became embedded in the patients' brain circuits and their body image
map was anatomically revised. After amputation, the brain's body image map
retained a paralyzed phantom limb complete with a memory of pain signals. A
mirror is placed in such a way that reflection of an intact limb creates the illusion
that it is a continuation of the amputated limb. Patients are then told to move
both limbs simultaneously. Amazingly, patients claim that they can feel the phantom limb move. By repeatedly doing this for a month, they feel the phantom limb
shrink and the painful sensations disappear. With people who have BIID, a mirror is used to create the illusion that the normal limb seems to be a continuation
of the affected limb. When this is done, in conjunction with injecting an anes-

thetic drug that blocks sensations in the affected limb, patients seem to lose the desire to have the limb amputated (Colapinto 2009). One theory about how all this works is that the brain contains a system of mirror neurons. By simply observing another person's actions, observers' mirror neurons become active as if they were performing the actions themselves. Through magnetic resonance imaging, it is thought that the mirror neuron system may exist in the inferior frontal cortex and the superior parietal lobe of the brain. Transcranial magnetic stimulation seems to enhance mirror neuron functioning. How all this new information about deep brain stimulation, transcranial magnetic stimulation, optical illusions, and the mirror neuron system plays out in regard to NSSI remain to be seen. It might open up entirely new types of treatment.

Psychological and Social Treatments

The literature, circa 1990, provided good advice and general principles for the treatment of self-injury. Tantam and Whittaker (1992), for example, proposed the following:

1. Making and maintaining a relationship: understanding, staying calm, reframing self-mutilation as an expression of feeling, avoiding threats or promises, sticking to limits, leaving the responsibility with the patient, sticking with the patient;
2. Breaking the habit: coping with withdrawal symptoms, increasing determination to change;
3. Maintaining change: rewards for new behavior, minimizing medicalization, resolving emotional conflicts, tackling coercion, training in intimacy.

The authors note that self-mutilation should be understood in the context of persistently disordered relationships "but do not consider that terming these a 'personality disorder' is particularly illuminating." They also warn against trying to save patients from themselves or from their families.

Hawton (1990) also considers principles of management:

1. Analyze the precipitating events, such as arguments or rejection. Identify thoughts ("I hate myself," "I am a failure," etc.), emotions (anger, low mood, tension), associated behaviors (seeking isolation and a cutting implement), factors that increase the likelihood of cutting (such as alcohol or isolation), and factors that delay or prevent cutting (such as contacting a friend or exercising). Note where the act of self-mutilation occurs, implement used,

extent and number of wounds, emotional state, and presence or absence of pain. Consider the goals of the act (e.g., to reduce tension or manipulate others) the benefits (e.g., tension reduction and a sense of well-being), and the negative consequences (e.g., disgust, guilt, scars, need to conceal cuts).

2. Gain control over cutting. Can precipitating events or aggravating factors (e.g., alcohol) be avoided? Emphasize factors that decrease the likelihood of self-mutilation. Initially focus on controlling the cutting through a change in thinking, ventilation of emotions, relaxation techniques (although they work better later in the treatment), physical exercise, physical contact with another person, and medications.

3. Once the cutting is controlled, examine the underlying problems. Focus on improving the patient's self-esteem and mood disturbances. Cognitive therapy is especially useful. The patient's communication problems may be helped by individual therapy, including role-playing and role reversal, group therapy, and assertiveness training. For this phase of treatment, at least six months may be required.

4. Inpatient treatment should be brief. A written contract with the patient and a clear policy about the treatment approach and restrictions should be known by all ward staff. Excessive restrictions are unhelpful "because the patient will often find a means of cutting in spite of them and they can become a major focus of dispute." If cutting occurs, it should be tended to with minimal fuss. If the cutting behavior spreads to other patients, discuss this at a ward community meeting; sometimes a patient (or two) central to the epidemic may need to be transferred to another unit.

Self-injuring patients on inpatient units have most of their contacts with nursing staff. Pawlicki and Gaumer (1993) discuss nursing interventions. The nurse coordinator should collaborate with the patient in developing a plan of care, and the patient should be assigned a different "shift associate" for each work shift. The nursing staff should help patients use self-soothing techniques "such as listening to a relaxation tape, taking a warm bath, holding a teddy bear." The staff can also teach anger management skills such as writing in a journal, exercising, asking for medication, talking, using a safe place on the ward, or asking to be put in restraints. Patients should collaborate with the nursing staff in identifying high-risk times for NSSI, early warning signs, and precipitating events. A plan is then developed, written down, and posted by patients in their rooms. The plan lists methods for helping patients to feel in control and to avoid self-harm and includes increasing involvement with others, physical activity such as vigorous walking, self-soothing activities, and the processing of feelings by talking or by writing in a journal. *Short-term* contracts should be developed (e.g., the patient agrees not to self-injure while taking a shower). "Longer term contracts are usually unrealistic for the patient and reflect wishful thinking by the staff." Patients should be taught how to care for their own wounds. Nursing staff should also constantly monitor patients' suicide potential. Providing "an atmosphere for appropriate ventilation of staff feelings is essential because it allows for validation and explanation of nurse-patient dynamics."

It is important to note that all the therapies that I discuss in the following sections do not preclude the use of psychotropic medications. In addition, while the therapies implicitly address various types of positive and negative reinforcements, a full consideration of the four function model can help to focus treatment.

Psychodynamic Therapy

Individual psychodynamic psychotherapy is probably the most used long-term outpatient treatment for NSSI, although the number of therapists trained in this approach is decreasing. Expressive (insight-oriented) therapy is the form most written about. To illustrate what may transpire during the course of intensive psychotherapy with habitual self-injurers and which issues may need to be dealt with and interpreted, several cases will be presented.

The first published psychoanalytic study of a self-injurer dealt with a 23-year-old woman (Emerson 1933). As a child she was frightened of her cruel father. At age 8, she was seen trampling her father's garden by her uncle. He threatened to report her unless she agreed to his sexual advances, and for five years she allowed him to masturbate her. At age 13, her periods began but were irregular, and she thought they caused her headaches.

Her headaches persisted. At age 20, while she had a severe headache, a cousin sexually assaulted her. In the scuffle she accidentally cut herself with a knife and noticed that her headache vanished. She said, "After I had let blood my headache went away, and I thought that the cutting of my wrist, and letting the blood flow had cured it." From that time on, she cut herself to relieve headaches.

She wanted to have a baby but, because of her shameful childhood experiences, she thought marriage an impossibility. In a moment of agony over this conflict, she cut her breast with a razor, thinking that her breasts were useless if she could not have a baby. "My head began to ache. I could not stand it. I thought a moment, then I cut over the left breast as deeply as the razor would go in, and I laughed." She decided to have a child out of wedlock but was unable to become pregnant. Later a suitor wished to marry her. She felt it necessary to reveal her past to him. He rejected her angrily and called her a whore, whereupon she carved the letter *W* on her leg with a razor. Eight months later, she gashed her vagina with a knife, feeling that if she would only menstruate, she would be all right. She continued to cut herself at various times. "The feeling I always had whether I had a headache or not was: What does it matter? Nobody cares enough to stop you. Of course there were people who did help me."

Emerson interpreted the cutting and its pain as a symbolic substitute for masturbation. When her uncle first masturbated her she experienced pain, and then the pain and sexual stimulation became intimately related. The pain also was a form of self-punishment for her acquiescence in her misdeeds. Her cutting, too, symbolized menstruation and her desire to be like other little girls. Emerson thought that because cutting is a masculine, aggressive act, "her sadistic impulses, probably strongly inherited from her father, got satisfaction while she satisfied her masochistic inclinations, inherited from her mother." In treatment, "she analyzed her own complexes and thereby gained much self-control. And most important of all, opportunity for sublimation was obtained for the patient and she was given a chance." When the article was written, the patient had not mutilated herself for fourteen months.

Crabtree (1967) provided an account of his successful therapy with a 16-year-old habitual self-injurer named Jane. Her mother was a cold, logical, dominant woman who had "tremendous underlying destructive urges toward Jane." She displayed affection only when Jane was ill or terrified because of recurrent nightmares and fears of death.

At age 13, Jane became infatuated with a male schoolteacher and began to scratch her arms, neck, and face with pins. She confessed her behavior to him. "At first he seemed very understanding but then became angry and I did it all the more. I don't know why but this scratching had something to do with my feelings about him." Because of this behavior she was hospitalized for over a year. Intensive individual psychotherapy, group therapy, and medications failed to control her self-injury. She deeply cut on her arms, broke windows, attacked other patients, eloped from the hospital, took an overdose of aspirin, and swallowed a needle. Her symptoms were worse during menstruation. After six months in a school for the mentally ill she was rehospitalized and began twenty months of psychotherapy.

Crabtree noticed that focusing on feelings and fantasies served to stimulate her and to aggravate her inclination to cut herself. "Jane was no longer cutting herself simply in response to an array of external events. She was now cutting herself in relation to me, a fact both disquieting and exasperating."

Although Jane's unabated self-injury gained her close physical contact with staff, Crabtree maintained his distance. He told her that she was responsible for her behavior and for its consequences. He urged her to experiment with alternative solutions, for example, to take warm milk instead of medications. He encouraged the staff to follow his lead by becoming "more spontaneously and directly expressive of the actual feelings aroused by her—especially angry ones." He insisted that she handle her feelings in a non-destructive way. She then stopped her cutting, as she realized that while it once forced people to react to her with feeling, it now caused people pain and pushed them away. For Crabtree, the turning point in therapy was his communication to Jane of his genuine experience of their relationship and of his feelings of being torn apart by her self-injury. As caveats for the treatment of self-injurers, he warned against an initial introspective approach with a focus on fantasy and feelings because this fostered regression and might lead to increased self-injury. He also warned against becoming too nurturant or "maternal" because this might also increase the patient's need for self-punishment.

Another report of successful intensive psychotherapy with a borderline, habitual self-injurer was the case of a 23-year-old woman named Gloria (Kwawer 1980). She was seen four times weekly in a residential hospital, and during an eighteen-month period she cut herself with broken glass, razor blades, pins, and knives.

Her cutting often occurred when she feared being abandoned—for example, when her therapist was on vacation. She became preoccupied with her blood and even saved it, "allowing it to drip into a small receptacle which was kept hidden in her closet and treasured especially during stressful times when it had a calming effect." She regarded her menstruation as particularly loathsome and disgusting. Her feelings of powerlessness were intense, and she had frequent fantasies of tying strings on her therapist and pulling on them like a puppet. She attempted to "blackmail" the staff and therapist, threatening that her blood would be shed on their behalf. She tried to polarize the staff by sharing "secrets" with certain people and then pledging them to secrecy.

Self-injury was constantly presented to her as a symptom of underlying problems. When she complained of night terrors and begged for drugs to dull her senses, she was offered people instead. She was encouraged to use the nursing staff to assist her during difficult times and to use psychotherapy "to continue self-exploration." Boundaries were reinforced and firm limits set to provide her with consistent and predictable reality experiences. Her conflicts over her relationship with her psychotic mother, her fears of separation and individuation, and her faulty perception of sexuality and of womanhood were explored and resolved. Therapy consisted of factual sex education in addition to exploration of her fantasies about homosexuality, prostitution, and masturbation. As Gloria improved she became more actively involved in the ward community, learned to drive, secured a part-time job, and planned to live outside of the hospital.

Michael Stone (1987) is a psychoanalyst who has done much work with patients who have borderline personality disorder. He notes that when self-injury is mostly related to traumatic loss, such as a death of a parent, therapy "should consist of partial compensation of the loss through the human relationship with the therapist." This long-term process with several sessions weekly "will diminish the need for symbolic replay of the trauma and fantasied revival of the dead" through self-injury. A different situation occurs when the patient has been abused by a sadistic parent or sibling. The capacity for trust is demolished, and supposedly helpful persons (including the therapist) are seen as malicious and dangerous. It may take years for the therapist "to establish his or her basic innocence, let alone helpfulness." The next step is "to enable the patient to believe in the possibility of tenderness" in a love partner. The final task is "helping the patient develop new habits of sexual excitement (ones less chaotic and violent; more able to fit in with the patterns of more ordinary and less harmful partners)."

Nelson and Grunebaum's (1971) follow-up study of ten patients found that improvement was associated with increased verbal capacity to express angry, sad, or anxious feelings during a long-term relationship with an accepting therapist. "Insight into the genesis of slashing behavior was not helpful." Psychodynamically oriented supportive therapy does not emphasize insightful interpretations of transference or of unconscious conflicts. It is more widely used than expressive (insight-oriented) therapy. Rockland (1987) notes the supportive techniques used in treating self-injurers; maintaining a positive rapport and therapeutic alliance with the patient; providing education, reassurance, an attitude of hopefulness, encouragement, and praise; giving suggestions and advice; clarifying and, when appropriate, confronting; setting limits and prohibitions; emphasizing the patient's strengths and talents; intervening in the patient's environment; encouraging sublimations; using medications and somatic treatments liberally; helping patients develop a more objective view of their life situation. In this approach the therapist is "real" (rather than a neutral blank screen), offers advice while encouraging patients to make their own decisions, and accentuates the positive.

Cognitive Behavioral Therapy

Cognitive behavioral therapy (CBT) has replaced dynamic psychotherapy as the treatment of choice for many patients who have depression and/or anxiety. It is less expensive because it requires fewer visits and is highly focused on targeted behaviors. There is good literature attesting to its efficacy in suicide prevention which, by extrapolation, may apply to NSSI. Although there are few studies about CBT and NSSI, many therapists use CBT techniques without realizing it, often in an informal but effective way. Newman's chapter (2009) on cognitive therapy for NSSI contains relevant references. He points out that CBT targets and attempts to modify the maladaptive automatic thoughts and core beliefs of self-injurers and also teaches them "alternative, more adaptive ways to cope with emotional distress, to use positive self-instruction to delay acting on urges to self-harm, to think about themselves and their relationship with their bodies in ways that are not conducive to NSSI, and to be more hopeful and self-efficacious." He also warns about some faulty assumptions that therapists may hold e.g., patients who seek help are totally committed to stopping their NSSI, patients will always report their acts of NSSI and their self-disclosure will be accurate, and NSSI is merely a way of getting attention and exerting control over others. This last assumption usually arises when therapists feel frustrated and manipulated.

A noncomplicated and useful explanation of cognitive therapy for NSSI is Walsh's *Treating Self-Injury* (2006). Among the most common maladaptive thoughts (cognitions) about self-injury are: It is acceptable because it always provides quick relief; it doesn't hurt anybody but me; It's my friend; It's my way of communicating what I feel inside; I deserve to be punished; I'm unlovable, a bad person, and a loser in life; It keeps people away; My body is my enemy; I'm ugly and my body is disgusting; I can't stop cutting myself; I'm addicted to cutting; It's what keeps me from killing myself.

Therapy consists of challenging these maladaptive thoughts, modifying them, and presenting adaptive behaviors to replace NSSI. Patients are taught to speak about rather than indulge in NSSI, to communicate feelings, and to think about a lifestyle without NSSI. They need to understand that NSSI is unacceptable and that they should respect their bodies. They need to learn how to manage relationships constructively, not always to anticipate failure, and to find ways to elevate their self-esteem and to improve their body image. There are techniques for

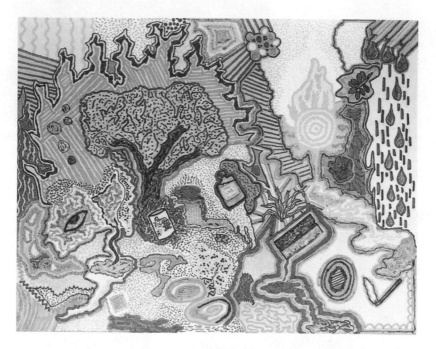

a

The drawing above and on pages 261 and 262 were made by a 21-year-old female patient during six months of intensive psychotherapy. When treatment began, she was cutting or burning her arms, chest, abdomen, and legs several times a week. Previous therapists had diagnosed her as having a variety of mental disorders, including manic-depressive psychosis and borderline personality disorder. In reality, her illness was hysterical in nature and was dominated by unresolved oedipal conflicts. (a) The histrionic (hysterical) nature of her illness is evident in her colorful and crowded drawings during this period. Depicted in this drawing are her cutting paraphernalia (razor, salt solution, gauze, trash can with Mickey Mouse on it for collecting her blood) and frightening figures, present in her mind since childhood, who urged her to harm herself. (b) After three months, the patient depicted herself as a wooden figure held together by stitches. She is tortured, trapped, and devoured by monsters representing her family members. (c) A week later, she vented her anger graphically by chopping up the monsters while Mickey Mouse laughed at them. (d) Shortly afterward, she portrayed herself as an innocent, sexless child surrounded by confusion. She is trying to see herself as a real person, different from the monsters and hopeful about the future. (e) After six months of therapy, she drew her "mixed-up" family (the Scrabble tiles). She is a pawn and a frightened cat in a game dominated by her parents. She is the Joker, caught between her father, the King of Hearts, and her mother, the Queen of Clubs.

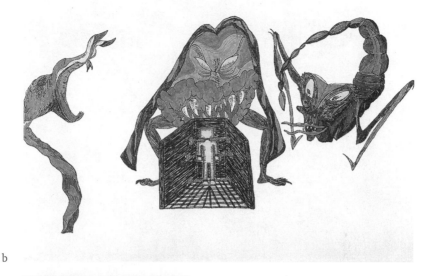

b

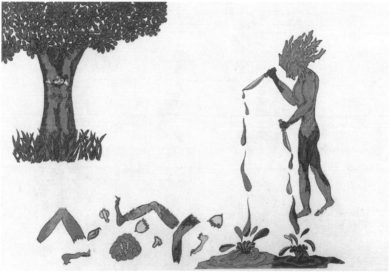

c

accomplishing all these things that involve much hard intellectual work by patients, written assignments, and experience trial runs that incrementally lead from fear of change to a desire for a harm-free life. Although cognitive therapists do not talk about it much, there are times when their trusting and caring relationship with a patient adds to, and may often even trump, all the formal techniques.

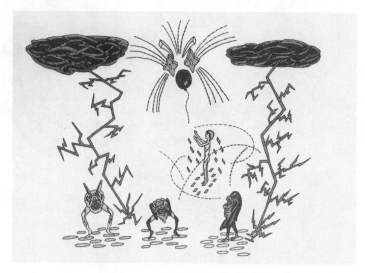

d

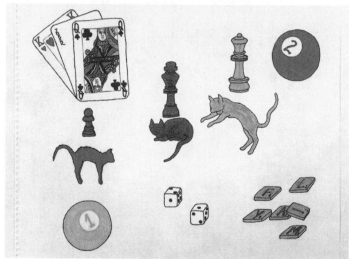

e

Dialectical Behavior Therapy

Therapists who practice dialectical behavior therapy (DBT) correctly are not at all like psychoanalysts but each goes through intensive training, reveres seminal texts or manuals, uses a distinctive language, and has a need for continuing supervision/consultation. DTB, founded by the psychologist Marsha Linehan, has grown enormously in the two decades since its inception but it still is available only in the larger cities. It requires a team to experience its full effect but individual therapists are now using DBT principles. The most concise, albeit technical, summary of DBT for NSSI is Lynch and Cozza's well-referenced chapter (2009). It explains DTB's roots in behavioralism, dialectical philosophy, and Zen Buddhism. From behavioralism, DBT uses established concepts such as conditioning and reinforcement that maintain NSSI, but with the added twist that changing self-injurious behaviors involves acceptance of what is and validation of patients' attempts to change. From dialectical philosophy, DBT examines the reasons for and contradictions contained in self-injurious behaviors (e.g., it may provide brief relief from troublesome thoughts and emotions, but they also have negative consequences such as medical and social morbidity); the goal is to synthesize these opposing forces into a more functional and healthier new way of life. This new way is akin to the "middle path" espoused by Buddhism; it is a path of moderation from the extremes of self-indulgence and self-mortification in which persons are obliged to investigate and analyze a problem in an unbiased way, to attempt to understand the truth, and to lead their lives based on a reasonable conclusion.

DBT is highly organized with manuals on just about everything, and all patients participate in both individual and group sessions. It demands a great deal of time, and real devotion and commitment by patients. The reduction or elimination of NSSI is the highest priority of DBT but this is coupled with learning better skills for leading a better life. A great deal of attention is devoted to identifying situations and cues associated with urges to self-injure (being alone during certain times of the day, razor blades or box cutters in plain view, specific social situations, etc.) and then taking steps to minimize being in those situations and to deal with and avoid cues. In DTB, biological vulnerabilities to self-harm urges are addressed by emphasizing healthy activities such as having proper nutrition, adequate sleep, physical exercise, avoidance of street drugs, and being compliant with treatments for medical illness. When emotional arousal becomes problematic patients are taught to dampen their nervous system through the dive reflex (holding one's breath and placing one's face in a container of cold water), through muscle relaxation exercises and engaging in periods of "mindfulness." The latter is a widely used practice in which persons quietly "observe" what thoughts and feelings they are experiencing without making judgments or responding to them. When done enough times, people come to realize thoughts or feelings related to self-harm are fleeting and do not have to be acted on. In DBT, persons who do commit an act of self-harm pay the painful price of reporting, in exquisite detail, all the chain of events regarding their act to their therapist and their group so it can be analyzed, over and over again. One patient described it to me as "like Chinese water torture!" The reason for this approach (beyond the fact that some patients may avoid NSSI rather than endure the tiresome process of analysis and reanalysis) is that by fully understanding the sequence of events associated with their NSSI, patients will become aware of the pattern that is being set into motion, and then will apply all the helpful techniques and skills that they have learned so as to stop the sequence from progressing. Because "soothing" patients after an act of NSSI has negative consequences (the behavior is reinforced and even amplified so the patients seek even more soothing), DBT has a rule that patients must wait twenty-four hours before contacting their therapist.

I have not done full justice to a complete explanation of DBT. It remains the only therapy that has been proven effective for NSSI when it is done properly. It remains to be seen if attenuated adaptations of the full procedure will also be effective.

The S.A.F.E. Alternative

S.A.F.E. is an acronym for self-abuse finally ends. It was coined by Karen Conterio, a therapist who, through her many media appearances over the past three decades, has been the single strongest advocate for raising public consciousness about the plight of self-injurers (Favazza and Conterio 1988). She, along with the psychologist Wendy Lader, ran the first and most successful inpatient program for self-injurers for many years, and has now switched her attention to outpatient programs such as S.A.F.E. Expressions (for adolescents), S.A.F.E. Focus (groups run by self-injurers and a therapist), S.A.F.E. Choice (adult individual therapy), and S.A.F.E. Alternatives (widely used manuals for school professionals and workbooks for student self-injurers).

The S.A.F.E. philosophy about self-injury and treatment approaches uses both psychodynamic and CBT principles but mainly derives from extensive and intensive clinical experience. It is a no-nonsense, highly practical, tough but caring, and efficacious but non-academic approach. My confidence in its efficacy is based on my personal observations rather than on published reports, although preliminary results of a self-report study of 123 patients that completed S.A.F.E. residential treatment program indicate a highly significant decrease in self-injurious behavior at three- and twelve-month follow-ups.

The book *Bodily Harm* (Conterio and Lader 1998) explains the S.A.F.E. philosophy and treatment in detail. Basically, self-injurers are not viewed as victims and their behavior is not considered an addiction. Patients should not enter therapy unless they have a strong, heartfelt desire to stop self-injuring, and must accept personal responsibility for keeping themselves safe. They can expect attention for *not* injuring themselves and they will be discouraged from displaying their scars (this avoids contests to see who can produce the biggest ones) or describing the mechanics of their self-injury (this eliminates shock value). They must refer to their behavior as "self-injury" rather than "cutting" or "burning" so that they do not substitute a description of the behavior for the behavior itself. Similarly, they should refer to themselves as "self-injurers" rather than "cutters" or "burners." They must learn to tolerate their mood swings, learn to verbalize their thoughts and feelings, and realize that every thought or emotion does not need to have a physical response. They must develop capacities to slow down, to delay acting on urges, to think, reflect, and problem solve. Unlike the Twelve Step recovery model, the S.A.F.E. model emphasizes that self-injurers are not powerless, that they can be cured of self-injury forever, and that relentlessly sharing stories about their self-injury may not be inspirational but rather may prevent them from moving forward.

These things can be accomplished in therapy by using the S.A.F.E. "toolbox." It starts with a realistic, written, no-harm *contract*, or *treatment participation agreement*, developed by the patient collaborating with the therapist. This document can contain such items as agreements not to self-injure for twenty-four hours before the session, to regularly attend sessions on time, to complete all written therapy assignments, etc. The second tool is the use of an *Impulse Control Log* that requires patients to briefly write down the following: time, date, location, situation and feelings, and thoughts when experiencing an urge to self-harm (even if no act of self-harm occurs). Additionally, they should write down what their self-harm would accomplish and what it would communicate. Finally, they should note what action they took and the outcome. The third tool is to *complete a list of at least five comforting activities or temporary distractions that are safe alternatives to self-injury* (e.g., writing in a journal, talking with a trusted person, just sitting and experiencing feelings, taking a walk, listening to music, working on an arts and crafts project, cooking a meal). Patients should use these alternative behaviors when they feel urges to self-harm. The final difficult and essential tool is *completing fifteen sequential writing assignments* for discussion in therapy. Because of their importance in S.A.F.E. therapy, I will list all the assignments.

1. Autobiography (in five to ten pages) from childhood to the present. "Writing a chronology of your life's events helps you synthesize them and place them in perspective. Putting difficult memories on paper can not only vent anger, but also lead to realizations or discoveries you may not have made before. Recalling happy times can give hope and solace and can lend promise of joy in the future."

2. How do I see myself? (e.g., emotionally, intellectually, behaviorally; roles you play in life; strengths and weaknesses).

3. The female most influential to me (e.g., What is significant about her? How has she influenced you positively and negatively? How does she react to your self-injury?).

4. The male most influential to me (see above).

5. The emotions surrounding self-injury (e.g., feelings and fantasies before, during, and after self-injury).

6. The anger inside me (e.g., What situations evoke your anger? What does it feel like to be angry? How can I handle my anger?).

7. What I can't stand about the people in my life.

8. Compensation for life's injuries (e.g., Identify the ways you have been hurt, abused, or victimized). What compensation would really make up for these injuries? What compensation that is actually available would make you feel at least a little repaid?

9. Nurturing myself (e.g., What gives you a lift and makes you feel good? hot baths? talking with friends? a massage?).

10. A time I was comfortable in someone else's presence (e.g., What factors make you feel comfortable with another person?).

11. The person I want to be (e.g., How do you want your life to be like, and what keeps you from achieving this goal?).

12. How do I feel about being a woman (for women): How do I feel about being a man (for men)?

13. Saying good-bye to self-injury (e.g., Imagine a life without self-injury. What will you miss about your old ways?).

14. What I have learned about myself through these assignments (e.g., What important, surprising, or unpleasant things have you learned about yourself?).

15. Future plans (e.g., List specific six-month goals. Describe where you see yourself in five years).

The voluminous information gathered from all these writing assignments is grist for the therapeutic mill, and elements from CBT, DBT, and psychodynamic therapy can be applied over the course of many sessions. This method allows for flexibility in treatment.

Behavioral Therapy

Straightforward behavioral therapy is mainly used for stereotypic self-injuries, especially those with developmental disabilities. In the old days punishment (more nicely labeled aversive therapy) was used (e.g., shocking patients with a cattle prod whenever they self-injured). Positive reinforcement in its various guises (e.g., paying attention to patients when they do not self-injure but withholding attention when they do, or rewarding patients with attention and/or objects that they desire when they do not self-injure for a specified period of time) remains the mainstay of treatments that can be refined after performing a functional or behavior assessment as described earlier. Mechanical devices, such as goggles for patients who gouge their eyes, can be used as a form of sensory extinction. Usually several behavioral techniques are used simultaneously. For a detailed and well-referenced description of behavioral therapy in stereotypic self-injury, see Luiselli (2009). In my experience, medications seem to enhance behavioral treatments.

It's not fashionable to write case reports nowadays, so it is worth describing a 1973 case of a 20-year-old man who had schizophrenia and a sixteen-month history of severe eye poking and a six-month history of lip and tongue biting (Cautela and Baron 1973). He had received inpatient psychiatric treatment, electroconvulsive therapy, multiple medications, and psychotherapy with no improvement. At one point, his eyes were sewn shut to prevent further damage, and he was kept in restraints almost constantly. By the time he entered into a behavioral treatment program, he was completely blind, and his mouth opening was reduced in size because of the buildup of scar tissue from constant biting.

In the first phase of treatment, both the patient and the hospital staff were told that his self-mutilative behavior was a learned habit that he needed to unlearn. Because this behavior was preceded by restlessness and by an urgent thought or feeling that he must injure himself, he was taught how to relax whenever he felt tense or had an urge to self-injure. He also was instructed in "thought-stopping," that is, he consciously forced himself to resist the thought of self-mutilation. He was instructed also to imagine a sequence of events leading to lip biting; when he clearly imagined having an "urge" to bite, he then imagined feeling sick to his stomach. Covert reinforcement was used to promote periods of feeling calm and relaxed. He made a therapeutic contract to practice these techniques. If he did them as assigned and did not injure himself for two months, then he would be evaluated for surgical repair of his lips. Because the patient was afraid of social contacts with new people, systematic desensitization was used to eliminate this fear. When he yelled for help to keep from biting, he was quietly escorted to his room and encouraged to use self-control techniques. This phase of treatment lasted two and a half months, during which both threatened and actual self-mutilative behavior continued at a high rate.

The second phase of treatment, lasting five months, emphasized more practice in self-control techniques, especially in regard to "convulsive-like" behaviors that preceded and accompanied his self-injury. The patient underwent behavioral rehearsals to handle social problems better and reinforcement sampling to strengthen behaviors incompatible with self-mutilation. Staff paid extra attention to him when his behavior was appropriate and when he carried out his ward jobs. In this phase no new injuries to his eyes or mouth occurred, the number of convulsive-like episodes decreased, and the patient experienced only occasional "urges" to harm himself.

During phase three, lasting three months, all destructive or disruptive behavior ceased. Treatment consisted of elimination of maladaptive thoughts, continued reinforcement sampling, and corrective plastic surgery. The patient was discharged from the hospital, completed a vocational rehabilitation program, entered college, and married. He seemed happy and enthusiastic about the future and no longer mutilated himself during a two-and-a-half-year follow-up period.

Not all cases turn out so well. Romanczyk and Goren (1975) reported their attempts to treat a 6-year-old child who had mental retardation and autism. In various social contexts and in response to any stimulus, the child would scratch himself, slap his face, or bang his head at a rate of 5,400 times an hour (this remarkable head-banging case was noted in chapter 9). The major treatment approach was punishment with an apparatus that delivered an electric shock. However, other techniques such as time out, shaping, and reinforcement were needed to modify the child's problematic screaming, fear of loud noises, and inability to feed himself. While his self-mutilative behaviors were suppressed briefly in the controlled hospital environment, they could not be controlled in any other setting. After more than one thousand therapy hours over a ten-month period, the child was placed permanently in an institution. He had improved somewhat, however, and at last count indulged in self-injurious behavior "only" five to fifteen times per hour.

Administrative Therapy

Changes in policy on inpatient units and in correctional and psychiatric facilities can reduce high rates of NSSI. A locked adolescent inpatient unit, for example, had a high incidence of NSSI, patient elopements, and disruptive behaviors. Crabtree and Grossman (1974) associated the locked doors with "the breeding of institutional mistrust, the development of staff mistrust and rigidity, and the promotion of regressive behaviors," although they provided some measure of containment, safety, and security in dealing with acutely psychotic, suicidal, and impulsive patients. After numerous preparatory meetings among staff and patients, the unit's doors were unlocked. The results were astounding. In the first month there was a 94 percent decrease in NSSI, as well as a 73 percent decrease in elopements and a 69 percent decrease in disruptive incidents. Over the course of a year, the decrease in NSSI episodes was 67 percent. Additionally, these episodes were fairly well separated and there were far fewer "epidemics" of NSSI. Also see Offer and Barglow's account (1960) of how NSSI was reduced on a general hospital ward by changing some hospital policies.

The most detailed report dealing with administrative therapy is a "carving study" at a Canadian correctional facility for girls. Of the 136 girls in the institution, 86 percent had carved their bodies. The administration, unable to cope with the situation with traditional remedies such as solitary confinement, medications, lectures, threats, counseling, and increased recreational activities, brought in Ross and McKay (1979). They tried intensive psychotherapy but noted that this approach increased carving among the girls tenfold. Then they tried various behavior modification programs. In a token economy program, the girls earned poker chips for good behavior and could purchase goods and privileges with the chips. In addition, staff responded to the carving in a matter-of-fact way. This approach failed, so a new factor was added: "Girls in the token economy were provided with specific training in reinforcement therapy principles and encouraged to utilize these principles in attempting to modify the behavior of their peers." In this new program, 66 percent of the girls in the program still carved themselves.

What finally worked was a strategy of co-opting in which they reassured the girls that they had some mastery over their fate. Co-opting involved persuading the girls that their carving played into the hands of institutional personnel whose control they opposed (i.e., the carving made life exciting and interesting for the staff). Ross and McKay convinced the girls "that they could better proclaim their autonomy by refusing to carve." The girls were converted from research subjects to research assistants; the most influential girls became paraprofessional therapists and, finally, program directors for a cadre of girls. Immediately after girls were proclaimed "therapists," their adjustment to the institution improved markedly. In using this approach on one troublesome girl, her pathology was relabeled by referring to "her manipulativeness as social skill, her unreliability as flexibility, her domineering as leadership, her histrionics as creativity, her callousness as pragmatism, her suspiciousness as insight." She became a "therapist" and convinced her friends into working for her. She trained them in simple behavioral techniques for use not only with girls but also with staff whose behavior was thought to be in need of modification. Throughout the co-opting program not one incident of carving occurred among the girls who acted as therapists.

After five months, however, the co-opting program was stopped. Ross and McKay attributed this to disgruntled staff and noted that "perhaps acceptance of our recommendations meant rejecting traditional roles, accepting reduced authority and responsibility, and living with lessened status. Implied by our comments was the conclusion that clinicians were not needed." The old programs of individual and group psychotherapy and behavior modification were reinstituted along with some new programs. According to Ross and McKay, however, "there also followed a resurgence of carving. We should have co-opted our colleagues."

The Internet

Just about all self-injurers as well as a large number of their families and friends nowadays use the Internet to find information about self-harm and to exchange messages or to "chat" with other self-injurers for support. It's anonymous, free, and easy. It can be accessed from the privacy of one's home. Unfortunately, there is so much information available that it is difficult to separate the wheat from the chaff. I typed "self-harm" into the Google search engine. I got 9.3 million hits! I cannot say that I have reviewed each one (my lifespan is limited), but I can recommend the following sites. My approval is based on the quality of the information they provide and, if they are interactive, the quality of the rules for posting information, and of the oversight of what self-injurers report, and of the links provided (e.g., local help, emergency hot-lines, other websites). Two of the sites that I recommend are based in England.

My favorite sites are "secret shame," www.palace.net/~llama/selfinjury/, and self-injury.org. Deb Martinson, longtime champion for the cause of self-injurers and author of the "Bill of Rights for People Who Self-harm," is a central figure behind these sites. They provide an amazing amount of useful information about self-harm and its treatment both for self-injurers and their families. "Secret shame" has a BUS (Bodies under Siege) chat room and message board that is tightly monitored and also will e-mail a daily digest. Self-injury.org is a clearinghouse for information about self-harm.

Lifesigns.org.uk and siari.co.uk are excellent British sites. Both offer a lot of good information and closely moderated message boards. Lifesigns has a free newsletter and good fact sheets for parents, guardians, friends, teachers, males, school personnel, and others. It even has a section for healthcare professionals with its own message board, specific resources, and articles. Siari (self-injury and related issues) is run by Jan Sutton, an experienced counselor who has written much about self-harm. Along with the usual solid information and a moderated message board, this lively site also offers a constantly updated section on media reports about self-harm from 2002 to the present.

Selfinjury.com, a site for the S.A.F.E. alternatives program which I previously discussed, is run by Karen Conterio and Wendy Lader. Their hotline number is 800-DONTCUT. It is a catchy number and has helped thousands of self-injurers over the years. The entire S.A.F.E. organization is responsive to personal messages. Selfinjuryfoundation.org is a site that provides up-to-date information and resources on self-injury as well as news about the Self-Injury Foundation that provides funding "for research, advocacy support and education for self-injurers, their loved ones and the professionals who work with them."

If you stick with the sites that I have recommended, you won't go wrong. They contain most everything you need from the Internet. *However, be advised that the Internet is a place to begin and does not replace face-to-face professional therapy.* The human touch is needed for adequate evaluation and treatment.

It is with some trepidation that I list bmezine.com, which is the major Web site among the more than 27 million (!) listed in a Google search under body modification. Among its goals are "to let people know that they are not alone and to help them understand who they are and what they are going through," and "to educate the public about body modification and manipulation for the purposes of safety, history, culture, and good will." The site states that BME "has documented (and experienced) the positive effect that body modification has had on the lives of many young people and will continue to do what it can to protect and embrace their right to modify their bodies as they see fit in a positive and affirming fashion." In fairness, the site posts warnings that it contains documentation of dangerous and/or life threatening activities of sometimes questionable legality, and that attempts to replicate the acts that are described can result in serious injury and/or death. So much for goodwill! Although the site provides much good information and does post warnings, it *really* is extreme and many of its photographs and "how to" sections are beyond the pale and deeply troubling. I encourage self-injurers to avoid this site, although I am not naive enough to believe that many will heed my advice. There is nothing wrong with basic piercings or tattoos but the decidedly deviant material presented on this site in gruesome detail may trigger unhealthy behavior in vulnerable persons.

CHAPTER TWELVE

Personal Reflections

I identify myself professionally as a cultural psychiatrist. In practical terms, this means that I ply my clinical craft by using psychological, biological, and social principles but with an understanding that they all exist within the overarching web of culture. Culture is not a thing that a person has but rather is an ongoing and historical process, created by shared interpersonal experiences, that reverberates throughout a society and affects its institutions and the daily life of its members. Matter is neutral; molecules, energies, and behaviors are meaningless until they are personally interpreted, explained, and accepted as reality through the cultural process.

Self-injury as I define it (the direct, deliberate alteration or destruction of body tissue with no intent to die, including both acts individuals inflict on themselves and acts that individuals voluntarily accept when done to them by others in culturally sanctioned ways) is a cultural category based on universal biological events and culturally diverse bodily experiences that may be interpreted and acted on differently. Cutting open the skin, for example, is an act of self-injury that can be understood only by considering the time, place, and circumstances of its occurrence. My greatest revelation regarding self-injury is that it is a personally meaningful behavior that I, as a clinician and cultural observer, need to understand in order to help persons who are in need of gaining control of a pathological process (Favazza 1998). Self-injury is a behavior that deserves to be studied in its own right, not simply passed off as an epiphenomenon of mental illness. However, some instances defy a search for meaning, as is the case with some automatic stereotypic behaviors that are completely driven by an incessant biological imperative.

As a clinician, I thrive on the stories, the life narratives, that patients tell me. From these stories, I try to extract some understanding, a process much more gratifying to me than trying to impose meaning on addled neurotransmitters or short-circuited neural networks (although I am glad that there are psychiatrists whose lives revolve around biology). Even patients who cannot tell stories can, through their behavior, provide understanding for clinicians. I will never forget the burly African American man who was brought to my ward because he was growling and menacingly barking at people in the street. The staff and patients on the ward felt threatened by his behavior. When the psychiatric resident on duty presented the case to me, I asked why the patient was barking. The resident attributed the behavior to the patient's bipolar psychiatric illness. I asked the question again, only to receive the same reply. I then asked if the resident had seen other patients who had bipolar psychosis. He said that he had, whereupon I asked if any of them had ever barked. His response, of course, was no. So I told him to find out what the barking meant. He was perplexed until, on physical examination, he discovered a crude brand on the patient's arm. Luckily, a staff member recognized it as a mark made during initiation into a college fraternity. We contacted the president of the local branch of this fraternity, who came to see the patient. He told us that barking was a secret signal signifying that a fraternity member was in distress and needed help. The mystery was solved, the tension on the ward receded, and the patient was treated successfully.

There once was something pure, perhaps even naively noble, about psychiatry's focus on the ethereal mind. Nowadays, our thoughts turn to the magisterial brain. The body has never really been our thing. It bleeds when stuck. It excretes foul substances. It oozes puss when infected. It is prone to hideous malformations, hairy moles, crusty growths. We tend to ascribe a higher value, a greater purpose, to our "inner" life of thoughts and feelings and spirituality, but our "outer" life is more than just a shell or a vessel or a machine. A net of nervous tendrils enmesh the brain with the entire body. Typically, we believe that the mind-brain gives meaning to the body, but the relationship is reciprocal. In fact, the body must endure the insults of twisted thoughts, chaotic emotions, and demonic spirituality when the mind-brain sputters and writhes. The body must have its due and the wounded body its respect.

For decades, I have been a connoisseur of self-inflicted wounds, some pathological and some culturally sanctioned. Dennis Slattery (1993) wrote a book that examines all sorts of wounds—accidental, naturalistic, and self-inflicted— described in literary works. His premise is that "the wound is where something bruised or hidden splits open, breaches, and reveals a memory, a site of pain, of suffering and death, but it can also include a joyful sense of new freedom as well. . . . Our wounds, scars, and markings may be the loci of a place that put us in the most venerable and vulnerable contact with the world, with divinity, with one another, and with ourselves. As such, the body may invoke an entire cosmology; it is cosmic in its symbolic nature" (p. 16).

Just after being named by his grandfather, Odysseus was gored deeply on the thigh by a wild boar. Like a rite of passage that marks the end of innocence, receiving the boar's gore opened Odysseus to the world of animal appetites and set his destiny. After twenty years of adventure, plunder, and deceit (Dante placed him in hell), Odysseus matured and wove his way home to find a group of suitors lusting after his wife. So greatly had he changed that his identity was established only when an old maidservant recognized his scarred thigh as she washed him. The suitors called him a "wild pig," and then he killed them all.

The "wound" of Jean Jacques Rousseau, whose *Confessions* mark the first full modern literary expression of self-consciousness, was a congenitally malformed bladder. Rousseau's purpose in writing was to display a word portrait of himself that was in every way true to nature and to bare his secret soul and character. Although he exposed his own imperfections, he also exposed the imperfections of others. He was repelled by the imperfection of a beautiful prostitute when she removed her clothes: "I saw as clear as daylight that instead of the most charming creature I could possibly imagine I held in my arms some kind of monster rejected by nature, men, and love. I carried my stupidity so far as to speak to her about her malformed nipple." Embarrassed by this cruel honesty, the prostitute told him to forget women and to study mathematics instead. In truth, Rousseau was terrified of dying an agonizing death because of the gravel and stones in his bladder that polluted him. He had to catheterize himself often to open up his system and purify his body, just as his confessions purified his soul. Interestingly, Rousseau's attempts to cleanse himself of his waste occurred at the same time that the city of Paris was constructing its sewer system.

Patients have always been my best teachers. Years ago, just as I was about to throw away my psychoanalytic texts, along came a patient reared in the cornfields of Iowa who would have been at home in turn-of-the-century Vienna. Janet was a severe repetitive cutter and burner caught up in a clear-cut oedipal drama. Her father was a man with characterological as well as depressive problems. He and Janet had formed a strong alliance against the rest of the family. The special attention he devoted to her during childhood continued to the present; for example, during a hospital visit, he carved their initials in a wooden bench and kissed her. He convinced her that they had special magical powers and that their lives were mysteriously entwined. Her greatest fantasy was to run off with her father, care for him, and protect him against the cruel world.

The sexualized aspect of her love for father, however, created enormous conflicts for Janet that were central to her nonsuicidal self-injury (NSSI). She cut herself as a punishment for her incestuous guilt and for her hateful feelings toward her mother and sister. The hatred she had for the female aspects of her body resulted from the recognition that, had she been a boy, she would not have to endure so many tribulations. In fact, she regarded her vagina as a "disgusting wound" and believed that she really possessed a penis; supposedly, it was once external but was pushed inside of her when she had an accident while riding her brother's bicycle. During a session in which we were trying to understand why she seemed to enjoy rubbing the scar tissue of her cuts, she blushed and said, "It's because it is hard and gets red like a penis." She detested her menstrual periods, and sometimes she cut herself in the hope of diverting blood away from her vagina. To my surprise, she exclaimed that the cuts on her skin were like little vaginas and that she liked to have her cuts sewn closed just as she would like to have her vagina sewn closed. She felt particularly "proud" of her stitches and lavished great care over them. Her tender descriptions of how she kept the wound area clean, used powder, and applied fresh bandages sounded much like the words of a mother changing a baby's diaper. If my interpretation is correct, the cuts, representing a vagina, were "impregnated" by the sutures, representing her father's sperm, resulting in scar tissue, which represented a baby. Thus, a "simple" cut created a complex scenario. It created a symbolic vagina, which, she imagined, her father lusted after. Her guilt over incest was resolved by sewing shut her "vagina," rendering it inaccessible. But, with the formation of scar tissue, which symbolized a baby, she was able to fulfill her fantasy of bearing her father's child. As she matured, she decreased her NSSI and married a man who was the same age as her father and had the same first name. My diagnosis was that she suffered from histrionic personality disorder. However, when she moved to another state she was diagnosed with schizophrenia and thus was able to receive psychiatric disability payments.

The self-injury literature has paid practically no attention to scars. Aside from their physiological importance, they may hold special meanings. A scar obtained from doing something stupid can be a reminder not to do it again. Scars can exemplify how we feel deep inside. The great Mexican painter Frida Kahlo had polio and lived a painful life as a result of a trolley car accident in which her pelvis and spinal column were broken and her uterus perforated. She had thirty-five operations on her back and leg and was bedridden for months at a time. Her marriage was tumultuous and confused with many bisexual extramarital affairs. Her physical and emotional pain can be seen in many of her self-portraits, in which she showed herself as cut open with gaping wounds and huge scars. In some African tribes, ritual scars can signify social status, tribal membership, bravery in men, and potential fertility in women. In Austria, at the turn of the twentieth century, socially elite students engaged in fencing duels; the winner was the person who acquired a "bragging scar," which was thought to be a sexy and masculine sign of courage and a good education. When we see people who have scars, we usually can't help but wonder how they occurred. Web sites are even devoted to the "mysterious" scar on the neck of the actress Sharon Stone. The scars of self-injurers come in all shapes and sizes. Some are faint and delicate, while others are red and angry. Some are covered by clothing, while others are on display. It is an ominous sign when they appear on the face. When patients inquire about plastic surgery to remove or minimize these scars, it means that they feel that they are in control and no longer plan to cut themselves. In the Christian tradition, the flawless and unscarred female body was the ideal. Mary conceived and gave birth to Jesus but retained her status as an immaculate (unstained) virgin with an intact hymen. She also was Jesus's virgin bride and symbolized the glorious Church that was married to Jesus, "not having spot or wrinkle or any such thing, but that she should be holy and without blemish" (Ephesians 5:27). An exception was made for martyrs and saints who zealously mortified their bodies.

At the turn of the century, for reasons that I do not fully comprehend (self-analysis *is* difficult), I became fascinated with the Bible and spirituality, although I was reared in a secular Catholic home and have never been a believer or a churchgoer. In 2004 I published *PsychoBible: Behavior, Religion, and the Holy Book,* and, in 2009, the first chapter on spirituality to appear in a major psychiatric textbook. Perhaps, after dealing intensively with injured bodies for so long, I needed a respite. *PsychoBible* won an award from the Society for the Study of Psychiatry and Culture, and it gave me a deeper, fuller perspective on religion, spirituality, and, oddly enough, self-harm. Churches may take aim at being unblemished, but their role model is the bloodied Suffering Servant. At any rate, my intensive studies invigorated me to return to my first love, the study and care of self-injurers.

I came to realize that self-injury is a complicated act, the meanings of which cannot be inferred by simple observation of the behavior itself. The presence of sanctioned self-mutilative practices across latitudes, longitudes, and centuries reflects the dynamic process of social life. With each marriage, birth, and death, with each change of season, with the ascendancy of each pathogen, with each covetous glance, are sown the seeds of social disruption. Mutilative rituals acknowledge disruptions within the social body and provide a mechanism for the reestablishment of harmony and equilibrium. Through the spilling of blood and the removal of limbs, the garden of relationships among humans, god, and nature is watered, pruned, and cultivated. Through the myths and personal dramas of dismemberment and reassembly, of wounding and healing, are played out the eternal struggles between men and women, parents and children, friends and enemies, humankind and the environment, the world of the flesh and the world of the spirit.

The individual human body mirrors the collective social body, and each continually creates and sustains the other. Misperceptions of reality, feelings of guilt, negative self-images, antisocial acts, and all the other symptoms we associate with personal mental illness defy understanding without reference to the psychological, social, cultural, and physical integrity of the communal "body."

So I have come full circle. Self-injury cannot be understood and dealt with without recourse to psychology, biology, and culture. When dealing with patients, I recognize self-injury not only as a pathological behavior but also as an expression of a struggle to reenter a "normal" life and achieve a psychophysiological homeostasis (Favazza 2008). A cut in the skin may let out "bad blood" but also provides an opening to the interior. Everyday life is primarily a surface phenomenon, but the examined life—getting to the heart of things—involves the painful process of dissection. For most of us, dissection is a metaphor for intellectual examination, but for others it is a physical act. Intellectually can we not at least entertain the notion that extirpation of a "bad seed" might be accomplished as well by cutting its roots as by poisoning it with drugs or chanting psychomantras and interpretive insights? It is easy to forget that dripping blood may accompany birth as well as death. The scars of the process are more than the artless artifacts of a twisted mind. They signify an ongoing battle and that all is not lost. As befits one of nature's greatest triumphs, scar tissue is a magical substance, a physiological and psychological mortar that holds flesh and spirit together when a difficult world threatens to tear them apart. Self-injurers seek what we all seek: an ordered life, spiritual peace—and maybe even salvation—and a healthy mind in a healthy body. Their desperate methods are upsetting to those of us who try to achieve these goals in a more tranquil manner, but the methods rest firmly on the dimly perceived bedrock of the human experience.

I have said that I like stories, so I shall end this book with a great one. Many women who harm themselves seem to find some measure of relief by writing poems that are typically poignant, heartbreaking, visceral, and laced with bitter anger. Such poems derive from the horrific childhood physical and sexual betrayal and abuse that can be found in up to 60 percent of impulsive self-injurers. But what about the other 40 percent? What sort of stories do they have to tell?

Caroline Kettlewell, the author of *Skin Game* (1999), is part of that other 40 percent, and, to my knowledge, she is the first to present a detailed personal account of cutting herself in which abuse and anger are supplanted by reasoned insight. Her astute observations and brilliant writing style keep the blood from spattering the pages. In her case, it is easy to hate the cutting but admire the cutter.

Hers is the story of a bright girl who grew up in a Virginia boarding school for boys where her father taught. Her childhood was fairly normal; yet, she writes, "I needed to kill something in me, this awful feeling like worms tunneling along my nerves. So when I discovered the razor blade, cutting, if you'll believe me, was my gesture of hope. That first time, when I was twelve, was like some kind of miracle, a revelation. The blade slipped easily, painlessly through my skin. As swift and pure as a stroke of lightening, it wrought an absolute and pristine division between before and after. All the chaos, the sound and fury, the uncertainty and confusion and despair—all of it evaporated in an instant, and I was for the moment grounded, coherent, whole. Here is the irreducible self. I drew the line in the sand, marked my body as mine, its flesh and its blood under my command" (p. 57).

Her family moved to Charlottesville, and her cutting, hidden from everyone, continued. In the seventh grade, she "tried one night to cut deeper, torn between the anticipated thrill of a deep slash and the body's organic mindless resistance to such assault. . . . To cut with conviction. To wound for the feverish beauty of the wound itself. I wanted blood—not the refined bubble of sundered capillaries, but a frantic spill, something beyond caution, beyond control" (p. 100).

I shall not take you through the frightful years of her life: the repetitive cutting, the anorexia, the failed first marriage, the psychiatrists, the therapy. Rather, let us jump to about age 30, when she fell in love with a man of determined good cheer. She explained to him that her cutting, unlike alcohol or doing drugs, was not destructive. He replied that it was destructive because it hurt him. "I was surprised, taken aback, then, by the expectation implicit in his stubborn refusal just to let the matter slide—the expectation that true love obligated me to consider *his* feelings in the issue" (p. 167).

She married and finally came to grips with her longstanding depression. After treatment with an average dose of a selective serotonin reuptake inhibitor, the anxiety and unhappiness that had clouded and wasted the preceding two decades of her life were lifted. She stopped the medication, however, when she decided to have a child. "I went through my entire pregnancy feeling I was trying to pull off a sham, pretending to the part of the ethereal Madonna when I was wholly unqualified for the part. And yet, when my son was born into the waiting shelter of my arms it was as though the shape and structure of me had been made precisely to the purpose of fitting him. I was shocked by the fierce and immediate entanglement of this bond, that my son should become to me like a chamber of my heart" (p. 174).

She stopped cutting "only because I could afford to, because my need for it had apparently run its natural course. . . . No matter how compelling the urge, the act itself was always a choice. I had no power over the flood tide of emotions that drove me to that brink, but I had the power to decide whether or not to step over it. Eventually I decided not to" (p. 177).

I have met with many hundreds of self-injurers, and some have told me stories similar to Kettlewell's. That is why I can still honestly offer hope to individuals whose lives have been overtaken by deliberate self-harm. *Skin Game* is a memoir and not an autobiography, so there is much about the author that is not revealed. Yet it is a solid book and marvelous read. I, for one, am gratified that the author's pen was mightier than her razor. And I am cautiously optimistic that in some small way *Bodies under Siege* will embolden self-injurers and those who care for them, both personally and professionally, to repair what has gone awry in their lives.

Body Play

My Journey

FAKIR MUSAFAR

Starting Ripples

Nearly fifteen years have gone by since I wrote an epilogue for the second edition of *Bodies under Siege*. Since then, the culture has changed, attitudes have changed, mindsets have changed. I take great satisfaction knowing that my early experiments in body play have had an influence on these changes.

What I pioneered and experienced from 1944 to 1996 become ripples sweeping over a budding subculture. And what was a subculture phenomenon in 1996 has become a mainstream tsunami in 2011. These days, what was rare is now "in-your-face" throughout most of mainstream society. For example: visible tribal-inspired tattoos; men and women with fully tattooed sleeves; women with delicate tattoos on the nape of the neck, small of the back, ankles, and feet; small waists in tight corsets; men and women shamelessly in the public eye with nose rings and enlarged ear lobe piercings with tribal plugs, hooks, and spirals. Twenty years ago, one could see such modifications only in *National Geographic* or *Piercing Fans International Quarterly*.

The role of these body modifications has gone beyond mere style. Their psychological impact has become, for some, a means of psychic expression and healing. Recently I watched a PBS documentary on American soldiers just back from or being deployed for tours in Iraq and Afghanistan. They had lots of psychological turmoil and internal conflict to resolve, PTSD. Where did they go for relief? The local tattoo shop near Fort Hood, Texas. In that nonjudgmental environment they told their truth. Seen-it-all tattoo artists were safe father confessors, sympathetic listeners to disturbing gut-level feelings. The tattoos they chose reflected the inner hurts of a cruel and alien war.

From my early experiments in body play, I had gained a new understanding of my own "body-spirit" relationship. And I couldn't find an expression of what I

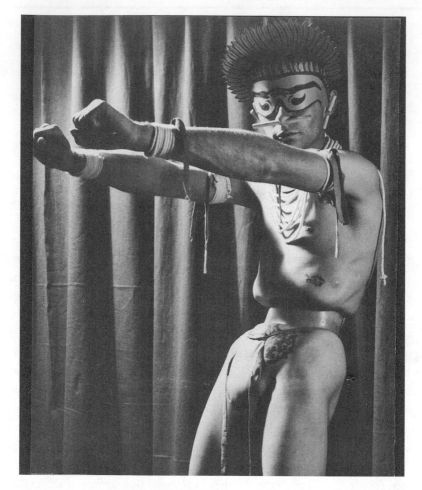

Fakir was inspired to modify his body by beauty ideals of natives on islands off the coast of New Guinea where small waists and well-spiked noses are the talk of the village. In this photo he has reduced his waist to twenty-two inches with a tight belt and pierced both nasal septum and ears with long spikes. (Photo courtesy of Fakir Musafar)

had learned anywhere else. By the 1950s I was so elated by what I had found that I felt compelled, out of altruism, to share with others. I wrote an article for John Willie's *Bizarre* magazine about my own physical emulation of the small-waisted boys of New Guinea. It was called "Is There an Ibitoe in the Crowd?" In the early 1940s and 1950s *Bizarre* magazine was an underground publication, published infrequently and sold only in the hundreds from under counters at smoke shops and offbeat book dealers. But it served as an outlet for mavericks, outcasts, and social nonconformists. In retrospect, it codified what has become the fetish fashion, BDSM and body modification phenomena of today.

Ibitoe is the name given to a boy of the Roro, Waima, and Elema tribes on islands off the coast of New Guinea. I first saw an image of an Ibitoe in *Compton's Pictured Encyclopedia* in my seventh-grade study hall. The sight almost stopped my heart. The caption read: "This Melanesian youth from one of the islands near New Guinea must be the talk of his village. For above all things, his people admire small waists and well-spiked noses." This was encouraged and socially sanctioned body modification.

However, I had to experience the esoteric mysteries of body modification mostly in private and underground for thirty years. Society was not ready to accept "body play" as a sane and potentially healing experience. I knew if I exposed myself I would probably be locked up and the key thrown away. Such was the state of psychological awareness in the 1930s, 1940s, and 1950s. So my teenage explorations continued in secret: self-applied tattoos, temporary and permanent piercings, branding, extreme waist reduction with belts, and prolonged dancing with weighted flesh hooks (which later became known as a "Ball Dance"). And in 1948, extreme self-bondage and sensory deprivation that led to a conscious out-of-body experience. Several years later, I wrote about this, my first transformative experience, in the first issue of *BodyPlay* magazine.

By the late 1950s and early 1960s, I had served two draft-induced years in the Army and moved from the vast inland plains of South Dakota to San Francisco. Now I was able to fulfill more sophisticated visions and find a few counterculture friends. First vision was evolvement of the wasp-waisted Ibitoe ideal. As a graduate of San Francisco State University with an M.A. in drama, I became a skilled costume designer with a solid background in fashion history. The Ibitoe in me found great possibilities for body modification in the revival of the hourglass corset. Unfortunately, none of the corset patterns of the hourglass period was suitable for modern figures, and no new patterns had been designed for some ninety years. My passion for the next few years then became the design of new patterns and techniques to make small waists on contemporary bodies, mine included.

I succeeded and soon founded the Hourglass Corset Company to serve like-minded devotees. In several years time (from 1958 to 1961), my handiwork spread through the small and exclusive world of corset fanciers. I advertised in "girlie" magazines of the day (the Internet was still thirty years away). Soon scores of body modifiers responded with corset orders and requests for more information. I devoted half of my day to corset construction. The other half was spent writing long letters on a portable typewriter. I made new friends like Will and Ethel

Granger, of England. Ethel had figure-trained since 1939 and achieved a 13-inch waist. She also had a pierced septum, pierced nostrils, pierced nipples, and tattooed lips. Meanwhile, I systematically reduced my own waist to 19 inches and pierced my nipples. Life was sweet, but the universe of body modifiers 1958 to 1961 was too limited and widespread to support me. I had to move on to other ventures until the ripples of desire for small waists had become more widespread.

The 1960s brought new adventures and new opportunities to expand a network of bodymod friends and supporters. I traveled to Japan, met Mr. Morishita, and found a culture with its own styles and fans of body modification, especially large all-body allegorical tattoos. In 1963 I met Davy Jones in Oakland, California. At last a tattoo artist who understood my desire to get the large blackwork tattoo I had envisioned since I was seventeen. For years prior, I had taken my visionary design to artists in Saint Louis, Kansas City, and Minneapolis. They had never been faced with a request for a large geometric and purely symbolic blackwork tattoo. The response I usually got was, "That's nice, sonny, but how about a panther on your shoulder?"

Davy had been a merchant seaman who spent time in western Samoa, where he had gotten the islanders' geometric "Flying Fox" tattoo on his thigh. He understood that tattoos are more than decoration. They are magic marks that impart certain changes in one's life. In 1963, over a three-month period, I got my magic mark from Davy Jones. He said he was honored to do this work. As far as I know, it was the first tattoo of its kind in Western culture. And with it came shamanic powers. Turns out a similar magic tattoo was recorded in a watercolor painting by Karl Bodmer in 1883. It was on a Yanktonai medicine man in eastern South Dakota, about 90 miles from where I was born. It represents fire coming up from the earth and denotes workers of fire energy. A few years later I met Leo Zulueto at Bob Roberts Spotlight Tattoo in Los Angeles. When he saw my tattoo, he said, "If you have the balls to get such big tribal blackwork, I'll get one too!" He did, and Leo continues to be a major champion of blackwork tattoos, which have become extremely popular.

In the next few years, Davy Jones turned out to be more than just an understanding tattooist. We became friends. I shared my body play desires with him. He, in turn, encouraged me and offered his assistance in the more complex body rituals to come. In 1961, by a strange twist of fate, Mr. Morishita guided me to a seller of rare books in the Kanda section of Tokyo. There I found and bought a treasure: a leatherbound original copy of George Catlin's 1867 Trubner & Co. London edition of *O-Kee-Pa: A Religious Ceremony and Other Customs of the Mandans, With Thirteen Illustrations*. How did this rare book get to Japan? Perhaps in

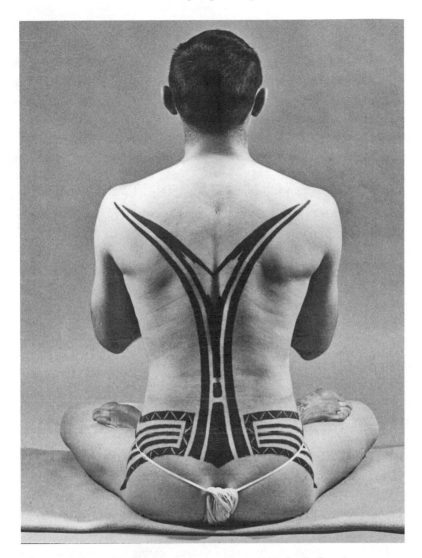

After many years of seeing this design in visions, Fakir finally found a sympathetic and understanding tattoo artist, Davy Jones, who gave him this "magic
mark" over a three-month period. The tattoo represents fire coming up from the
earth. (Photo courtesy of Fakir Musafar)

some 1800s diplomat or missionary's trunk? My heart raced at the sight of men
suspended by body piercings. What did this mean? The text documented what I
had long suspected. This was a deeply spiritual body ritual, initiation, and journey
to unseen worlds. In intent, it was similar to the more familiar Sioux Sun Dance
but with a physical and psychic guide called a Ka-See-Ka.

For the next few years I pleaded with Davy Jones to help me experience the O-Kee-Pa suspension ritual with two deep piercings in my chest, to be my Ka-See-Ka. In 1967 he finally relented. Because there were no pure-blood Mandan Indians or culture left (mostly lost to smallpox back in the 1830s), we had to improvise and recreate the ritual based primarily on Catlin's lengthy description. I fasted and prepared myself with other austerities for two days prior. At 6 a.m., with the sun just rising, I pierced two deep holes in my chest. We departed for an empty garage that was arranged to be similar to the lodge where Mandan initiation rituals were performed. I stood on a stool and Davy hooked my chest piercings to a rope in the ceiling. Inch by inch he lifted me up until I was standing on tiptoes. With about 80 percent of my weight on the piercings, the sensation was so intense I had to either give up or swing free suspended only by flesh. I took the gamble, stepped off my support, and let my entire weight hang on body piercings.

Within ten seconds, I zoomed out of my body and floated upward. No more pain. Only a warm, pleasant, floating sensation. I looked above and saw a blinding white light. It spoke to me: "Hello, I am you and you are me and I'm as close to God as you'll ever be." The light radiated unconditional love, a love I'd never felt before. I asked, "Do you always appear as a white light?" "No," was the reply, "I appear like you think I will appear." I wanted to go closer to the light, be consumed by its radiance. But I was told I couldn't come closer or be absorbed. That meant death of the physical body still hanging limp on body piercings below. I had a long telepathic conversation with the white light and it told me many things. I call this my second transformative experience.

Later that same year, 1967, I asked Davy Jones to again be my Ka-See-Ka for a Hindu body ritual: taking the Kavadi. When I first saw an image of Kavadi bearing in an old *National Geographic*, I was transfixed. Men were locked in portable cages with hundreds of long irons spears pierced into their chests and back. My emotions burned with the fire of that experience. A few years later I saw a scene of the Hindu Thaipusam Festival with Kavadi bearing in a 1945 documentary called *Dangerous Journey*. The scene was only three minutes long, but I sat through the whole movie three more times to relive the passion of that vicarious experience that flung a fourteen-year-old boy into a trance state right there in the Lyric Theater. Davy said he would put me in a Kavadi if I made one and signed a statement releasing him from liability in case I was injured.

We settled on 48 long spears. After an hour or so, the multiple hot sensation of many rods pierced into my body merged into one overall sensation of warmth and euphoria. I started to float and fly as I spun around and danced in a joyous

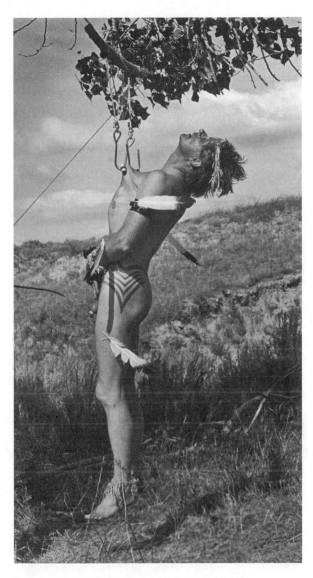

In the spirit and style of the Ogalala Sioux, Fakir is suspended by two deep chest piercings near Devil's Tower, Wyoming. He claims he leaves his body and zooms out into the cosmos during this twenty-minute body ritual. This Wyoming suspension was filmed for the documentary movie *Dances Sacred and Profane*. (Photo courtesy of Charles Gatewood and Fakir Musafar)

frenzy. The spears rattled in their sockets and thrust themselves deeper into my flesh. I lost all track of time. I was totally engulfed in flame, a ball of fire. My consciousness floated up into the rafters of the building. I watched my robot body trapped inside the Kavadi cage running around in crazy circles below. A friend of Davy shot pictures. I danced like this for two hours.

Spreading Ripples

A new phase of body play ripples started in the 1970s. I had sent small ripples through a few underground communities with extensive correspondence, circulation of photos, and a few articles in publications like *Bizarre* magazine. Now I longed to connect with a wider community and create even more ripples. I wanted to share my ecstatic discoveries. It started in 1972, when I first connected with a fetish group in southern California. These uninhibited folks were eager to try some of my body play practices: small waist training in corsets, bondage, body piercings, tattoos, and branding. On one of my visits, a strange and curious man showed up: Doug Malloy. He was intrigued by my stories and photos and wanted to know me better. We saw eye-to-eye on our respective feelings about body modification: the experience and potential transformations were of paramount importance; the visual and artistic ramifications were secondary. So I invited him to visit me in San Francisco. When he arrived, we talked for hours on end about our passions, but I still didn't know who he was until several weeks later, when my southern California friends told me he was a kinky multimillionaire.

Doug Malloy (a pseudonym) turned out to be a super patron of the body modification experience. He brought together everyone he could find who had a body piercing, large tattoo, or unusual body play practice. In my mind, Doug was the godfather of the contemporary body piercing movement. From 1972 to 1979 he went to great lengths to assemble a core group, which eventually developed all the techniques, tools, and styles of body piercing that are in common use today. He encouraged us to share our experiences at regular tattoo and piercing parties and jointly explore and develop modern ways to apply what we learned. Over a period of five years, what had been the secret passion of a few blossomed into an underground network. At first, we practiced our newly formed skills on each other and by individual appointments. Soon, demand forced us to hold private group piercing sessions in Los Angeles and San Francisco. By 1977, Doug's vision helped us open the first body piercing studio on Santa Monica Boulevard in Los Angeles. This was the first public door in the United States, Canada, and Europe that one could enter and get any kind of body piercing, from ears to genitals. This one-of-a-kind shop was called Gauntlet, was operated by Jim Ward, and for many years enjoyed a virtual monopoly on body piercing.

Word spread quickly about this unique shop. During those early summers when the traffic for body piercing was at its peak at the Gauntlet, I honed my craft by flying from San Francisco every weekend to pierce. In the beginning, only three of us could do all the piercings: Doug Malloy, Jim Ward, and me. Doug Malloy was always busy, so at first the shop was just Jim and me with a bench full of waiting piercees. We also started a publication called *Piercing Fans International*. I wrote extensively on my pet body play subjects, with lots of photos of my own adventures and those of the handful of friends whom I dubbed "modern primitives" in a 1978 issue. Our humble fan magazine soon developed a growing international circulation. Ripples were spreading.

More ripples spread from a 1977 public event. Doug Malloy arranged for Jim Ward and me to attend the First International Tattoo Convention, in Reno, Nevada. Doug encouraged me to show everything I had learned in my explorations and assume a new and more memorable identity. Because I had long identified with the twelfth-century Sufi mystic Fakir Musafar, whose credo was "piercing the body brings you closer to the Divine," I adopted his name as my new identity for a closing show in the hotel ballroom. The "Reno Fakir" received a standing ovation and special section in the *Reno Gazette* for stunts like lying on a bed of nails, inserting daggers in his chest, and pulling a hotel baggage cart around the ballroom (with tattooed belly dancer passenger) via deep chest piercings. The show was widely publicized. The Fakir namesake stuck! Unfortunately, our mentor and patron, Doug Malloy, passed away unexpectedly in 1979.

Going Public

The 1980s started a new era for the popularization of body modifications. In 1981 I met New York film producers Mark and Dan Jury. They were in the process of making a documentary about American subcultures being explored by anthropologist Charles Gatewood. Charles had photographed me in New York in the 1970s. So while speaking at the San Francisco Art Institute in 1981, Charles introduced me to the Jurys as well as publisher V. Vale. It was a love affair of offbeat artists and explorers. We spent many hours getting to know each other in the back room of a Chinatown restaurant. The result was an agreement to include Fakir's adventures and impact on modern subcultures in the as-yet-unnamed documentary film. V. Vale also expressed interest in producing a popular book on modern primitives. Big ripples to come!

In the summer of 1982, I took a month off to prepare for the fulfillment of an old vision: to do a Sun Dance and Ogalala-style suspension (outdoor variation of the Mandan O-Kee-Pa ritual) as close to the tribal versions as possible. Traveling alone, I scouted remote locations in western Wyoming. I found "good vibes" on the Thunder Basin National Grasslands, near Devil's Tower and Sun Dance, Wyoming. I phoned the Jurys and my piercing friend Jim Ward. I asked if we could all meet several weeks later in nearby Rapid City, South Dakota. I asked Jim if he would do the Sun Dance with me and be my Ka-see-Ka for the suspension. He said yes. Then I gave permission to the Jurys to film the rituals, but with the understanding they had to be virtually invisible, out-of-sight, while filming on the National Grasslands. The Jurys agreed.

Wyoming was a marvelous experience. Jim Ward and I did the Sun Dance together and were joined by blood. The Jurys came away with some sensitive and remarkable film. I had a third life-changing transformative experience: a trip to and through the physical sun and out into the cosmos. The closest I can describe that journey was its similarity to the final scenes in Stanley Kubrik's movie *2001*. The Jurys' film took three years to edit and finally got its name: *Dances Sacred and Profane*. It premiered at the Roxie theater in San Francisco in 1986, was shown in film festivals worldwide, was seen by thousands of mainstream people, but never became a commercial success. The film was way ahead of its time. At the premiere, however, I met my life partner and spiritual companion, Carla. She fell in love with the man hanging suspended by piercings in a Wyoming cottonwood tree! We are still together after twenty-four years.

Three years later, in 1989, V. Vale and Andrea Juno came through with their promise to publish a book on modern primitives. I started the project by suggesting the title and giving them twenty-seven hours of interview plus several hundred photographs. They expected a modest success for the book, titled *Modern Primitives: An Investigation of Contemporary Adornment and Ritual*. The first print run sold out in a matter of months. Since then, it has been reprinted many times. This one publication has had an astounding impact on contemporary culture, and I am proud I suggested it back in 1982.

The 1980s also saw the blooming of a number of kinky special interest educational groups, like the Society of Janus in San Francisco and Eulenspiegle in New York. They were open to all kinds of explorations in fetishism, erotic sex, sadomasochism, BDSM relationships, and sensation seeking. I wrote articles for their publications and became a regular presenter at their programs. At one of these meetings in 1985, I met a couple who wanted to learn how to make hourglass corsets. For the next year, I trained Ruth Johnson of BR Creations in the art of corset construction and let her use my unique corset patterns on a royalty basis. In the years that followed, figure-modifying corsets became popular again. For the next 25 years, Ruth Johnson made some of the best. She just retired.

Passing the Torch

By the 1990s, the wheels of culture had turned so far that the shy, isolated boy of the 1940s who had practiced "self-mutilation" in secret was now becoming a public darling. "Body Is the Door to Spirit" resonated with larger and larger segments of society. Fakir, as he was now known, was invited to demonstrate and pass this message on worldwide. There was that fortunate meeting with Dr. Favazza in 1990 on a CBS talk show. And travels to speak and facilitate workshops in Los Angeles, Chicago, Washington, DC, Minneapolis, Portland, Phoenix, Houston, Dallas, and Vancouver. By the mid-1990s, European art and culture festivals extended invitations: the Institute of Contemporary Arts (ICA) in London, the Body Ritual/Manipulation Conference in Copenhagen, Festival Atlantico in Lisbon. There was even another trip to Japan with shows in Tokyo and Osaka. However, I was not interested in doing "shows," just educational programs and spiritually oriented body rituals.

To further my educational mission, I was inspired to start two new projects in 1991. First was a magazine called *BodyPlay and Modern Primitives Quarterly*. Second was a body piercing school to pass on what we, the founders of the contemporary body piercing movement, had learned by trial and error. The magazine was in tune with the zeitgeist and started out with mainstream distribution through such outlets as Borders and Tower Records. For nine years it gave me the opportunity to document and photograph the budding body modification and body ritual movements. Also, what was gaining popularity in the mainstream culture was increasingly being covered by the mainstream media: news outlets and television shows like Learning Channel, Discovery Channel, and even National Geographic television. I appeared on many. And then came the Internet.

The body piercing school, however, was the biggest surprise. It turned out to be a magnet for those disenfranchised body modifiers who felt alone and isolated—the pierced, the cutters, the heavily tattooed. They were true modern primitives who had abandoned the outdated notion that their bodies belong to others. They lived their lives like their bodies belonged to them, the person living inside. In

2004, I started an informal survey of piercing school students. I asked three simple questions:

1. How many of you, past or present, have deliberately pierced yourself?
2. How many of you, past or present, have deliberately cut yourself?
3. How many of you, past or present, have deliberately burned yourself?

I kept a record of results, which showed that approximately 80 percent of the students had pierced themselves, approximately 60 percent had been cutters, and 60 percent had burned themselves. That is not the result one could expect of a random sample of people on the street. In fact, at one advanced piercing class I had students actually take a random sample of people in the nearby café where we ate lunch; same questions. We found no one who had done any of the three acts of self-mutilation. In some of my most recent classes, the number of self-mutilators was even higher, like 100 percent self-piercers, 80 percent self-cutters, 70 percent self-burners. It seems "self-mutilators" are drawn to sanctioned havens like my school.

Beginning with the turn of the millennium, I became conscious that what I had started was not just a fad. It was here to stay. But as these practices were now spreading rapidly through the culture, primarily by the Internet, they were being diluted and diffused. The origin and intent was being lost. What had started out as an avenue of personal exploration and healing had frequently become mere show business, expression of ego. What I had done with Jim Ward as a spiritual ritual in the Wyoming Sun Dance and suspension had become "fun and games" for many others—something to amuse a crowd in a night club, a carnival act designed for shock and awe.

To counteract this trend, I focused my energies on education and the training of protégés to carry the torch. I gathered a core group of devoted instructors to pass on the techniques, commonsense principles, and spiritual aspects of the body piercing and body branding, not just as an art form, but as a way to experience shifts in consciousness. Now there is an established institution known as "Fakir Intensives," organized and self-sustaining even if Fakir himself is no longer there to guide it.

A public message was also needed to express and reinforce the basic truths behind body rituals and modifications. So I gave permission to French film producers in Paris (with financial support from Canal+) to craft a brief film, *Fakir Profile*, for the European event called La Nuit du Cyclone. The profile film was shown widely in most European countries on New Year's Eve 1999. I was invited to Paris with my partner to speak and be part of the event in Montmartre. In 2004,

Self-mutilator Survey, Students, Fakir Piercing School,
January 2004–September 2007

Class (Mo./Yr.)	Students (Total: M/F)	Self-piercing	Self-cutting	Self-burning
1/04	9:4/5	8	5	4
3/04	9:5/4	7	4	5
5/04	8:6/2	6	6	5
7/04	10:6/4	7	7	7
1/05	11:7/4	9	8	6
3/05	8:5/3	8	7	8
3/05	10:7/3	9	6	5
5/05	10:4/6	7	4	6
7/05	7:3/4	4	2	3
9/05	9:4/5	8	8	7
3/06	10:4/6	8	5	8
5/06	10:3/7	8	5	6
7/06	11:5/6	9	7	7
9/06	10:7/3	8	5	9
11/06	10:1/9	6	7	7
6/07	11:5/6	9	3	2
8/07	10:5/5	6	4	6
9/07	10:5/5	10	7	5
Total	173:86/87	137 (79.1%)	100 (57.8%)	106 (61.2%)

I had another opportunity to present these ideas on National Geographic's television series *Taboo: Body Modification.*

Fakir's private group rituals with Ball Dances, the Kavadi, Hook Pulls, and Spiritual Suspensions have been around since 1980. But with the spreading of ripples since 2000, people worldwide desired a chance to experience them, not as unique pastimes but as serious transformative ritual. I started what I call "Spirit + Flesh Workshops." These collaborative daylong events with trained protégés and my spiritual partner, Carla, include: background on the cultural origins of the rituals, contemporary adaptation, spiritual intent, physical exercises, psychic purification, and opening circle, invocation and altar to Divine energy and spirits and the ritual dance itself with tribal drumming. Spirit+Flesh workshops/rituals are being held on a regular basis in the United States, Canada, and Europe. The torch has been passed.

Why Modify?

Why was I obsessed to modify my body? Why would I abandon the comfort of the status quo for the unknowns of body modification and ritual? I did it primarily because I was curious and bored with the status quo—probably for the same reasons early explorers risked the hazards of sailing uncharted seas. And like explorers of the past, present, and future seeking rewards of some kind: treasure or knowledge. In my journey, I sought to explore the seas of consciousness, my own inner self. The most personal and accessible vehicle was my own body. During my more than fifty years of sailing via body ritual, I have found some of the same reasons in the body rituals of other cultures.

1. As a rite of passage
2. For creation of life-long peer bonding
3. As a sign of respect or honor for elders and ancestors
4. As a symbol of status, belonging, bravery, or courage
5. For initiation into greater mysteries or entry to unseen worlds
6. As protection from evil spirits and dark energy
7. As an opening for beneficial spirits and positive energy
8. For rebalancing body and/or spirit energies
9. For healing of a diseased body, self, and others
10. For healing of a wounded psyche, self, and others
11. For healing of tribal disorders and creation of tribal bonding
12. To promote tribal/community connection to greater forces, especially in times of chaos, disaster, or war

In contemporary Western culture I've found maladies not usually found in tribal and non-Western cultures. These disorders deal with inhumanity, excess, and abuse of others. They are traumas inflicted through the body: gross sexual, physical, emotional, and substance abuse resulting in alienation of the body. A large majority of the students who come to my school, to our Spirit+Flesh rituals and S/M workshops are survivors of abuse. They are seeking to *reclaim* their bodies, take back their bodies. Physical body rituals and body modifications often help and are therapies worthy of exploration.

Why do we continue to alter, change, adjust, adopt, amend, revise, reshape, refashion, restyle, revamp, and refine our bodies? There seem to several intents. One is superficial: to be different, to stand out, to be noticed, or to fit a cultural stereotype. The other is to experience a transformation of some kind, a nonvisual as well as a three-dimensional change. This kind of modification requires a ritual. That means forethought, a solemn ceremony based on wisdom and a prescribed order. Many of the body modifications we see in contemporary culture are based on adaptations from other cultures: the tattoos, body piercings, cuttings, suspensions, etc. But they are mostly adopted *without* the rituals that are integral to their originators. So meaning gets lost. The rich rewards of a transformative experience get lost. Body and spirit do not always connect!

However, I am not entirely pessimistic about the sea contemporary culture is sailing. I have seen some marvelous transformations in the students who come to my schools and in the bold ones who have the courage to venture forth and participate in our Spirit+Flesh rituals. Even those who've experienced a number of body modifications without ritual eventually discover the precious value of the unseen experience that naturally follows. They discover that body is the door to spirit!

Abrahams BS, Geschwind DH. 2008. Advances in autism genetics. *Natl Rev Genetics* 9:341–55.

Abu-Salieh SA. 1994. To mutilate in the name of Jehovah or Allah. *Medicine and Law* 13: 575–622.

Adam J. 1883. Cases of self-mutilation of the insane. *J Ment Science* 29:213–19.

Adams WL. 2007. Quirky minds: Amputee wannabees. *Psychology Today* July/August.

Ajape A, Issa B, Buhari O, Adeoye P, Bobata A, Abiola O. 2010. Genital self-mutilation. *Annals African Medicine* 9:31–34.

Alao AO, Yolles JC, Huslander W. 1999. Female genital self-mutilation. *Psychiatric Services* 50:971.

Al-Dargazelli S. 1993–94. New findings in healing research. *Doctor-Healer Network Newsletter* (England) (Winter): 12–17.

Alexander HB. 1967. *The World's Rim: Great Mysteries of the North American Indians.* Lincoln: University of Nebraska Press.

Ali AH. 2007. *Infidel.* London: The Free Press.

Al-Qattan MM. 1999. Self-mutilation in children with obstetric brachial plexus palsy. *J Hand Surg Brit* 24:547–49.

Alroe CJ, Gunda V. 1995. Self-amputation of the ear. *Aust New Zeal J Psychiatry* 29:508–12.

Amandan S, Wigg C. 2004. Psychosurgery for self-injurious behavior in Tourette's disorder. *J Child Adol Psychopharmacol* 14:531–38.

Anaclerio AM, Wicker HS. 1970. Self-induced solar retinopathy by patients in a psychiatric hospital. *Am J Ophthalmology* 69:731–36.

Ananth J, Kaplan HS, Lin K-M. 1984. Self-enucleation of the eye. *Can J Psychiatry* 29: 145–46.

Anderson W, Lenz F. 2009. Lesioning and stimulation as surgical treatments for psychiatric disorders. *Neurosurg Quarterly* 19:132–43.

Anumonye A. 1973. Self-inflicted amputation of the penis in two Nigerian males. *Nigerian Med J* 3:51–52.

Arens W. 1979. *The Man-Eating Myth.* New York: Oxford University Press.

Arons BS. 1981. Self-mutilation: Clinical examples and reflections. *Am J Psychotherapy* 25: 550–58.

Arora M, Praharaj S, Prakash R. 2008. Electroconvulsive therapy for multiple major self-mutilations in bipolar psychotic depression. *Turk Psikiyatri Derg* 19:209–12.

Asch SS. 1971. Wrist scratching as a symptom of anhedonia. *Psychoanalytic Quar* 40:630–37.

Axelrod F, Gold-von-Simson G. 2007. Hereditary sensory and autonomic neuropathies. *Orphanet J Rare Diseases* 2:39–47.

Axenfeld T. 1899. Über Luxation, Zerstörung und Herausreissung des Augapfels als Selbstuerstummelung bei Geisteskranken. *Z für Augenheilkunde* 1:128–51.

Bach-Y-Rita G. 1974. Habitual violence and self-mutilation. *Am J Psychiatry* 131:1018–20.

Baek S, Lee M, Choi H. 1992. Radiography, US, and CT of acupucture needles in the abdominal organs. *J Comput Assit Tomog* 16:834–35.

Balduzzi E. 1961. Contributo alla psicopatologia degli stati ossessivi. *Riv Sper Freniat* 85: 314–31.

Ballard CG. 1989. Benign intracranial hypertension and repeated self-mutilation. *Br J Psychiatry* 155:570–71.

Barber ME, Marzuk PM, Leon AC, Portera L. 1998. Aborted suicide attempts. *Am J Psychiatry* 155:385–89.

Baroff GS, Tate BG. 1968. The use of aversive stimulation in the treatment of chronic self-injurious behavior. *J Am Acad Child Psychiatry* 7:454–70.

Barr MW. 1920. Some notes on asexualization. *J Nerv Ment Disease* 51:231–41.

Basedow H. 1927. Subincision and kindred rites of the Australian aboriginal. *J Roy Anthropol Institute* 57:123–56.

Bates WJ, Smeltzer DJ. 1982. Electroconvulsive treatment of psychotic self-injurious behavior in a patient with severe mental retardation. *Am J Psychiatry* 139:1355–56.

Bauer L. 1879–80. Infibulation as a remedy for epilepsy and seminal losses. *St. Louis Clinical Record* 6:163–65.

Baumeister AA, Frye GD. 1985. The biochemical basis of the behavioral disorder in the Lesch-Nyhan syndrome. *Neurosci Biobehav Review* 9:169–78.

Bayne T, Levy N. 2005. Amputees by choice: Body integrity disorder and the ethics of amputation. *J Applied Philosophy* 22:75–86.

Beilin LM, Gruenberg J. 1948. Genital self-mutilation by mental patients. *J Urology* 59: 635–41.

Benezech M, Bourgeois M, Boukhabza D, Yesavage. 1981. Cannibalism and vampirism in paranoid schizophrenia. *J Clin Psychiatry* 42:290.

Benjamin LS. 1987. An interpersonal approach. *J Personality Disorders* 1:334–39.

Benn JA. 2007. *Burning for Buddha: Self-immolation in Chinese Buddhism.* Honolulu: Kuroda Institute / University of Hawaii Press.

Beresford TP. 1980. The dynamics of aggression in an amputee. *Gen Hosp Psychiatry* 3: 219–25.

Bergmann GH. 1846. Ein Fall von religioser Monomanie. *Allgemeine Z für Psychiatrie* 3: 365–80.

Bergua A, Sperling W, Kuchie M. 2002. Self-enucleation in drug-related psychosis. *Ophthalmologica* 216:269–71.

Berndt R. 1962. *Excess and Restraint.* Chicago: University of Chicago Press.

Bettelheim B. 1955. *Symbolic Wounds.* London: Thames and Hudson.

Betts WC. 1964. Autocannibalism. *Am J Psychiatry* 121:402–3.

Bhatia M, Aurora S. 2001. Penile self-mutilation. *Br J Psychiatry* 178:86–87.

Bhattacharya SK, Jaiswal AK, Mukhopadhyay M, Datla KP. 1988. Clonidine-induced auto-mutilation in mice as a laboratory model for clinical self-injurious behavior. *J Psychiatric Research* 22:43–50.

Bigot A. 1938. Recherches sur le penis des Tonkinois, suivies d'une note sur les auto-mutilations genitales. *Rev Med France d'Extreme-Orient* 16:717–23.

Bille-Brahe V. 1982. Persons attempting suicide in the Danish welfare system. *Social Psychiatry* 17:181–88.

Biven B. 1977. A violent solution: The role of skin in severe adolescent regression. *Psychoanal Stud Child* 32:327–52.

Blacker KH, Wong N. 1963. Four cases of autocastration. *Arch Gen Psychiatry* 8:169–76.

Bliss EL. 1980. Multiple personalities. *Arch Gen Psychiatry* 37:1388–97.

Blondel C. 1906. Les automutilateurs. Medical thesis, Paris.

Boardman R, Smith R. 1997. Dental implications of oral piercing. *J Calif Dent Assn* 25: 20–207.

Boddy J. 1982. Womb as oasis: The symbolic context of Pharaonic circumcision in rural Northern Sudan. *Am Ethnol* 9:682–98.

Boecker H, Sprenger T, Spilker M. 2008. The runners high: Opioidergic mechanisms in the human brain. *Cerebral Cortex* 18:2523–31.

Boehm C. 1984. *Blood Revenge: The Anthropology of Feuding in Montenegro and Other Tribal Societies.* Lawrence: University Press of Kansas.

Bohannon P. 1956. Beauty and scarification among the Tiv. *Man* 51:117–21.

Bonnard A. 1960. The primal significance of the tongue. *Intl J Psychoanalysis* 41:301–7.

Bourdillon MFC, Fortes M (eds.). 1980. *Sacrifice.* New York: Academic Press.

Bowen DI. 1971. Self-inflicted orbitocranial injury with a plastic ballpoint pen. *Br J Ophthalmology* 33:427–30.

Bowker J. 1970. *Problems of Suffering in Religions of the World.* Cambridge, England: Cambridge University Press.

Bowman KM, Engle B. 1957. Medicolegal aspects of transvestism. *Am J Psychiatry* 113: 583–88.

Bradford DT. 1990. Early Christian martyrdom and the psychology of depression, suicide and bodily mutilation. *Psychotherapy* 27:30–41.

Bradley JM. 1933. A case of a self-made eunuch. *Weekly Bulletin St. Louis Med Soc* 28: 133–54.

Brain R. 1979. *The Decorated Body.* New York: Harper and Row.

Breece GR, Knapp DJ, Chriswell HE. 2005. The neonate-6-hydroxydopamine-lesioned rat: A model for clinical neurosciences and neurobiological principles. *Brain Research Reviews* 48:57–73.

Breslauer J. 1994. The body politics. *Los Angeles Times,* 2 July, pt. F, p. 1, col 4.

Bridy A. 2004. Confounding extremities: Surgery at the medico-ethical limits of self-modification. *J Law Medicine Ethics* 32:148–58.

Bromberg W, Schilder P. 1933. Psychologic considerations in alcoholic hallucinosis-castration and dismembering motives. *Intl J Psychoanalysis* 14:206–24.

Brown BZ. 1970. Self-inflicted injuries of the eye. *Trans Pacific Coast Oto-ophthalmol Soc* 51:267–76.

Brown J. 1963. A cross-cultural study of female initiation rites. *Am Anthropol* 65:837–53.

Brown K. 1993. Blood-letting in bulimia nervosa. *Br J Psychiatry* 163:129.

Brown P, Tuzin D. 1983. *The Ethnography of Cannibalism*. Washington, DC: Society for Psychological Anthropology Special Publication.

Burkert W. 1983. *Homo Necans*. Berkeley: University of California Press (originally published in German in 1972).

Burnham RC. 1969. Symposium on impulsive self-mutilation. *Br J Med Psychology* 42: 223–27.

Burstyn L. 1996. Female circumcision comes to *America*. *Atlantic Monthly* 276 (4): 28–35.

Burton-Bradley BG. 1976. Cannibalism for cargo. *J Nervous Ment Disease* 163:428–31.

Byman S. 1978. Ritualistic acts and compulsive behavior: The pattern of Tudor martyrdom. *Am Historical Rev* 83:625–43.

Byrnes VA. 1949. A case of self-mutilation involving both eyes. *Am J Ophthalmology* 32: 268–69.

Cain AC. 1961. Presuperego turning-inward of aggression. *Psychoanalytic Quar* 30:171–208.

Cameron N. 1963. *Personality Development and Psychopathology*. Boston: Houghton Mifflin.

Carroll J, Schaffer C, Spensley J, Abramowitz SI. 1980. Family experience of self-mutilating patients. *Am J Psychiatry* 137:852–53.

Carroll MP. 1982. The rolling head. *J Psychoanalytic Anthropol* 5:29–56.

Carson DI, Lewis JM. Ocular auto-enucleation while under the influence of drugs: A case report. 1971. *Adolescence* 6:397–403.

Cautela JR, Baron MG. 1973. Multifaceted behavior therapy of self-injurious behavior. *J Behav Therapy Exp Psychiatry* 4:125–31.

Cawte J. 1974. *Medicine Is the Law*. Honolulu: University Press of Hawaii.

Cawte J, Djagamara N, Barrett MG. 1966. The meaning of subincision of the urethra to aboriginal Australians. *Br J Med Psychology* 39:245–53.

Chabukswar YV. 1921. A barbaric method of circumcision among some of the Arab tribes of Yemen. *Indian Med Gaz* 56:48–49.

Channing W. 1877–78. Case of Helen Miller. *Am J Insanity* 34:368–78.

Christensen W. 1989. A fashion for ecstasy: Ancient Maya body modifications. In Vale V, Juno A. *Modern Primitives*. San Francisco: Research Publications.

Christenson GA, Popkin MK, Mackenzie TB, Realmuto GM. 1991. Self-harming behaviors in incarcerated male delinquent adolescents. *Am Acad Child Adolescent Psychiatry* 30: 202–7.

Christie R, Bay C, Kaufman IA, Babey B, Borden M, Nyhan WL. 1982. Lesch-Nyhan disease. *Dev Med Child Neurology* 24:293–306.

Claes L. 2004. Self-injury in Eating Disorders. Doctoral thesis, Catholic University of Leuven, Belgium.

Clark RA. 1981. Self-mutilation accompanying religious delusions: A case report and review. *J Clin Psychiatry* 42:243–45.

Cleckley H. 1964. *The Mask of Sanity*. St. Louis: Mosby.

Clendenin WW, Murphy GE. 1971. Wrist cutting: New epidemiological findings. *Arch Gen Psychiatry* 25:465–69.

Cleveland SE. 1956. Three cases of self-castration. *J Nerv Ment Disease* 123:386–91.

Coccaro EF, Astill JL, Szeeley PJ, Malkowica DE. 1990. Serotonin in personality disorders. *Psychiatric Annals* 20:587–92.

Coccaro EF, Siever LJ, Klar HM. 1989. Serotonergic studies in patients with affective and personality disorders: Correlates with suicidal and impulsive aggressive behavior. *Arch Gen Psychiatry* 46:587–99.

Cohen Y. 1964. *The Transition from Childhood to Adolescence*. Chicago: Aldine.

Cohn N. 1958. *The Pursuit of the Millennium*. New York: Essential Books.

Coid J, Allolio B, Rees CH. 1983. Raised plasma metenkephalin in patients who habitually mutilate themselves. *Lancet*, 3 Sept., 545–46.

Coid J, Wilkins J, Coid B, Everitt B. 1992. Self-mutilation in female remanded prisoners II: A cluster analytic approach towards identification of a behavioral syndrome. *Criminal Behavior Mental Health* 2:1–14.

Colapinto J. 2009. Brain Games. *New Yorker*, 11 May, pp. 76–87.

Collins DT. 1965. Head banging: Its meaning and management in the severely retarded adult. *Bull Menninger Clin* 29:205–11.

Conacher GN, Westwood GII. 1987. Autocastration in Ontario federal penitentiary inmates. *Br J Psychiatry* 150:565–66.

Conacher N, Villeneuve D, Kane G. 1991. Penile self-mutilation presenting as rational attempted suicide. *Can J Psychiatry* 36:683–85.

Conklin BA. 1995. Mortuary cannibalism in an Amazonian society. *Am Ethnologist* 22: 75–101.

Conn JH. 1932. A case of marked self-mutilation presenting a dorsal root syndrome. *J Nerv Ment Disease* 75:251–62.

Conrad K, Bers N. 1954. Die Chronischer taktile halluzinose. *Fortschrift Neurol* 22:254–70.

Conterio K, Lader W. 1998. *Bodily Harm*. New York: Hyperion.

Conze E, Horner IB, Snellgrove D, Waley A. 1995. *Buddhist Texts through the Ages*. Oxford: Oneworld Publications.

Coons PM. 1992. Self-amputation of the breasts by a male with schizotypal personality disorder. *Hosp Comm Psychiatry* 43:175–76.

Coons PM, Ascher-Svanum H, Bellis K. 1986. Self-amputation of the female breasts. *Psychosomatics* 27:667–68.

Coons PM, Milstein V. 1990. Self-mutilation associated with dissociative disorders. *Dissociation* 3:81–87.

Cooper SN. 1968. Self-inflicted ocular injuries. *J All India Ophthal Soc* 16:213–16.

Cooper WW. 1859. *On Wounds and Injuries of the Eye*. London: John Churchill.

Couts CA, Gleason OC. 2006. Self-mutilation of fingers after cervical spinal cord injury. *Psychosomatics* 47:269–70.

Coxon A. 1962. The Kisii art of trephining. *Guy's Hospital Gaz* 76:263–66.

Crabtree LH. 1967. A psychotherapeutic encounter with a self-mutilating patient. *Psychiatry* 30:91–100.

Crabtree LH, Grossman WK. 1974. Administrative clarity and redefinition for an open adolescent unit. *Psychiatry* 37:350–59.

Crapanzano V. 1973. *The Hamadsha*. Berkeley: University of California Press.

Cross HA, Harlow HF. 1965. Prolonged and progressive effects of partial isolation on the behavior of macaque monkeys. *J Exp Res Personality* 1:39–49.

Cross L. 1993. Body and self in feminine development: Implications for eating disorders and delicate self-mutilation. *Bull Menninger Clinic* 57:41–68.

Crowder JE, Gross CA, Heiser JF, Crowder AM. 1979. Self-mutilation of the eye. *J Clin Psychiatry* 24:420–23.

Crowell S, Beauchaire T, McCauley E. 2008. Parent-child interactions, peripheral serotonin, and self-inflicted injury in adolescents. *J Consult Clin Psychol* 76:15–21.

Cummings JF, de Lahunta A, Winn SS. 1981. Acral mutilation and nocioceptive loss in English pointer dogs: A canine sensory neuropathy. *Acta Neuropathology* 53:119–27.

Curran W. 1886. The making of eunuchs. *Provincial Med J*, 1 April, 149–51.

Cyr PR, Dreher GK. 2001. Neurotic excoriations. *Am Fam Physician* 64:181–84.

Dabrowski E, Smathers S, Ralstrom C. 2005. Botulinum toxin as a novel treatment for self-mutilation in Lesch-Nyhan syndrome. *Developmental Med Child Neurol* 47:636–39.

Daldin H. 1990. Self-mutilating behavior in adolescence with comments on suicidal risk. *Bull Anna Freud Centre* 13:279–93.

Darnton R. 1984. *The Great Cat Massacre*. New York: Basic Books.

Davenport MD, Lutz CK, Tiefenbacher S. 2008. A rhesus monkey model of self-injury: Effects of relocation stress on behavior and neuroendocrine function. *Biol Psychiatry* 15:990–96.

Deacon J, Rowan M, Hartmann P. 2009. Association of nipple piercing with abnormal milk production and breastfeeding. *JAMA* 301:2550–51.

Dean C. 2001. Repeated self-mutilation and ECT. *Am J Psychiatry* 158:1331.

Dearborn GVN. 1932. A case of congenital pure analgesia. *J Nerv Ment Disease* 75:612–15.

de Lissovoy V. 1961. Head-banging in early childhood. *J Pediatrics* 58:803–5.

DeMuth GW, Strain JJ, Lombardo-Maher A. 1983. Self-amputation and restitution. *Gen Hosp Psychiatry* 5:25–30.

Dennis SG, Melzak R. 1979. Self-mutilation after dorsal rhizotomy in rats. *Exp Neurol* 65:412–21.

Desoff J. 1943. The eye and related functional disturbances. *Med Ann District Columbia* 12:97–101.

Dingman CW, McGlashan TH. 1988. Characteristics of patients with serious suicidal intentions who ultimately commit suicide. *Hospital Community Psychiatry* 39:295–99.

Dingwall EJ. 1925. *Male Infibulation*. London: John Bale, Sons and Danielson.

———. N.d. *Very Peculiar People*. London: Rider (year of publication not listed in book, probably 1930s).

———. 1931. *Artificial Cranial Deformation*. London: John Bale, Sons and Danielson.

Diniz B, Krelling R. 2006. Self-mutilation of fingers and lips in a schizophrenic patient. *Res Psiquiat Clinica* 33:272–75.

Dolfus M-A, Michaux L. 1957. Un cas d'oedipisme suivi d'un double décollement de retine. *Bull Soc Ophthal France* 3:161–63.

Dollard J, Doob L, Miller N, Mowrer OH, Sears RR. 1939. *Frustration and Aggression*. New Haven: Yale University Press.

Dubovsky SL. 1978. "Experimental" self-mutilation. *Am J Psychiatry* 135:1240–41.

Dubovsky SL, Groban S. 1975. Congenital absence of sensation. *Psychoanalytic Study Child* 30:49–73.

Duggal HS, Jagadheesan K, Nizamie SH. 2002. Acute onset of schizophrenia following autocastration. *Can J Psychiatry* 47:283–84.

Dupeyrat A. 1954. *Savage Papua*. New York: Dutton.

Durham ME. 1928. *Some Tribal Origins, Laws and Customs of the Balkans*. London: Allen and Unwin.

du Toit PL, van Kradenburg J, Nichaus D, Stein DJ. 2001. Comparison of obsessive-compulsive disorder patients with and without comorbid putative obsessive-compulsive spectrum disorders using a structured clinical interview. *Comprehensive Psychiatry* 42: 291–300.

Egan J. 1997. The thin red line. *NY Times Mag*, 27 July, 20–25, 34, 40, 43–44, 48.

Eibl-Eibelsfeldt I. 1972. *On Love and Hate*. New York: Holt Rinehart Winston.

Eigner EH. 1966. Self-induced solar retinitis. *Am J Ophthalmology* 61:1546–47.

Eisenberg L. 1973. The human nature of human nature. In Montague A. *Man and Aggression*. New York: Oxford University Press.

Ekc E, Elcnwo S. 1999. Male genital mutilation. *J Clin Forensic Med* 6:246–48.

El Dareer A. 1982. *Women, Why Do You Weep?* London: Zed Press.

Eliade M. 1960. *Myths, Dreams and Mysteries*. New York: Harper and Row.

———. 1974. *Shamanism*. Princeton: Princeton University Press.

———. 1975. *Rites and Symbols of Initiation*. New York: Harper and Row.

Elkin AP. 1945. *Aboriginal Men of High Degree*. Sydney: Angus and Robertson.

Elliott C. 2000. A new way to be mad. *Atlantic Monthly* 286 (6): 72–84.

Elwin V. 1943. Vagina dentata legend. *Br J Med Psychology* 19:439–53.

Emerson LE. 1933. The case of Miss A: A preliminary report of a psychoanalytic study and treatment of a case of self-mutilation. *Psychoanalytic Rev* 1:41–54.

Engelman ER, Polito G, Perley J, Bruffy J, and Martin, DC. 1974. Traumatic amputation of the penis. *J Urology* 112:774–78.

Engle BS. 1936. Attis: A study of castration. *Psychoanalytic Rev* 23:363–72.

Erickson E. 1950. *Childhood and Society*. New York: W. W. Norton.

Esman AH. 1954. A case of self-castration. *J Nerv Ment Disease* 120:79–82.

Evans C, Lacey JH. 1992. Multiple self-damaging behavior among alcoholic women. *Br J Psychiatry* 161:643–47.

Evans-Pritchard EE. 1956. *Nuer Religion*. Oxford: Clarendon Press.

Fan A, Fink S. 2007. Autoenucleation: A case report and literature review. *Psychiatry* 4: 30–36.

Fauber J. 2008. Method detects self-injury: Teens embedding objects under skin. *Milwaukee Journal Sentinel*. 4 December, pt. A, p. 5.

Favazza A. 1989a. Normal and deviant self-mutilation. *Transcultural Psychiatric Research Review* 26:113–27.

———. 1989b. Why patients mutilate themselves. *Hosp Community Psychiatry* 40:137–45.

———. 1991. Masturbation or mutilation? *Medical Aspects Human Sexuality* (May): 45–46.

———. 1992. Repetitive self-mutilation. *Psychiatric Annals* 22:60–63.

———. 1998. The coming of age of self-mutilation. *J Nerv Ment Dis* 186:259–68.

———. 2004. *PsychoBible: Behavior, Religion, and the Holy Book.* Charlottesville, VA: Pitchstone.

———. 2006. Self-injurious behavior in college students. *Pediatrics* 117:2283–84.

———. 2008. Self-injurious behavior. In Grunewald M. *Human Haptic Perception.* Basel: Switzerland.

———. 2009. Spirituality and psychiatry. In Sadock B, Sadock V, Ruuiz P. *Comprehensive Textbook of Psychiatry* (9th ed.). Baltimore: Lippincott Williams & Wilkins.

Favazza A, Conterio K. 1988. The plight of chronic self-mutilators. *Community Mental Health J* 24:22–30.

———. 1989. Female habitual self-mutilators. *Acta Psychiatrica Scandinavica* 79:283–89.

Favazza A, DeRosear L, Conterio K. 1989. Self-mutilation and eating disorders. *Suicide Life-Threatening Behavior* 19:352–61.

Favazza A, Dos Santos E. 1985. Depersonalization episodes in self-mutilation. *Am J Psychiatry* 142:1390.

Favazza A, Rosenthal R. 1990. Varieties of pathological self-mutilation. *Behavioral Neurology* 3:77–85.

———. 1993. Diagnostic issues in self-mutilation. *Hosp Community Psychiatry* 44:134–40.

Favazza A, Simeon D. 1995. Self-mutilation. In Hollander E, Stein D. *Impulsivity and Aggression.* New York: Wiley.

Featherstone M (ed.). 2000. Body modification. *Body and Society* 5 (1–2).

Female circumcision. 1983. *Lancet,* 12 March, 569.

Ferguson G. 1954. *Signs and Symbols in Christian Art.* New York: Oxford University Press.

Ferguson-Rayport SM, Griffith RM, Straus EW. 1955. The psychiatric significance of tatoos. *Psychiatric Quar* 29:112–31.

Fichter MM, Quadflieg N, Rief W. 1994. Course of multi-impulsive bulimia. *Psychological Medicine* 24:592–604.

Figueroa MD. 1988. A dynamic taxonomy of self-destructive behavior. *Psychotherapy* 25: 280–87.

First MB. 2005. Desire for amputation of a limb. *Psychol Med* 35:919–28.

Fisch RZ. 1987. Genital self-mutilation in males: Psychodynamic anatomy of a psychosis. *Am J Psychotherapy* 41:453–58.

Fleischer K. 1980. Uvula-excision in Afrika. *Curare* 3:19–22.

Fleming JB. 1960. Clitoridectomy: The disastrous downfall of Isaac Baker Brown. *J Ob Gyn Br Empire* 67:1017–34.

Flory R, Jensen D. 2000. Marked for Jesus: Sacred tattooing among a new generation of Evangelicals. In Flory R, Miller D. *GenX Religion.* New York: Routledge.

Flugel JC. 1925. A note on the phallic significance of the tongue and of speech. *Intl J Psychoanalysis* 6:209–15.

Fountas K, Smith J, Lee G. 2007. Bilateral stereotactic amygdalotomy for self-mutilation disorder. *Stereotact Funct Neurosurgery* 85:121–28.

Frances A. 1987. Introduction [to the section on self-mutilation]. *J Personality Disorders* 1:316.

Frances A, Gale L. 1975. The proprioceptive body image in self-object differentiation. *Psychoanal Quarterly* 44:107–28.

Frances A, Munro A. 1989. Treating a woman who believes she has bugs under her skin. *Hospital Community Psychiatry* 40:1113–14.

Frazer JG. 1958. *The Golden Bough.* New York: Macmillan (originally published in 1922).

French AP, Nelson HL. 1972. Genital self-mutilation in women. *Arch Gen Psychiatry* 27: 618–20.

Freud A. 1946. *The Ego and the Mechanisms of Defense.* New York: International Universities Press.

Freud A, Burlingham DT. 1944. *Infants without Families.* New York: International University Press.

Freud S. 1917. *Mourning and Melancholia. Standard Edition of the Complete Psychological Works of Sigmund Freud,* vol. 14, 243–58. London: Hogarth Press.

———. 1919. *The Uncanny. Standard Edition of the Complete Psychological Works of Sigmund Freud,* vol. 12, 243–58. London: Hogarth Press.

———. 1920. *A General Introduction to Psychoanalysis.* London: Boni and Liveright.

———. 1930. *Civilization and Its Discontents.* London: Hogarth Press.

———. 1939. *Moses and Monotheism.* New York: Vintage Books.

———. 1950. *Totem and Taboo.* New York: W.W. Norton (original work published in 1913).

Freudenmann R, Lepping P. 2008. Second-generation antipsychotics in primary and secondary delusional parasitosis. *J Clin Psychopharm* 28:500–508.

Fromm E. 1973. *The Anatomy of Human Destructiveness.* New York: Holt Rinehart Winston.

Furth G, Smith R. 2000. *Apotemnophilia: Information, Questions, Answers, and Recommendations about Self-demand Amputation.* Bloomington, IN: 1st Books

Gaddini E. 1982. Early defensive fantasies and the psychoanalytic process. *Int J Psychoanalysis* 63:379–88.

Gadoth N, Mass E. 2004. Hereditary neuropathies with self-mutilation. *J Pediatric Neurol* 2:205–11.

Galt J. 1884. Suicidal amputation of the penis. *Med Herald* 6:225–28

Gardiner M. 1971. *The Wolf-Man.* New York: Basic Books.

Gardner AR, Gardner AJ. 1975. Self-mutilation, obsessionality, and narcissim. *Br J Psychiatry* 127:127–32.

Gardner R, Heider KG. 1968. *Gardens of War.* New York: Random House.

Gerard P, Wilck E, Schiano T. 1993. Imaging implications in the evaluation of permanent needle acupuncture. *Clin Imaging* 17:36–40.

Gerhard M. 1968. A propos des automutilations oculaires. *Bull Soc Ophthal France* 68: 622–26.

Ghaffari-Nejad A, Kerdegari M, Reihani-Kermeni H. 2007. Self-mutilation of the nose in a schizophrenic patient with Cotard's syndrome. *Arch Iranian Med* 10:540–42.

Gifford ES. 1955. Psychogenic ocular symptoms. *Arch Ophthalmology* 53:318–29.

Gillette PJ. 1966. *The Complete Marquis de Sade.* Los Angeles: Holloway House.

Gillman MA, Sandyk R. 1985. Opiatergic and dopaminergic functions and Lesch-Nyhan syndrome. *Am J Psychiatry* 142:1226.

Girard R. 1977. *Violence and the Sacred.* Baltimore: Johns Hopkins University Press (originally published in French as *La Violence et Le Sacre,* 1972).

Glenn J. 1960. Circumcision and anti-Semitism. *Psychoanalytic Quar* 29:395–99.

Gluckman M. 1962. *Essays on the Ritual of Social Relations.* Manchester, England: Manchester University Press.

Goffin. 1887. Ein Fall von schwerer Selbstverummelung. *Bull Med Mentale de Belgique* 3:8.

Goldberg BZ. 1930. *The Sacred Fire (Skoptsi).* New York: Horace Liveright.

Golden S, Chosak A. 1964. Oral manifestations of a psychological problem. *J Periodentology* 35:349–50.

Goldenberg E, Sata LS. 1978. Religious delusions and self-mutilation. *Curr Concepts in Psychiatry* (September/October): 2–5.

Goldfield MD, Glick IA. 1970. Self-mutilation of the female genitalia. *Dis Nerv System* 31: 843–45.

———. 1973. Self-mutilation of the genitalia. *Med Aspects Human Sexuality* 7:219–32.

Goldney RD, Simpson IG. 1975. Female genital self-mutilation, dysorexia and the hysterical personality: The Caenis syndrome. *Can Psychiatric Assn J* 20:435–41.

Goldstein IC, Dragan AI. 1967. Self-inflicted oral mutilation in a psychotic adolescent. *J Am Dental Assn* 74:750–51.

Goldstein N. 1979. Psychological implications of tatoos. *J Dermatol Surg Oncology* 5: 883–88.

Goldstein N, Sewell M. 1979. Tatoos in different cultures. *J Dermatol Surg Oncology* 5: 857–64.

Goodhart S, Savitsky N. 1933. Self-mutilation in chronic encephalitis. *Am J Med Science* 185:674–84.

Gorin M. 1964. Self-inflicted bilateral enucleation. *Arch Ophthalmology* 72:225–26.

Gould GM, Pyle WL. 1956. *Anomalies and Curiosities of Medicine.* New York: Julian Press (originally published in 1896).

Gould RA. 1969. *Yiwara: Foragers of the Australian Desert.* New York: Scribner's.

Grabman JM. 1975. The Witch of Mallegem; print by Bruegel the Elder. *J Hist Med Allied Sciences* 30:385.

Graff H, Mallin R. 1967. The syndrome of the wrist cutter. *Am J Psychiatry* 124:36–42.

Graillot H. 1912. *Le Culte de Cybele.* Paris.

Grant J, Odlaug B, Kim S. 2009. N-acetylcysteine, a glutamate modulator, in the treatment of trichotillomania. *Arch Gen Psychiatry* 66:756–63.

Gratz K, Roemer L. 2008. The relationship between emotion dysregulation and deliberate self-harm among female undergraduate students at an urban commuter university. *Cogn Behav Therapy* 37:14–25.

Graver D. 1995. Violent theatricality. *Theatre Journal* 47:43–64.

Green C, Kaysz W, Tsuang M. 2000. A homeless person with bipolar disorder and a history of serious self-mutilation. *Am J Psychiatry* 157:1392–97.

Green E, Green A. 1977. *Beyond Biofeedback.* New York: Melroyd Lawrence.

Greenacre P. 1926. The eye motif in delusion and fantasy. *Am J Psychiatry* 82:553–79.

Greenberg J. 1981. *I Never Promised You a Rose Garden*. New York: Holt Rinehart Winston.

Greenspan GC, Samuel SE. 1989. Self-cutting after rape. *Am J Psychiatry* 146:789–90.

Gregor JT. 1998. *Circus of the Scars*. Seattle: Dalsgard Publishers.

Gregurek-Novak T, Novac-Bilic G, Vicic M. 2005. Dermatitis artefacta: Unusual appearance in an older woman. *J Eur Acad Dermatol Venereol* 19:223–25.

Greilsheimer H, Groves JE. 1979. Male genital self-mutilation. *Arch Gen Psychiatry* 36: 441–46.

Griffin JA. 1971. Is a cannibal a criminal? *Melanesian Law Journal* 1:79–81.

Griffin JC, Williams DE, Stark MT. 1985. Self-injurious behavior: A statewide prevalence survey. *Applied Research Mental Retardation* 7:105–16.

Griffin N, Webb MGT, Parker RR. 1982. A case of self-inflicted eye injuries. *J Nerv Ment Diseases* 170:53–56.

Gruenbaum E. 1982. The movement against clitoridectomy and infibulation in Sudan: Public health policy and the women's movement. *Med Anthropol Newsletter* 13:4–12.

Grunebaum HV, Klerman GL. 1967. Wrist slashing. *Am J Psychiatry* 124:527–34.

Gunderson JG, Zanarini MC. 1987. Current overview of the borderline diagnosis. *J Clin Psychiatry* 48 (Suppl.): 5–11.

Haberman MA, Michael RP. 1979. Autocastration in transsexualism. *Am J Psychiatry* 136: 347–48.

Hahn DS, Hahn DS. 1967. A case of penis amputation. *Korean Med J* 12:113–16.

Haines J, Williams CL, Brain KL, Wilson GV. 1995. The psychophysiology of self-mutilation. *J Abnormal Psychology* 104:471–89.

Hall DC, Lawson BZ, Wilson LG. 1981. Command hallucinations and self-amputation of the penis and hand during a first psychotic break. *J Clin Psychiatry* 42:322–24.

Hama Y, Kaji T. 2004. A migrated acupuncture needle in the medula oblongata. *Arch Neurol* 61:1608.

Hare RD. 1970. *Psychopathy Theory and Research*. New York: Wiley.

Harrer VG, Urban HJ. 1950. Zur Selbstblendung und Selbstverstummelung. *Wiener Medizinische Wochenschrift* 100:37–40.

Hartley B, Rowe-Jones J. 1994. Uvulectomy to prevent throat infections. *J Laryngol Otology* 108:65–66.

Hartman DE, Powander SM. 1987. Identification with a brain-damaged parent: Theoretical considerations on a case of self-mutilation. *Psychoanalytic Psychology* 4:171–78.

Hartmann H. 1926. Self-mutilation. *Arch Neurol Psychiatry* 15:384–86.

Hawton K. 1990. Self-cutting. In Hawton K, Cowen P. *Dilemmas and Difficulties in the Management of Psychiatric Patients*. Oxford: Oxford University Press.

Hays HR. 1964. *The Dangerous Sex*. New York: Putnam.

Hays TE, Hays PH. 1982. Opposition and complementarity of the sexes in Ndumba initiation. In Herdt GH. *Rituals of Manhood*. Berkeley: University of California Press.

Hemphill RE. 1951. A case of genital self-mutilation. *Br J Med Psychology* 24:291–95.

Herdt GH. 1982. Sambia nosebleeding rites and male proximity to women. *Ethos* 10: 189–231.

Herpertz S. 1995. Self-injurious behavior. *Acta Psychiatrica Scandinavica* 91:57–68.

Herpertz S, Sass H, Favazza AR. 1997. Impulsivity in self-mutilative behavior: Psychometric and biological findings. *J Psychiat Res* 31:451–65.

Hibbard SK. 1994. The mechanisms and meanings of self-cutting. *Modern Psychoanalysis* 19:45–54.

Hillbrand M, Krystal JH, Sharpe KS, Foster HG. 1994. Clinical predictors of self-mutilation in hospitalized forensic patients. *J Nerv Mental Disease* 182:9–13.

Hochman B. 2009. Nuggets making their mark in ink. *Denver Post*, 19 May.

Hoffman HA, Baer PN. 1968. Gingival mutilation in children. *Psychiatry* 31:380–86.

Hogbin HI. 1970. *The Island of Menstruating Men*. Scranton, PA: Chandler.

Hollender MC, Abram HS. 1973. Dermatitis factitia. *Southern Med J* 66:1279–85.

Hong CC, Ediger RD. 1978. Self-mutilation of the penis in C57BL/6N mice. *Laboratory Animals* 12:55–57.

Horn F. 2003. A life for a limb: Body integrity identity disorder. *Social Work Today*, 24 February.

Hosken FP. 1978. The epidemiology of female genital mutilations. *Tropical Doctor* 8: 150–56.

Howden JC. 1882. Mania followed by hyperaesthesia and osteomalacia: Singular family tendency to excessive constipation and self-mutilation. *J Ment Sci* 28:49–53.

Hrdlicka A. 1939. Trepanation among prehistoric people. *CIBA Symposia* 1:170–77.

Hubert H, Mauss M. 1899. Essai sur la nature et la fonction du sacrifice. *L'Année sociologique* 2 (published in English as *Sacrifice: Its Nature and Function*. London: Cohen and West, 1964).

Hunter A, Kennard AB. 1982. Mania operativa: An uncommon, unrecognized cause of limb amputation. *Can J Surgery* 85:96–98.

Hussein JN, Fatooki LJ, Al-Dargazelli S, Almuchtar N. 1993. The deliberately caused bodily damage phenomena: Mind, body, energy, or what? Paramann Programme Laboratories, Amman, Jordan.

Huxley J. 1931. *Africa View*. London: Chatto and Windus.

Hyneck RW. 1932. *Konnersreuth: A Medical and Psychological Study of the Case of Therese Neumann*. New York: Macmillan.

Isaac E. 1967. The enigma of circumcision. *Commentary* 43:51–56.

Jacobi W. 1923. *Die Stigmatisiertia: Bertrage für Psychologie der Mystik*. Munich: Bergmann.

Jacobs BW, Isaacs S. 1986. Pre-pubertal anorexia nervosa. *J Child Psychology Psychiatry* 27:237–50.

Jacobs J, Scaravilli F, Duchen LW. 1981. A new neurological rat mutant "mutilated foot." *J Anatomy* 132:525–43.

Jacobson CM, Gould M. 2007. The epidemiology and phenomenology of non-suicidal self-injurious behavior among adolescents. *Arch Suicide Res* 11:129–47.

Jagmeet P, D'Silva S, Lokhandwala Y. 1992. Intercardiac needle in a man with self-injurious behavior presenting with only a cardiac murmur. *Thorac Cardiovasc Surg* 40:231–33.

James EO. 1962. *Sacrifice and Sacrament*. London: Thames and Hudson.

Jamieson RA. 1882. Self-mutilation in China. *Br Med J* 1:397–98.

Jankovic J. 1988. Orofacial and other self-mutilations. In Jarkovic J, Tolsa E. *Advances in Neurology*, vol. 49, *Facial Dyskinesias*. New York: Rowen Press, pp. 365–81.

Janssens PA. 1957. Medical views on prehistoric representations of human hands. *Med History* 1:318–22.

Jilek WG, Jilek-Aall L. 1978. Initiation in Papua–New Guinea. *Papua–New Guinea Med J* 21:252–63.

Jinnah HA, Yitta S, Drew T. 1999. Calcium channel activation and self-biting in mice. *Proc Natl Acad Sci* USA 96:15228–32.

Johnson EH, Britt B. 1967. *Self-mutilation in Prison: Interaction of Stress and Social Structure.* Carbondale: Southern Illinois University Center for the Study of Crime, Delinquency, and Corrections.

Joiner T, Brown J, Wingate L. 2005. The psychology and neurobiology of suicidal behavior. *Annual Rev Psychol* 56:287–314.

Jonaitis A. 1988. Women, marriage, mouths and feasting: The symbolism of Tlingit labrets. In Rubin A. *Marks of Civilization.* Los Angeles: Museum of Cultural History, UCLA.

Jones A. 1986. Self-mutilation in prison. *Criminal Justice and Behavior* 13:286–96.

Jones IH, Barraclough BM. 1978. Auto-mutilation in animals and its relevance to self-injury in man. *Acta Psychiatrica Scandinavica* 58:40–47.

Jones IH, Congiv L, Stevenson J, Frei B. 1979. A biological approach to two forms of human self injury. *J Nerv Ment Disease* 167:74 78.

Jones R. 1961. Flagellants. In Hasting J. *Hasting's Encyclopedia of Religion and Ethics*, vol. 6. New York: Scribner's.

Jordan J. 2004. The rhetorical limits of the "plastic body." *Quart J Speech* 90:327–58.

Kafka JS. 1969. The body as a transitional object: A psychoanalytic study of a self-mutilating patient. *Br J Med Psychology* 42:207–12.

Kahan J, Pattison EM. 1984. Proposal for a distinctive diagnosis: The Deliberate Self Harm Syndrome. *Suicide and Life Threatening Behavior* 14:17–35.

Kalin NH. 1979. Genital and abdominal self-surgery. *JAMA* 241:2188–89.

Kasim S, Jinnah H. 2003. Thresholds for self-injurious behavior in a genetic mouse model of Lesch-Nyhan disease. *Pharmacology Biochemistry Behavior* 73:583–92.

Kehoe AB. 1979. The Sacred Heart: A case for stimulus diffusion. *Am Ethnol* 6:763 71.

Keleman P. 1967. *Baroque and Rococco in Latin America.* New York: Dover.

Kennedy BL, Feldman TB. 1994. Self-inflicted eye injuries. *Hosp Community Psychiatry* 45:470–74.

Kenyon HR, Hyman RM. 1953. Total autoemasculation. *JAMA* 151:207–10.

Kernberg O. 1987. A psychodynamic approach. *J Personality Disorders* 1:344–46.

Kettlewell C. 1999. *Skin Game.* New York: St. Martin's Press.

Kies SD, Devine DP. 2004. Self-injurious behavior: A comparison of caffeine and pemoline models in rats. *Pharmacol Biochem Behavior* 79:587–98.

Kim Y, Kim J, Choi B. 2006. Right ventricular acupuncture needle embolism detected on coronary computed tomography angiography. *Circulation* 114:623–26.

King BH, Au D, Poland RE. 1993. Low dosage naltrexone inhibits pemoline-induced self-biting in prepubertal rats. *J Child Adol Psychopharmacology* 3:71–79.

Kirtley M, Kirtley A. 1982. The Ivory Coast. *Nat Geographic* 162:94–124.

Klauder JV. 1938. Stigmatization. *Arch Dermatology Syphilology* 37:650–59.

Klonsky E, Moyer A. 2008. Childhood sexual abuse and nonsuicidal self-injury: Meta-analysis. *Brit J Psychiatry* 192:166–70.

Klonsky E, Weinberg A. 2009. Assessment of nonsuicidal self-injury. In Nock M. *Understanding Nonsuicidal Self-Injury*. Washington, DC: American Psychological Association Press.

Koblenzer CS. 2000. Dermatitis artefacta. *Am J Clin Dermatol* 1:47–55.

Koenig LM, Carnes M. 1999. Body piercing medical concerns with cutting-edge fashion. *J Gen Intern Med* 14:379–85.

Koh K, Yeo B. 2002. Self-enucleation in a young schizophrenic patient. *Singapore Med J* 43:159–60.

Konicki E, Schulz C. 1989. Rationale for clinical trials of opiate antagonistic in treating patients with personality disorder and self-injurious behavior. *Psychopharmacology Bulletin* 25:556–63.

Kramrisch S. 1981. *Manifestations of Shiva*. Philadelphia: Philadelphia Museum of Art.

Krieger MJ, McAninch JW, Weimer SR. 1982. Self-performed bilateral orchiectomy in transsexuals. *J Clin Psychiatry* 43:292–93.

Kroll JL. 1978. Self-destructive behavior on an inpatient ward. *J Nerv Ment Disease* 166: 429–34.

Kuhn J, Lenartz D, Mai J. 2008. Disappearance of self-aggressive behavior in a brain-injured patient after deep brain stimulation of the hypothalamus. *Neurosurgery* 62:E1182.

Kushner AW. 1967. Two cases of auto-castration due to religious delusions. *Br J Med Psychology* 40:293–98.

Kwawer JS. 1980. Some interpersonal aspects of self-mutilation in a borderline patient. *J Am Acad Psychoanalysis* 8:203–16.

Lacey JH. 1982. Anorexia nervosa and a bearded female saint. *Br Med J* 285:1816–17.

Lacey JH, Evans CDH. 1986. The impulsivist. *Br J Addictions* 81:641–49.

Lagercrantz S. 1935. Fingerverstummelungen und ihre Ausbreitung in Afrika. *Z für Ethnologie* 67:129–55.

———. 1938. Zur Verbreitung der Monorchie. *Z für Ethnologie* 70:199–208.

Landwirth J. 1964. Sensory radicular neuropathy and retinitis pigmentosa. *Pediatrics* 34: 519–24.

Larbig W. 1982. *Schmerz und Schmerzbehandlung*. Stuttgart: Kohlhammer.

Large M, Babidge N, Andrews D. 2009. Major self-mutilation in the first episode of psychosis. *Schizophr Bulletin* 35:1012–21.

Lea HC. 1973a. *The Ordeal*. Philadelphia: University of Pennsylvania Press (originally published in 1866).

———. 1973b. *Torture*. Philadelphia: University of Pennsylvania Press (originally published in 1866).

Leach ER. 1976. *Culture and Communication*. Cambridge, England: Cambridge University Press.

Lechler A. 1933. *Das Rätsel von Konnersreuth in Lichte eines neuer Falles von Stigmatisation*. Munich: Elberfeld.

Lena SM, Bijoor S. 1990. Wrist cutting: A dare game among adolescents. *Can Med Assn J* 142:131–32.

Lennon S. 1963. Genital self-mutilation in acute mania. *Med J Australia* 50:79–81.

Lepping P, Russell I, Freudenmann R. 2008. Antipsychotic treatment of primary delusional parasitosis: Systematic review. *Br J Psychiatry* 191:198–205.

Leung CM, Lee TS, Chan Ho MW. 1996. A case of unrelenting pursuit of castration. *Aust NZ J Psychiatry* 30:150–52.

Levison CA. 1970. Development of head banging in a young rhesus monkey. *Am J Ment Deficiency* 75:323–28.

Levitt J, Sansone R, Cohn L. 2004. *Self-Harm Behaviors and Eating Disorders*. New York: Brunner-Routledge.

Levy HS. 1968. *Chinese Footbinding*. New York: Bell.

Lewis NDC. 1927, 1928. The psychobiology of the castration reaction. *Psychoanalytic Rev* 14:420–46; 15:53–94, 174–209, 304–23.

———. 1931. Additional observation on the castration reaction in males. *Psychoanalytic Rev* 18:146–65.

Lidz RW, Lidz T. 1977. Male menstruation. *Intl J Psychoanalysis* 58:17–31.

Liebenluft E, Gardner DL, Cowdry RW. 1987. The inner experience of the borderline self-mutilator. *J Personality Disorders* 1:317–24.

Lim E, Ng T-H, Seet R. 2005. A woman whose radiographs showed subcutaneous metallic objects. *Canad Med Assn J* 173:150–51.

Lim YC, Seng BK. 1985. Self-mutilation in a family. *Singapore Med J* 26:482–84.

Lincoln B. 1975. The Indo-European myth of creation. *History Religion* 15:121–45.

———. 1981. *Emerging from the Chrysalis*. Cambridge, MA: Harvard University Press.

Lloyd-Richardson E, Perrine N, Dierker L. 2007. Characteristics and function of non-suicidal self-injury in a community sample of adolescents. *Applied Preventive Psychol* 37:1183–92.

Lorenz K. 1954. *Man Meets Dog*. Cambridge, MA: Riverside Press.

———. 1966. *On Aggression*. New York: Harcourt Brace World.

Lowry FH, Kolivakis TL. 1971. Autocastration by a male transsexual. *Can Psychiatric Assn J* 16:399–405.

Lubin AJ. 1961. Vincent Van Gogh's ear. *Psychoanalytic Quar* 30:351–84.

Luiselli JK. 2009. Nonsuicidal self-injury among people with developmental disabilities. In Nock M. *Understanding Nonsuicidal Self-injury*. Washington, DC: American Psychological Association.

Lynch T, Cozza C. 2009. Behavior therapy for nonsuicidal self-injury. In Nock M. *Understanding Nonsuicidal Self-Injury*. Washington, DC: American Psychological Association.

MacKinlay JG. 1887. Complete self-enucleation of eyeball. *Trans Ophthalmological Soc U.K.* 7:298–300.

MacLean G, Robertson BM. 1976. Self-enucleation and psychosis: Report of two cases and discussion. *Arch Gen Psychiatry* 33:242–49.

Majno G. 1975. *The Healing Hand*. Cambridge, MA: Harvard University Press.

Malavitis A, Arapis D, Stamatinis C. 1967. A case of auto-enucleation. *Bull Soc Hellenique Ophtalmologie* 23:200–201.

Malcove L. 1933. Bodily mutilation and learning to eat. *Psychoanalytic Quar* 2:557–61.

Maloney C. 1976. *The Evil Eye*. New York: Columbia University Press.

Marano L. 1982. Windigo psychosis. *Current Anthropology* 23:385–412.

Margetts EL. 1960. Subincision of the urethra in the Samburu of Kenya. *East African Med J* 37:105–8.

Margo GM, Newman JS. 1989. Venesection as a rare form of self-mutilation. *Am J Psychotherapy* 43:427–32.

Markowitz PI, Coccaro EF. 1995. Biological studies of impulsivity, aggression, and suicidal behavior. In Hollander E, Stein, DJ. *Impulsivity and Aggression*. New York: John Wiley & Sons.

Martin P. 2005. Unusual devastating self-injurious behavior in a patient with a severe learning disability: Treatment with citalopram. *Psychiatr Bull* 29:108–10.

Marx P, Brocheriou J. 1961. Automutilation oculaire chez un malade atteint de schizophrénie. *Bull Soc Ophthal France* 2:98–101.

Master V, Santucci R. 2003. An American hijra. *Urology* 62:1121–22.

Matthews PC. 1968. Epidemic self-injury in an adolescent unit. *Intl J Social Psychiatry* 14:125–33.

McCallum D. 1988. Historical and cultural dimensions of the tattoo in Japan. In Rubin A. *Marks of Civilization*. Los Angeles: Museum of Cultural History, UCLA.

McCann ME, Berde CB, Gourmnerova LC, Waters PM. 2002. Self-mutilation in young children following neonatal brachial plexus injury. *Anesthesiology* 96:A1221.

McGeoch P, Brang D, Song T. 2009. *NeuroReport* 19:1305–6.

McHenry LC. 1985. Neurological disorders of Dr. Samuel Johnson. *J Royal Soc Medicine* 78:485–91.

McKinney WT. 1974. Primate social isolation: Psychiatric implications. *Arch Gen Psychiatry* 31:422–26.

Mellon CD, Barlow C, Cook J, Clark LD. 1989. Autocastration and autopenectomy in a patient with transsexualism and schizophrenia. *J Sex Research* 26:125–30.

Menninger K. 1935. A psychoanalytic study of the significance of self-mutilation. *Psychoanalytic Quar* 4:408–66.

———. 1938. *Man against Himself*. New York: Harcourt Brace World.

Meyer-Holzapfel M. 1968. Abnormal behavior in zoo animals. In Fox FW. *Abnormal Behavior in Animals*. Philadelphia: Saunders.

Michael KD, Beck R. 1973. Self-amputation of the tongue. *Intl J Psychoanalytic Psychotherapy* 2:93–99.

Mihmanli I, Kurugoglu S, Kantarci F. 2002. Intercardiac needle in a 12-year-old girl with self-injurious behavior. *Pediatr Radiol* 32:209–10.

Miller F, Baskhin E. 1974. Depersonalization and self-mutilation. *Psychoanalytic Quar* 43:638–49.

Mintz IL. 1964. Autocannibalism: A case study. *Am J Psychiatry* 120:1017.

Mitchell J. 1984. *Eccentric Lives and Peculiar Notions*. London: Thames and Hudson.

Mitchell JE, Boutacoff CI, Hatsukami D, Pyle RL, Ekert ED. 1986. Laxative abuse as a variant of bulimia. *J Nerv Ment Disease* 174:174–76.

Money J, DePriest M. 1976. Three cases of genital self-surgery and their relationship to transsexualism. *J Sex Rsch* 12:283–94.

Money J, Jobsris R, Furth G. 1977. Apotemnophilia: Two cases of a self-demand amputation as a paraphilia. *J Sex Rsch* 13:115–25.

Money-Kryle R. 1930. *The Meaning of Sacrifice.* London: Hogarth Press.

Montagu A. 1946–47. Ritual mutilation among primitive people. *CIBA Symposia* 8:421–36.

———. 1973. *Man and Aggression,* 2d ed. London: Oxford University Press.

Moodie RL. 1920. The amputation of fingers among ancient and modern primitive peoples and other voluntary mutilations indicating some knowledge of surgery. *Surgical Clinic Chicago* 4:1299–1306.

Morgan HG. 1979. *Death Wishes?: The Understanding and Management of Deliberate Self-Harm.* New York: Wiley.

Mori T, Ito S, Kita T. 2007. Oxydative stress in methamphetamine-induced self-injurious behavior in mice. *Behav Pharmacology* 3:239–49.

Morinis A. 1985. The ritual experience. *Ethos* 13:150–74.

Morris D. 1967. *The Naked Ape.* New York: McGraw-Hill.

Morton A. 1992. *Diana: Her True Story.* New York: Simon and Schuster.

Moskovitz RA, Byrd T. 1983. Rescuing the angel within: PCP-related self-enucleation. *Psychosomatics* 24:402–6.

Mucci M, Dalgalarrondo P. 2000. Self-mutilation: Report of six cases of enucleation. *Rev Brazil Psiquiatria* 22:80–86.

Muehlmann AM, Brown BD, Devine DP. 2008. Pemoline-induced self-injurious behavior: A rodent model of pharmacotherapeutic efficacy. *J Pharmacol Experimental Therapeutics* 324:214–23.

Mueller K, Hsiao S. 1980. Pemoline-induced self-biting in rats and self-mutilation in the deLange syndrome. *Pharmacol Biochem Behav* 13:627–31.

Mueller K, Nyhan WL. 1982. Pharmacologic control of pemoline-induced self-injurious behavior in rats. *Pharmacol Biochem Behavior* 16:957–63.

———. 1983. Clonidine potentiates drug induced self-injurious behavior in rats. *Pharmacol Biochem Behav* 18:891–94.

Mueller K, Saboda S, Palmour R, Nyhan WL. 1982. Self-injurious behavior produced in rats by daily caffeine and continuous amphetamine. *Pharmacol Biochem Behav* 17:613–17.

Murase J, Wu J, Koo J. 2006. Morgellons disease: A rapport-enhancing term for delusions of parasitosis. *J Am Acad Dermatol* 55:913–14.

Murphy GH. 1985. Self-injurious behavior in the mentally handicapped. *Newsletter Assn Child Psychology Psychiatry* 7:2–11.

Murray BJ. 1993. I never promised you a rose garden: Compulsive self-mutilation. In Goodwin JM. *Rediscovering Childhood Trauma.* Washington, DC: American Psychiatric Press.

Murray TJ. 1979. Dr. Johnson's movement disorder. *Br Med Journal* 1:1610–14.

Myers WC, Nguyen M. 2001. Autocastration as a presenting sign of incipient schizophrenia. *Psychiatric Services* 52:685–86.

Nadeau G. 1941. Indian scalping. *Bull Hist Med* 10:178–94.

Nagera H. 1967. *Vincent Van Gogh: A Psychological Study.* London: Allen and Unwin.

Nanda S. 1999. *Neither Man nor Woman: The Hijras of India*. Toronto: Wadsworth Publishing.

Nelson SH, Grunebaum H. 1971. A follow-up study of wrist slashers. *Am J Psychiatry* 127: 1345–49.

Nemiah J. 1985. Dissociative disorders. In Kaplan HI, Sadock B. *Comprehensive Textbook of Psychiatry*, 4th ed. Baltimore: Williams and Wilkins.

Newman CF. 2009. Cognitive therapy for nonsuicidal self-injury. In Nock M. *Understanding Nonsuicidal Self-injury*. Washington, DC: American Psychological Association.

Newman PL. 1965. *Knowing the Gururumba*. New York: Holt Rinehart Winston.

Newman PL, Boyd DJ. 1982. The making of men: Ritual and meaning in Awa male initiation. In Herdt GH. *Rituals of Manhood*. Berkeley: University of California Press.

Nielsen K, Jeppesen M, Simmelsgaard L. 2005. Self-inflicted skin diseases: A retrospective analysis of 57 patients with dermatitis artefacta. *Acta Dermatol Venereol* 85:512–15.

Nock M. 2009a. *Understanding Nonsuicidal Self-injury*. Washington, DC: American Psychological Association.

———. 2009b. Why do people hurt themselves? *Current Directions Psychological Science* 18:78–82.

Nock M, Cha C. 2009. Psychological models of nonsuicidal self-injury. In Nock M. *Understanding Nonsuicidal Self-Injury*. Washington, DC: American Psychological Association.

Nock M, Favazza A. 2009. Nonsuicidal self-injury: Definition and classification. In Nock M. *Understanding Nonsuicidal Self-Injury*. Washington, DC: American Psychological Association.

Nock M, Kessler R. 2006. Prevalence and risk factors for suicide attempts versus suicide gestures. *J Abnorm Psychology* 115:616–23.

Nock M, Mendes W. 2008. Physiological arousal, distress tolerance, and social problem-solving deficits among adolescent self-injurers. *J Consult Clin Psychology* 76:28–38.

Nock M, Prinstein M. 2005. Contextual features and behavioral functions of self-mutilation among adolescents. *J Abnormal Psychol* 114:140–46.

Nock M, Prinstein M, Sterba S. 2009. Revealing the form and function of self-injurious thoughts and behaviors: A real-time ecological assessment study among adolescents and young adults. *J Abnormal Psychology* 118:816–27.

Noel LP, Clarke WN. 1982. Self-inflicted ocular injuries in children. *Am J Ophthulmol* 94: 630–33.

Nor M, Yushar A, Razili R. 2006. Incidental radiological findings of susuk in the orofacial region. *Dentomaxillofac Radiol* 35:473–74.

Novak MA. 2003. Self-injurious behavior in rhesus monkeys. *Am J Primatology* 59:3–19.

Novotny P. 1972. Self-cutting. *Bull Menninger Clin* 36:505–14.

Nyhan WL. 1976. Behavior in the Lesch-Nyhan syndrome. *J Autism Childhood Schizophrenia* 6:235–52.

Offer D, Barglow P. 1960. Adolescent and young adult self-mutilation incidents in a general psychiatric hospital. *Arch Gen Psychiatry* 3:194–204.

Oliver C, Murphy GH, Corbett JA. 1987. Self-injurious behavior in people with mental handicap. *J Mental Deficiency Research* 31:147–62.

Pabis R, Mirla MA, Tozmans S. 1980. A case study of autocastration. *Am J Psychiatry* 137: 626–27.

Paivio S, McCulloch C. 2004. Alexithymia as a mediator between childhood trauma and self-injurious behaviors. *Child Abuse Neglect* 28:339–54.

Pao P-N. 1969. The syndrome of delicate self-cutting. *Br J Med Psychology* 42:195–206.

Parkin JR, Eagles JM. 1993. Bloodletting in bulimia nervosa. *Br J Psychiatry* 162:246–48.

Parry A. 1934. Tatooing among prostitutes and perverts. *Psychoanalytic Quar* 3:476–82.

Parry-Jones B, Parry-Jones WL. 1993. Self-mutilation in four historical cases of bulimia. *Br J Psychiatry* 163:394–402.

Patel SR, Thavaseelan S, Handel LN. 2007. Bilateral manual externalization of testis with self-castration in patient with prion disease. *Urology* 70:59.

Pattison EM, Kahan J. 1983. The deliberate self-harm syndrome. *Am J Psychiatry* 140: 867–72.

Patton D, McIntosh A. 2008. Head and neck injury risks in heavy metal: Head bangers stuck between rock and a hard bass. *Brit Med J* 337–43.

Pawlicki CM, Gaumer C. 1993. Nursing care of the self-mutilating patient. *Bull Menninger Clinic* 57:380–89.

Peters JM. 1967. Caffeine induced hemorrhagic automutilation. *Arch Intl Pharmacodynamics* 169:139–46.

Peterson J, Freedenthal S, Sheldon C. 2008. Nonsuicidal self-injury in adolescents. *Psychiatry* 5 (11): 20–26.

Philipsen A, Richter H, Schmahl C. 2004. Clonidine in acute aversive inner tension and self-injurious behavior in female patients with borderline personality disorder. *J Clin Psychiatry* 65:1414–19.

Phillips K, Didie E, Feusner J. 2008. Body dysmorphic disorder. *Am J Psychiatry* 165: 1111–18.

Pierloot RA, Wellens W, Houben ME. 1975. Elements of resistance to a combined medical and psychotherapeutic program in anorexia nervosa. *Psychotherapy Psychosomatics* 26: 101–17.

Pitman RK. 1990. Self-mutilation in combat related post-traumatic stress disorder. *Am J Psychiatry* 147:123–24.

Podvoll EM. 1969. Self-mutilation within a hospital setting. *Br J Med Psychology* 42:213–21.

Poems of Catullus. 1969. Translated by Michie J. New York: Random House.

Pompili M. Lester D, Tatarelli R. 2006. Incomplete oedipism and chronic suicidality in psychotic depression with paranoid delusions related to eyes. *Annals Gen Psychiatry* 5: 18–20.

Poole FP. 1983. Cannibals, tricksters, and witches: Anthropophagic images among Bimin-Kuskumin. In Brown P, Tuzin D. *The Ethnography of Cannibalism.* Washington, DC: Soc Psychological Anthropology.

Posner K, Oquendo MD, Gould M. 2007. Columbia classification algorithm of suicide assessment. *Am J Psychiatry* 164:1035–43.

Price B, Baral I, Cosgrove G. 2001. Improvements in severe self-mutilation following limbic leucotomy. *J Clin Psychiatry* 62:925–32.

Primeau F, Fontaine R. 1987. Obsessive disorder with self-mutilation. *Can J Psychiatry* 32: 699–701.

Prince R. 1960. Curse, invocation, and mental health among the Yoruba. *Can Psychiatric Assn J* 5:65–79.

Prinstein M, Guerry J, Browne C. 2009. Interpersonal models of nonsuicidal self-injury. In Nock M. *Understanding Nonsuicidal Self-Injury*. Washington, DC: American Psychological Association.

Procacci P, Maresca M. 1990. Autotomy. *Pain* 43:394.

Putnam FW, Guroff JJ, Silberman EK, Barban L, Post RM. 1986. The clinical phenomenology of multiple personality disorder: Review of 100 recent cases. *J Clin Psychiatry* 47: 285–93.

Rada RT, James W. 1982. Urethral insertion of foreign bodies: A report of contagious self-mutilation in a maximum-security hospital. *Arch Gen Psychiatry* 39:423–29.

Rado S. 1933. Fear of castration in women. *Psychoanalytic Quar* 2:425–75.

Rajathurai A, Chazan BI, Jeans JE. 1983. Self-mutilation as a feature of Addison's disease. *Br Med J* 287:1027.

Read KE. 1965. *The High Valley*. New York: Scribner's.

Reddy G. 2003. "Men" who would be kings. *Social Research* 70:163–98.

Rideout V, Roberts DF, Fochr UG. 2005. *Generation M. Media in the Lives of 8–18 Year-Olds*. Washington, DC: Kaiser Family Foundation.

Rinpoche G. 1975. *The Tibetan Book of the Dead*. Berkeley: Shambala.

Ristic D, Petrovic D, Ciric Z. 2008. Penile self-mutilation: Two cases in one family. *Psychiatr Danube* 20:332–36.

Rivers WHR. 1926. *Psychology and Ethnology*. London: Kegan Paul, French and Trubner.

Robertson MM, Trimbale MR, Lees AJ. 1989. Self-injurious behavior and the Giles de la Tourette syndrome. *Psychological Medicine* 19:611–25.

Rockland LH. 1987. A supportive approach: Psychodynamically oriented supportive therapy–treatment of borderline patients who self-mutilate. *J Personality Disorders* 1: 350–55.

Rodham K, Hawton K. 2009. Epidemiology and phenomenology of nonsuicidal self-injury. In Nock M. *Understanding Nonsuicidal Self-injury*. Washington, DC: American Psychological Association Press.

Rogers T, Pullen I. 1987. Self-inflicted eye injuries. *Br J Psychiatry* 151:691–93.

Roheim G. 1932. Psychoanalysis of primitive cultural types. *Intl J Psychoanalysis* 13:1–224.

———. 1949. The symbolism of subincision. *Am Imago* 6:321–29.

Romanczyk RG, Goren ER. 1975. Severe self-injurious behavior. *J Consulting Clin Psychology* 43:730, 739.

Rosen DH. 1972. Focal suicide. *Am J Psychiatry* 128:1009–11.

Rosenberg P, Krohel G, Webb R. 1986. Ocular Munchausen's syndrome. *Ophthalmology* 93:1120–23.

Rosenthal RJ, Rinzler C, Walsh R, Klausner E. 1972. Wrist-cutting syndrome: The meaning of a gesture. *Am J Psychiatry* 128:1363–68.

Ross RR, McKay HB. 1979. *Self-mutilation*. Lexington, MA: Lexington Books.

Ross S. 2000. Complications of body piercing. *Proc UCLA Health Care* (Winter).

Ross S, Heath N. 2002. A study of the frequency of self-mutilation in a community of adolescents. *J Youth Adolescence* 1:67–77.

Roy A. 1978. Self-mutilation. *Br J Med Psychology* 51:201–3.

Roy J. 1974. Acupuncture needle in the bladder. *Urology* 4:584.

Rozycki A. 2007. Prison tattoos as a reflection of the criminal lifestyle and predictor of recidivism. Counseling Psychology Dissertation. Lubbock: Texas Tech University.

Russ MJ. 1992. Self-injurious behavior in patients with borderline personality disorder: Biological perspectives. *J Personality Disorders* 6:64–81.

Russ MS, Roth SD, Lerman A, Kakuma T, Harrison K, Shindledecker RD, Hull J, Mattis S. 1992. Pain perception in self-injurious patients with borderline personality disorder. *Biol Psychiatry* 32:501–11.

Russell (Lord of Liverpool). 1954. *The Scourge of the Swastika*. London: Cassell.

Ryan C. 2008. Out on a limb: The ethical management of body integrity identity disorder. *Neuroethics* 2:21–33.

Sackett GP. 1968. Abnormal behavior in laboratory-reared rhesus monkeys. In Fox MW. *Abnormal Behavior in Animals*. Philadelphia: Saunders.

Saez-de-Ocariz M, Orozco-Covarrubias L, Mora-Magana I. 2004. Dermatitis artefacta in children. *Pediatr Dermatol* 21:205–11.

S.A.F.E. Alternatives. 2008. *S.A.F.E. (Self Abuse Finally Ends): A Manual for School Professionals*. Chicago: Virgin Ink Press.

S.A.F.E. Alternatives. 2008. *Student Workbook*. Chicago: Virgin Ink Press.

Sagan E. 1974. *Cannibalism*. New York: Harper and Row.

Saint Margaret Mary. 1931. *Gems of Thought from Saint Margaret Mary*. New York: Benziger.

Samantha S, Tweeten M, Rickman L. 1998. Haemophilius aphrophilus endocarditis after tongue piercing. *Clin Infect Dis* 26:735–40.

Sandman C. 2009. Psychopharmacologic treatment of nonsuicidal self-injury. In Nock M. *Understanding Nonsuicidal Self-injury*. Washington, DC. American Psychological Association.

Savely VR, Leitas MM, Stricker R. 2006. The mystery of Morgellons disease: Infection or delusion? *Am J Clin Dermatol* 7:1–5.

Schecter DC. 1962. Breast mutilation in the Amazons. *Surgery* 51:554–60.

Schele L, Miller ME. 1986. *The Blood of Kings*. Fort Worth, TX: Kimbell Art Museum.

Schiller G. 1972. *Iconography of Christian Art*, vol. 2: *The Passion of Jesus Christ*. Greenwich, CT: New York Graphic Society.

Schlossman HH. 1966. Circumcision as a defense: A study in psychoanalysis and religion. *Psychoanalytic Quar* 35:340–56.

Schlozman SC. 1998. Upper-extremity self-amputation and replantation. *J Clin Psychiat* 59:681–86.

Schneider SF, Harrison SI, Siegel BL. 1965. Self-castration by a man with cyclic changes in sexuality. *Psychosomatic Med* 27:53–70.

Schroeder SR, Schroeder CS, Smith B, Dalldorf, J. 1978. Prevalence of self-injurious behavior in a large state facility for the retarded. *J Autism and Developmental Disorders* 8:261–69.

Schweitzer I. 1990. Genital self-amputation and the Klingsor syndrome. *Austral New Zealand J Psychiatry* 24:566–69.

Segal P, Mrzyglod S, Alichniewicz-Czaplicka H, Dunin-Horkawicz W, Zwyrzykowski E. 1963. Self-inflicted eye injuries. *Am J Ophthalmology* 349–62.

Shah KN, Fried RG. 2006. Factitial dermatoses in children. *Curr Opin Pediatr* 18:403–9.

Shapira NA, Lessig MC, Murphy TK. 2002. Topiramate attenuates self-injurious behavior in Prader-Willi syndrome. *Int J Neuropsychopharmacol* 5:141–45.

Shapiro S. 1987. Self-mutilation and self-blame in incest victims. *Am J Psychotherapy* 41: 46–54.

Shaw S. 2002. The complexity and paradox of female self-injury. Doctoral thesis, Harvard University Graduate School of Education, Cambridge, MA.

Shea S. 1993. Personality characteristics of self-mutilating male prisoners. *J Clinical Psychology* 49:576–85.

Sher L, Stanley B. 2009. Biological models of non-suicidal self-injury. In Nock M. *Understanding Nonsuicidal Self-injury.* Washington, DC: American Psychological Association.

Shiraeshi S, Goto I, Kurolwa Y. 1979. Spinal cord injury as a complication of acupuncture. *Neurology* 29:1188–90.

Shore D, Anderson DJ, Cutler NR. 1978. Prediction of self-mutilation in hospitalized schizophrenics. *Am J Psychiatry* 135:1406–7.

Silva JA, Leong GB, Weinstock R. 1989. A case of skin and ear self-mutilation. *Psychosomatics* 30:228–30.

Silverman M, Berman A, Sandall N. 2007a. Rebuilding the Tower of Babel: A revised nomenclature for the study of suicide and suicidal behaviors. Part 1: Background, rationale, and methodology. *Suicide Life Threatening Behav* 37:248–63.

———. 2007b. Rebuilding the Tower of Babel: A revised nomenclature for the study of suicide and suicidal behaviors. Part 2: Suicide-related ideations, communications, and behaviors. *Suicide Life Threatening Behav* 37:264–77.

Simeon D, Stanley B, Frances A, et al. 1992. Self-mutilation in personality disorders. *Am J Psychiatry* 149:221–26.

Simpson CA, Porter GL. 1981. Self-mutilation in children and adolescents. *Bull Menninger Clin* 45:428–38.

Simpson MA. 1973. Female genital self-mutilation. *Arch Gen Psychiatry* 29:808–10.

———. 1975. Symposium-self injury: The phenomenology of self-mutilation in a general hospital setting. *Can Psychiatric Assn J* 20:429–34.

———. 1976. Self-mutilation and suicide. In Schneidman ES. *Suicidology: Contemporary Developments.* New York: Grune and Stratton.

Sinclair E. 1886–87. Case of persistent self-mutilation. *J Ment Science* 32:44–46.

Siomopoulos V. 1974. Repeated self-cutting: An impulse neurosis. *Am J Psychotherapy* 28: 85–94.

Slattery D. 1993. *The Wounded Body.* Albany: State University of New York Press.

Slawson PF, Davidson PW. 1964. Hysterical self-mutilation of the tongue. *Arch Gen Psychiatry* 11:581–88.

Soderstrom J. 1938. Die Rituellen Fingerverstummelungen in der Sudsee und in Australien. *Z für Ethnologie* 70:24–47.

Soebo J. 1948. Automutilation bulborum. *Acta Ophthalmologica* 26:451–53.

Solvang P. 2007. The amputee body desired: Beauty destabilized? Disability revalued? *Sexuality Disability* 25:51–64.

Somerset IJ. 1945. Self-inflicted conjunctivitis. *Br J Ophthalmology* 29:186–204.

Somerville-Large LB. 1947. Self-inflicted eye injuries. *Trans Ophthalmological Soc U.K.* 67: 185–201.

Spencer RJ, Haria S, Evans RD. 1999. Gingivitis artefacta. *Br J Orthodontics* 2:93–96.

Standage KF, Moore JA, Cole MG. 1974. Self-mutilation of the genitalia by a female schizophrenic. *Can Psychiatric Assn J* 19:17–20.

Stannard K, Leonard T, Holder G, Shilling J. 1984. Oedipism reviewed: A case of bilateral ocular self-mutilation. *Br J Ophthalmology* 68:276–80.

Stein DJ, Hutt C, Spitz J, Hollander E. 1993. Compulsive picking and obsessive-compulsive disorder. *Psychosomatics* 34:177–81.

Stewart C. 2001. Body piercing: Seductions and medical complications of a risky business. *Med Aspects Human Sexuality* (July): 45–50.

Stinnett JL, Hollender MH. 1970. Compulsive self-mutilation. *J Nerv Ment Disease* 150: 371–75.

Stone M. 1987. A psychodynamic approach. *J Personality Disorders* 1:347–49.

Storr A. 1968. *Human Aggression.* New York: Atheneum.

Strack HL. 1909. *The Jew and Human Sacrifice*, 8th ed. London: Cope and Fenwick.

Stroch D. 1901. Self-castration. *JAMA* 36:270.

Strong M. 1993. A bright red scream. *San Francisco Focus* (December), 58–144.

———. 1998. *A Bright Red Scream.* New York: Viking.

Suh-ho. 1915. In praise of footbinding. *New Republic* (18 December), 170–72.

Suk JH, Son BK. 1980. A study on male genital self-mutilation. *Neuropsychiatry* (Seoul, South Korea) 19:97–104.

Sullivan N. 2005. Integrity, mayhem, and the question of self-demand amputation. *Continuum: J Media Cult Studies* 19:325–33.

Swedo SE, Rapoport JL. 1991. Annotation: Trichotillomania. *J Child Psychology Psychiatry* 32:401–9.

Swedo SE, Leonard HL, Rapoport JL, Lenane MC, Goldberger EL, Cheslow DL. 1983. A double-blind comparison of clomipramine and desipramine in the treatment of trichotillomania. *N Eng J Med* 321:497–501.

Sweeny S, Zamecnik K. 1981. Predictors of self-mutilation in patients with schizophrenia. *Am J Psychiatry* 138:1086–89.

Taira T, Kobayashi T, Hori T. 2003. Disappearance of self-mutilating behavior in a patient with Lesch-Nyhan syndrome after bilateral chronic stimulation of the globus pallidus internus. *J Neurosurgery* 98:414–16.

Tantam D, Whittaker J. 1992. Personality disorder and self-wounding. *Br J Psychiatry* 161: 451–64.

Tapper CM, Bland RC, Danyluk L. 1979. Self-inflicted eye injuries and self-inflicted blindness. *J Nerv Ment Disease* 167:311–14.

Terson A. 1911. L'auto-enucleation des deux yeax dans la mélancolie avec délire religieux. *Ann d'Oculistique* 145–46:81–87.

Tharoor H. 2007. A case of elderly genital self-mutilation in an elderly man. *Prim Care Companion J Clin Psychiatry* 9:396–97.

Thomas EWP. 1937. Dermatitis artefacta: A note on an unusual case. *Br Med J* 1:804–6.

Thompson JN, Abraham TK. 1983. Male genital mutilation after paternal death. *Br Med J* 287:727–28.

Thurston H. 1952. *The Physical Phenomena of Mysticism*. London: Burns and Oates.

Tiefenbacher S, Novack M, Marinus L. 2004. Altered hypothalamic-pituitary-adrenocortical function in rhesus monkeys with self-injurious behavior. *Psychoneuroendocrinology* 29: 501–55.

Tinklepaugh DL. 1928. The self-mutilation of the male macacus rhesus monkey. *J Mammol* 9:293–300.

Toch H. 1975. *Men in Crisis*. Chicago: Aldine.

Trabert W. 1995. 100 years of delusional parasitosis: Meta-analysis of 1223 case reports. *Psychopathology*. 28:239–46.

Tsao CI, Negrette G, Riley A. 2009. Self-amputation of the nipples and penis in a non-psychotic, non-gender-dysphoric man. *Psychosomatics* 50:178–80.

Turner TH, Toffler DS. 1986. Indications of psychiatric disorders among women admitted to prison. *Br Med J* 292:651–53.

Turner V. 1968. *Drums of Affliction*. Oxford: Clarendon Press.

———. 1969. *The Ritual Process*. Ithaca: Cornell University Press.

———. 1977. Sacrifice as quintessential process. *History Religions* 16:189–215.

Tuwir I, Chako E, Brosnahan D. 2005. Drug-induced autonucleation with resultant chiasmal damage. *Brit J Ophthalmol* 89:121–22.

Ullroth J, Haines S. 2007. Acupuncture needles causing lumbar cerebrospinal fluid fistula. *J Neurosurg Spine* 6:567–69.

Urechia M. 1931. Autophagie des doits chez un paralytique en rapport avec une pachymeningite cervicale. *Revue Neurologique* 55:350–52.

Urgulu S, Bartley GB, Otley CC. 1999. Factitious disease of the periocular and facial skin. *Am J Ophthalmol* 128:196–201.

Vale V, Juno A. 1989. *Modern Primitives*. San Francisco: Research Publications.

van der Kolk BA, Perry C, Herman JL. 1991. Childhood origins of self-destructive behavior. *Am J Psychiatry* 148:1165–73.

van Gennep A. 1909. *The Rites of Passage*. London: Routledge & Kegan Paul.

Van Putten T, Shaffer I. 1990. Delirium associated with buproprion. *J Clin Psychopharmacology* 10:234.

Veale D. 2006. A compelling desire for deafness. *J Deaf Studies Deaf Education* 11:369–72.

Vermasseren MJ. 1977. *Cybele and Attis: The Myth and the Cult*. London: Thames and Hudson.

Verraes-Derancourt S, Derancourt C, Poot F. 2006. Dermatitis artefacta: Retrospective study in 31 patients. *Ann Dermatol Venereal* 133:235–38.

Verzin JA. 1975. Sequelae of female circumcision. *Tropical Doctor* 5:163–69.

Wachtel L, Contrucci-Kuhn S, Griffin M. 2009. ECT for self-injury in an autistic boy. *Eur Child Adoles Psychiatry* 18:458–63.

Wackenheim A, Becker Y, Nevers J. 1956. L'automutilation oculaire. *Cahiers de Psychiatrie* 11:108–18.

Waddell H. 1957. *The Desert Fathers*. Ann Arbor: University of Michigan Press.

Wakefield PL, Frank A, Meyers RW. 1977. The hobbyist: A euphemism for self-mutilation and fetishism. *Bull Menninger Clin* 41:539–52.

Walsh B. 2006. *Treating Self-injury*. New York: Guilford.

Walsh B, Rosen P. 1988. *Self-mutilation: Theory, Research, and Treatment*. New York: Guilford.

Warlomont E. 1875. *Louise Lateau: Rapport médical sur la stigmatisée de Bois-d'Haine, fait à l'Académie royale de médicine de Belgique*. Paris: Ballière.

Warrington. 1882–83. The case of Isaac Brooks. *J Ment Science* 33:69–74.

Waugaman RM. 1999. Genital self-mutilation. *Psychiatric Services* 50:1362.

Wehrli GA. 1939. Trepanation in former centuries. *CIBA Symposia* 1:178–86.

Weierich M, Nock M. 2008. Posttraumatic stress symptoms mediate the relation between childhood sexual abuse and nonsuicidal self-injury. *J Consult Clin Psychology* 76:39–44.

Weinstock R. 1988. Self-amputation of the ear. *Can J Psychiatry* 33:242–43.

Weiss C. 1962. A worldwide survey of the current practice of milah (ritual circumcision). *Conference on Jewish Social Studies*, 30–48.

Weissman MM. 1975. Wrist cutting: Relationship between clinical observations and epidemiological findings. *Arch Gen Psychiatry* 32:1166–71.

Weld KP, Mench JA, Woodward RA. 1998. Effect of tryptophan treatment on self-biting and central nervous system serotonin metabolism in rhesus monkeys. *Neuropsychopharmacology* 19:314–21.

Westermeyer J, Serposs A. 1972. A third case of self-enucleation. *Am J Psychiatry* 129:484.

Whiting JWM, Kluckhohn R, Anthony A. 1947. The functions of male initiation ceremonies at puberty. In Macoby E, Newcomb T, and Hartley E. *Readings in Social Psychology*. New York: Holt Rinehart Winston.

Whiting M. 1884. Self-castration. *Peoria Med Monthly* 5:297–300.

Whitlock FA, Hynes JV. 1978. Religious stigmatization. *Psychological Medicine* 8:185–202.

Whitlock JL, Eckenrode JE, Silverman D. 2006. Self-injurious behavior in a college population. *Pediatrics* 117:1939–48.

Whitlock JL, Lader W, Conterio K. 2007. The role of virtual communities in self-injury treatment. *J Clin Psychology: In Session* 63:1135–43.

Whitlock JL, Powers J, Eckenrode JE. 2006. The virtual cutting edge: Adolescent self-injury and the Internet. *Developmental Psychology* 42:407–17.

Whitlock JL, Purington A, Gershkovich M. 2009. Media, the internet, and nonsuicidal self-injury. In Nock M. *Understanding Nonsuicidal Self-injury*. Washington, DC: American Psychological Association Press.

Widick MH, Coleman J. 1992. Perichondral abscess resulting from a high ear-piercing. *Otolaryngol Head Neck Surg* 107:803–4.

Wilkins J, Coid J. 1991. Self-mutilation in female remanded prisoners I: An indicator of severe psychopathology. *Criminal Behavior Mental Health* 1:247–67.

Williams P. 1989. *Mahayana Buddhism: The Doctrinal Foundations*. London: Routledge.

Wilson J. 1992. *The Bleeding Mind*. London: Weidenfeld and Nicolson.

Wilson WA. 1955. Oedipism. *Am J Ophthalmology* 40:563–67.

Winchel RM, Stanley M. 1991. Self-injurious behavior: A review of the behavior and biology of self-mutilation. *Am J Psychiatry* 148:306–17.

Winnicott DW. 1949. Hate in the counter-transference. *Intl J Psychoanalysis* 30:69–74.

———. 1958. Transitional objects and transactional phenomena. In *Collected Papers.* New York: Basic Books.

Wise TN, Kalyanam RC. 2000. Amputee fetishism and genital mutilation. *J Sex Marital Therapy* 26:339–44.

Wurfler P. 1956. Selbstblendung eines cocainsuchtigen Betrugers. *Nervenartz* 27:325–26.

Yang HK, Brown GC, Magargal LE. 1981. Self-inflicted ocular mutilation. *Am J Ophthalmology* 91:658–63.

Yang JG, Bullard M. 1993. Failed suicide or successful male genital self-amputation. *Am J Psychiatry* 150:350–51.

Yaroshevsky F. 1975. Self-mutilation in Soviet prisons. *Can Psychiatric Assn J* 20:443–46.

Yaryura-Tobias JA, Neziroglu F. 1978. Compulsions, aggression, and self-mutilation: A hypothalamic disorder? *Orthomolecular Psychiatry* 7:114–17.

Yates T. 2009. Developmental pathways from child maltreatment to nonsuicidal self-injury. In Nock M. *Understanding Nonsucidal Self-injury.* Washington, DC: American Psychological Association.

Yellowlees AJ. 1985. Anorexia and bulimia in anorexia nervosa. *Br J Psychiatry* 146:648–52.

Young FW. 1965. *Initiation Ceremonies.* Indianapolis: Bobbs-Merrill.

Zaidens SH. 1951. Self-inflicted dermatoses and their psychodynamics. *J Nerv Ment Disease* 113:395–404.

Zillboorg G. 1939. The discovery of the Oedipus complex: Episodes from Marcel Proust. *Psychoanalytic Quar* 8:279–302.

ABOUT THE AUTHOR

Armando Favazza, M.D., is an emeritus professor of psychiatry at the University of Missouri–Columbia, which presented him with its Faculty-Alumni Award in 2008. He received his undergraduate degree from Columbia University, where he studied anthropology with Margaret Mead. He received his M.D. from the University of Virginia and his M.P.H. from the University of Michigan, where he also completed his psychiatry residency training. He has been a pioneer in the study of nonsuicidal self-injury since the 1980s and was cited in the *New York Times Magazine* as the first person to comprehensively study the topic. *Bodies under Siege* is generally regarded as the seminal book in the field. He is cofounder of the Society for the Study of Psychiatry and Culture and has published seven books and more than two hundred chapters, articles, and reviews with a special focus on self-injury, cultural psychiatry, and spirituality. He has lectured on self-injury at more than half of the medical schools in the United States and Canada as well as at many psychiatric congresses and international universities. His media presentations on self-injury and body modification include *20/20, Dateline*, MSNBC, the National Geographic and Discovery Health channels, the BBC, and National Public Radio. In 2010, he delivered the keynote address at the fifth annual meeting of the International Society for the Study of Self-injury.